Readings in

RESEARCH METHODOLOGY

Readings in RESEARCH METHODOLOGY

SECOND EDITION

FLORENCE S. DOWNS, EdD, FAAN
Former Editor, *Nursing Research*

Lippincott
Philadelphia • New York • Baltimore

Acquisitions Editor: Margaret Zuccarini
Developmental Editor: Sara Lauber
Production Editor: Virginia Barishek
Production Manager: Helen Ewan
Production Service: P.M. Gordon Associates, Inc.
Compositor: Circle Graphics
Printer/Binder: R.R. Donnelley & Sons/Crawfordsville
Cover Designer: Melissa S. Walter
Cover Printer: Lehigh Press

Second Edition

9 8 7 6 5 4 3 2 1

Library of Congress Cataloging-in-Publication Data

Readings in research methodology / [edited by] Florence S. Downs. — 2nd ed.
p. cm.
Rev. ed. of : Handbook of research methodology. c1988.
Includes bibliographical references.
ISBN 0–7817–1924–0
1. Nursing—Research—Methodology—Handbooks, manuals, etc.
2. Research—Methodology—Handbooks, manuals, etc. I. Downs, Florence S. II. Handbook of research methodology.
[DNLM: 1. Nursing Research collected works. WY 20.5 R2873 1999]
RT81.5.R416 1999
610.73′07′2—dc21
DNLM/DLC
for Library of Congress 98–40626
CIP

Care has been taken to confirm the accuracy of the information presented and to describe generally accepted practices. However, the authors, editor, and publisher are not responsible for errors or omissions or for any consequences from application of the information in this book and make no warranty, express or implied, with respect to the contents of the publication.

The authors, editor, and publisher have exerted every effort to ensure that drug selection and dosage set forth in this text are in accordance with current recommendations and practice at the time of publication. However, in view of ongoing research, changes in government regulations, and the constant flow of information relating to drug therapy and drug reactions, the reader is urged to check the package insert for each drug for any change in indications and dosage and for added warnings and precautions. This is particularly important when the recommended agent is a new or infrequently employed drug.

Some drugs and medical devices presented in this publication have Food and Drug Administration (FDA) clearance for limited use in restricted research settings. It is the responsibility of the health care provider to ascertain the FDA status of each drug or device planned for use in their clinical practice.

Preface

Answering research questions is difficult because it requires the investigator to construct a seamless set of logical techniques to answer a question. The less ambiguity there is in a research design, the more trust one can place in the information obtained. Since most of the research conducted in nursing involves the cooperation of human beings, eliminating ambiguity involves more than elegant design and statistical manipulations. The researcher must also take into account the effects of human behavior on the study findings.

Although many view research design as consisting of a rather dull set of mechanistic operations, nothing could be further from the truth. Research is about finding answers to pesky problems. In order to do that, ingenious people have found intriguing ways to go about it. Some of the means are based in research experience and some on mathematical and strategic reasoning. Taken together, they enable the modern researcher to approach problem solving at a higher level of competence than ever before, and to avoid blind alleys and the mistakes of others. It was with these ideas in mind that the "Methodology Corner" was initiated in *Nursing Research*.

Readings in Research Methodology is the second edition of articles derived from the "Methodology Corner." Authors of the articles were requested to avoid topics routinely covered in texts and to narrow their focus to allow in-depth coverage of the subject. All the articles were reviewed by experts and carefully edited before publication. The result was a set of highly readable pieces that are of great utility in designing and conducting a research project. I believe that bringing them together under one cover greatly enhances their usefulness.

If nursing is to stay abreast of the rapidly changing world of health care, we must give careful attention to the quality of the information we want to use for education and practice. In this regard, there is no substitute for a clear understanding of research methods and their efficacy. Although the researcher certainly bears a major responsibility for conducting research in a thorough and ethical manner, this does not exempt the consumer from the responsibility of evaluating the results in unabridged form. Thus, many who want to evaluate research and conduct it may find this volume a handy resource for judging the interpretations drawn from research findings.

Florence S. Downs, EdD, FAAN

Contents

PART FIVE
Measures and Measurement Issues

PART SIX
Special Analytic Techniques

Introduction

This edition of *Readings in Research Methodology* is an expanded and updated version of the first edition. Most of the articles included in the first edition remain. Although some references are dated, the richness of content makes these pieces "oldies but goodies." As in the first edition, most of the articles were drawn from the "Methodology Corner" section of *Nursing Research*. This feature has been a favorite of readers since its inception, because each article deals in depth with a select facet of the research enterprise. Articles in this volume do not include many topics routinely covered in research texts; one purpose of the "Methodology Corner" was to avoid such repetition. Therefore, this book is a supplement to standard texts that can help researchers and students gain a more thorough understanding of textual material.

The articles were written by experts and carefully reviewed for accuracy and clarity. The frequency with which these articles have been quoted is testimony to their usefulness and quality. References to previously published material in the "Methodology Corner" provide a continuity among the readings. The pieces are rich in the kind of real-life examples and commentary that textbook writers can rarely afford to include. As the editor of *Nursing Research,* I was often impressed by the way authors explicated complex subject matter. In compiling this handbook, my original impressions were reinforced many times over.

Research is often called an orderly process, which leads the novice to believe that there is some set way of going about the task. In fact, there is a great deal of redundancy in refining an idea or figuring out what is going on in a given research situation. The point of this redundancy is to shape a research project so that the results are as unambiguous as possible. It forces the investigator to constantly reevaluate the consistency among the parts of the entire project, e.g., how data are analyzed varies with sampling design and with the characteristics of the sample and data. To know one's data is to understand what they contribute to the results. However, the overlaps between research design and methods made it difficult to imagine how to partition the contents of this book sensibly. In compiling each section of the book, I tried to imagine where I would look for content if I had no directory. The result is an idiosyncratic organization based on the available material. Even so, I believe the individual parts have a coherence that is all their own, which will tempt the thoughtful reader to consider material in the adjacent works.

Part One of this publication deals with issues related to sampling, sample size, and sample assignment. This section opens with an article on pilot work because many hidden sampling problems can be revealed through preliminary work. The authors take note of other difficulties that may be uncovered, but emphasize the critical nature of pilot studies in avoiding later complications in data collection.

Elder subjects have been documented as especially difficult subjects to recruit and retain in research studies. Refusals by subjects in any age group to participate in a study can seriously jeopardize the integrity of the sample and introduce biases that are difficult to account for. Furthermore, subjects who enter a study in the belief that they are making a significant contribution to a scientific endeavor and are treated with respect are likely to be those who remain in the study until its conclusion. The authors of the article on a consumer approach to recruitment discuss methods to obtain this end in detail. Their thoughts and suggestions regarding this issue apply equally to all adult subjects and can be useful in obtaining an adequate, representative sample. You may wish to read this article together with "Strategies to Minimize Attrition in Longitudinal Studies," included in Part Three.

Much has been said on the importance of using a sample of sufficient size to detect important differences. Clearly, no funding agency wants to invest in a study that is unlikely to uncover important differences, if they exist. Everyone agrees that good research design should include some rational plan for determining an appropriate sample size. Samples that are too small put the researcher at risk of failing to find important differences that exist. On the other hand, overly large samples are not only expensive to recruit, but may produce significant differences that are unimportant. The critical nature of pilot work in establishing a data-based approach to sample size should not be underestimated, as is noted in the opening article.

Not everyone agrees on how to choose a proper sample size. Clearly, the rules vary for qualitative and quantitative work. There are also variations that are possible within quantitative designs. The group of articles devoted to power analysis is introduced by Thomas Knapp's commentary, "The Overemphasis on Power Analysis," which places the other pieces on this subject in perspective. As he notes, the objective is to obtain a sample that is "not too small, not too large, but just right." After reading the work included here on power analysis, one should be able to avoid writing, "This study should be replicated with a larger sample." That sentence stands as one of the most depressing I have ever read.

The last group of articles in this section deal with sampling and sample assignment. I remember my first encounter with randomization very well. Fresh from courses on research design and statistics, I was, naively, convinced that random assignment performed some sort of magic to equalize treatment and control groups. I was astounded when several crucial variables failed to be evenly distributed throughout the three groups we had recruited. Somewhere along the way, I had failed to heed the words "helps to balance." Although there is no foolproof method for selecting or assigning a sample, the articles provided here offer sophisticated suggestions for avoiding bias and achieving balance between groups.

Part Two of this collection is devoted to issues related to qualitative research. The first articles deal with the issues of integrating qualitative and quantitative methods. Today, there seems to be less controversy about the selective use of this approach. But there are still many who question the validity of an integrative approach. It seemed natural to follow these articles with those about triangulation, because triangulation often involves the use of both methods. The pieces provide excellent, clear, and detailed definitions and examples of the various forms of this procedure. The slight variations in definitions and applications simply emphasize that the last word has yet to be said on the topic.

Although interviewing is a necessary part of many types of research, it is at the heart of qualitative methods. Too often investigators in nursing assume that the interpersonal nature of the discipline is such that interviewing skills can be taken as a given. This is not so, as anyone who has listened to taped interviews done by novices recognizes. Much more attention needs to be given to this important topic, if respondents' reports are to be considered accurate. The articles included here cover not only interviewer training, but use of self-as-instrument and threats to the integrity of semistructured interviews. Last, but not least, I added the articles on interrater reliability. Although quantitative in nature, they deal with the use of subjective judgment and can be useful in content analysis.

Much of the research undertaken by nurses involves helping people to alter their behavior. In "Using Slopes to Measure Directional Change," Suter, Wilson, and Naqvi refer to the measurement and analysis of change as a "long-lived methodological puzzle." Part Three is about the intricacies of this puzzle, and how to measure effects in before and after longitudinal designs.

I began this part with "Know Thy Data," a simple injunction to examine data before jumping to conclusions. As the editor of *Nursing Research,* I often thought that researchers were so anxious to see the results of their analyses that they forgot to look at the descriptive data. Standard deviations of immense proportions were often ignored, as were statistically significant differences between values that would be meaningless in a clinical situation. Authors were also fond of the words *approached statistical significance.* Unfortunately, there is no such thing. The statement amounts to wishful thinking. Errors in the interpretation of statistical significance as an indicator of the strength of a relationship were common. The second article, "*, **, ***; Statistical Nonsense at the .00000 Level," deals with the interpretation of statistical significance in the light of its clinical meaning. The authors also point out the important link between power calculations and significance. Articles about power analysis are included as part of the content on sampling in Part One. This is a good example of the redundancy present in research design. Power is both part of sampling strategies and part of the interpretation of the results of the investigation.

The midsection of Part Three includes articles that deal with specific methods of statistical analyses of differences. It was once common to see multiple *t* tests and flagrant abuses of difference scores in nursing research. For the most part, those days are behind us. The choice of the proper method of statistical analysis of data, however, remains a knotty decision. "Testing for Experimental Effects in the Pretest-Posttest Design" can be of substantial help in unraveling the intricacies involved in making that decision. The articles that follow offer further suggestions for alternative analyses, including the use of slopes and handling noninterval data.

The next portion of Part Three contains articles that consider various designs that are appropriate for the study of changes that occur over time. Two of these articles contain information on designs rarely seen in the nursing literature: case-control design and the mixed-method approach. Case-control design is a method to assess the effects of exposure to risk. It is commonly used in the field of epidemiology. In the rapidly changing environment of health care, it is likely that nursing will become far more population-oriented than it has been in the past. Consequently, designs that expose factors that are antecedent to various conditions may become increasingly important.

In "A Mixed-Method Approach for Using Cross-Sectional Data for Longitudinal Inferences," the authors describe a way to circumvent some of the difficulties inherent in conducting longitudinal studies. In effect, cross-sectional data are combined with data from a subsample containing longitudinal data. Most studies require considerable time to accumulate the necessary sample. Consequently, it may be possible to follow some of the original participants over time with little additional effort. The general effect is to strengthen the inferences that can be made from cross-sectional data.

The essence of the articles that conclude Part Three is really a reiteration of the importance of understanding data regardless of the source. "Longitudinal Studies as Intervention" is an excellent case in point. The possibility of interviewer effects was anticipated, and open-ended questions were included in the last measure. Careful examination of the answers verified the investigators' suspicions that many participants had been affected by inclusion in the study. The surrounding articles feature many helpful suggestions about how to manage, examine, and clean your data. Handling large data sets for the first time can be an unexpectedly complicated process. Many of the recommendations for surmounting this daunting task are based on the experience of the authors. Following their suggestions may save you from developing the Penelope Syndrome. Victims must unravel each day's work and begin again on the day that follows. Penelope was successful in evading suitors by using this method, but if your suitors are from a funding agency, the effect could prove to be disastrous.

Part Four contains articles related to some of the most widely reported methods that employ sophisticated use of correlation. With the use of computers, modern correlational techniques used in nursing research have become far cries from what once prevailed. Early articles submitted for publication often contained hundreds of correlations involving all the variables used in the research. Obviously, investigators had a hard time trying to explain the findings in any meaningful way. Gradually, this misuse of correlation gave way to forms of regression analysis and causal models that are better suited to analyzing complex relationships. This created a different kind of problem: how to report the analyses in a concise and understandable manner. "Regression Analyses: What to Report" is a useful guide to solving this problem when preparing a research article.

There has been a great deal of discussion regarding the appropriate sample size for conducting a regression analysis. The general rule of thumb is ten subjects per variable. In clinical studies, obtaining a sample of the size required by the inclusion of even a moderate number of variables can be difficult. The statistical problem to be surmounted is the likelihood of chance associations among predictors. Prescott discusses this problem in "Multiple Regression Analysis with Small Samples: Cautions and Suggestions." Among her suggestions is the use of the jackknife procedure when sample sizes are considered too small to be reliable. In "The Rough and Ready Jackknife," Resnick develops this point in sufficient detail to make this little-used statistic an understandable means for analyzing small samples.

Although I was unable to include the article in this publication, I strongly recommend reference to the article, "Sex, Age, Height, and Weight as Predictors of Selected Physiologic Outcomes" by Brown, Knapp, and Radke. This article appeared in the March/April 1997 issue of *Nursing Research*. It deals with an issue that receives little attention by investigators when choosing predictors or determining sample size; namely, just how much variation in effects can I expect, given the amount of variance I really have to work with? It is a strong argument for not only knowing your data but also the clinical entity you are attempting to change.

Both moderation and mediation are important concepts that are indispensable in model construction. However, the similarity between moderation and mediation, both semantically and statistically, can be a source of confusion. Reference to "Theoretical and Methodological Differentiation of Moderation and Mediation" will resolve the confusion. The explanation is clear and accompanied by examples that I believe will be helpful in distinguishing between these two important entities.

The remainder of Part Four is concerned with discussions of modeling techniques. Sometimes readers of the research literature complain that the results of these methods are too complicated to understand. Given the complexity of human interactions and motivations, there is no simple method available to account for them. The days when the use of a single independent and dependent variable constituted acceptable research are gone. We need to resign ourselves to the fact that our research has proceeded beyond that point. Model construction is an important way to understand how events and variables are related and an indispensable component of theory building. The explanations provided in the articles included here are probably as simple as the discussion of model construction can be. They are excellent references for both researchers and those who wish to develop a basic understanding of the method.

Part Five is about measurement, a subject that is extensively covered in standard texts. Despite the attention given to the principles of reliability and validity, the concepts are still cloaked in a certain amount of ambiguity. Authors have sometimes argued that support of study hypotheses is evidence of validity for the instruments used; a classic case of getting the cart before the horse. The confusion that exists between stability of a construct and stability of a test is a good example of the somewhat elusive nature of reliability. "Validity, Reliability, and Neither" sets forth clear distinctions that are helpful in avoiding erroneous interpretations of the literature on reliability and validity. "Managing Measurement Error" augments the discussion of instrument reliability by placing emphasis on the importance of checking a measure's reliability each time it is used. The argument that the instrument was developed using a similar sample simply does not hold. Lynn's article, "Determination and Quantification of Content Validity," adds a thorough treatment of the intricacies of establishing content validity.

Given the thousands of measurement devices available to investigators, the choice of an appropriate measure can be a difficult decision. Many instruments that appear in the literature are poorly described or of questionable reliability. In her classic article, Norbeck argues that to aid potential consumers, minimal standards of psychometric testing should be met before publication. She explicitly describes those standards, which make the content helpful to both those who are considering an instrument for use and those who are developing an instrument.

In samples that are notably different, as they may be in cross-cultural research, measures may need a great deal of revision before they can be considered as reliable and valid. In "Instrumentation in Cross-Cultural Research," Jones and Kay review the basic points that need to be taken into account in preparing instruments for such use. I have paired this article with one describing visual analogue scales because they are often used in samples in which language presents a barrier. Additionally, visual analogue scales make handy, easily used measures in a variety of clinical situations.

Part Six consists of a group of alternative analytic techniques that are designed for special purposes. Meta-analysis, in particular, has gained considerable popularity as a method for integrating the findings from groups of studies. It can be especially useful for examining findings as indicators of clinical feasibility. Unfortunately, the method has been subjected to a number of abuses that have made its use controversial. Researchers have attempted to synthesize findings using too few studies, those of questionable quality, and those with mixed variable definitions. The articles included here augment the discussions that can be found in classic texts on the subject. The issue of determining the quality of primary studies, in particular, is dealt with in-depth in Brown's article, "Measurement of Quality of Primary Studies for Meta-Analysis."

Factor analysis is a familiar method for use in data reduction and calculating composite scores from several measures. However, it is an indispensable tool for examining the structure of an instrument and its validity. In "Factor Analysis Revisited," Ferketich and Muller present a detailed discussion of the analytic options available through the use of factor analysis and the assumptions underlying them. This discussion is greatly enhanced by analysis of data using each extraction method presented by Youngblut in "Comparison of Factor Analysis Options Using the Home/Employment Orientation Scale." Taken together, the two pieces provide a description of factor analysis techniques that is of unusual clarity.

I have completed Part Six with two articles, one on canonical analysis and one on discriminant analysis. Although neither technique is widely reported in the nursing literature, both have specific and useful purposes. Most textbook discussions are quite murky, since they lack the necessary detail and examples to be instructive. You will welcome the clear exposition of both methods of analysis in these pieces.

Indeed, I believe you will find this entire collection of articles a welcome relief from some of the tangled explanations that are often a deterrent to the use of efficient research methods. I took my first research and statistics courses many years ago. I still remember asking my professor to define a standard deviation. He answered my question by repeating the list of calculations necessary to derive the statistic. I said, "But what *is* it?" He seemed baffled by the question. Several years later, I came upon a book intended for the statistically retarded. The meaning of a standard deviation was demonstrated by crows in a bush. A boy frightened the crows and they flew to an overhead wire. "Ah," I said, "it's dispersion." It is of such stuff that research careers are made.

PART ONE

Samples and Sampling Issues

The Potential Uses of Pilot Work

Patricia A. Prescott ■ Karen L. Soeken

Despite the importance of pilot studies to the success of well-conducted research, a review of nursing research texts and published studies suggests that pilot studies are underdiscussed, underused, and underreported. This article discusses the potential of pilot studies for nursing research and compares this potential with actual practice.

Treatment in Research Texts and Journals

A review of a convenience sample of nine current introductory texts designed for undergraduate or master's level nursing students, published within the past 7 years (see Appendix), revealed that the majority (7) mentioned pilot studies. In general, pilot studies were defined as small-scale versions of the planned study, trial runs of planned methods/measures, or a miniature version of the anticipated research. These definitions imply that pilot work is to assess the (a) feasibility of the planned study, (b) adequacy of the instrumentation, and (c) problems in data collection strategies and proposed methods.

However, little discussion followed the definition of pilot work regarding how it could be designed or implemented to achieve these purposes, except in the case of assessing the reliability of proposed instrumentation. The definition given in the texts suggests that pilot studies are small-scale tests conducted after the research plan has been developed. Revisions then are made in the plan based on the results of the pilot study.

Although pilot studies can provide small-scale tests of a complete study plan, they also have other potential uses (Yaremko et al., 1982). In particular, pilot work can be thought of as work (a) designed to answer a methodological question(s) and (b) conducted prior to or as a part of the development of a research plan. For example, questions such as, "What is a reasonable estimate of the relative variance of my dependent variable?," "Which internal validity threats are likely in this setting and how might they be controlled?," or "How much missing data can I reasonably expect and what kind of follow-up procedures are possible?," are best answered with pilot study data. These questions are methodological in nature and their answers guide the researcher toward empirically determined nonarbitrary answers to many design issues that must be dealt with in preparing a research proposal. When used this way, pilot work serves to guide the development of a research plan instead of being a test of the already-developed plan.

Two hundred twelve studies published during the 3 years 1985–1987 in three research journals (*Nursing Research, Research in Nursing and Health,* and *Western Journal of Nursing Research*) were reviewed. Of these, only 18 (8.8%) reported pilot studies of any kind. In 13 of the 18 studies, the main purpose was related to assessment of instrument reliability. The remaining 5 articles described a ministudy of the sort congruent with the text definition, that is, a small-scale test of a completed research plan. No examples of pilot studies addressing methodological questions important to the development of a research plan were located.

Although we recognize that the phases of a study are interactive and often are developed simultaneously, with decisions regarding one phase affecting decisions made at other phases, this article focuses on the separate major components of a study to highlight the potential contributions of pilot work to each.

Problem Identification and Conceptualization of the Study

Whether a researcher is concerned with developing operational definitions of independent and dependent variables or translating the theoretical concepts of interest to the particular operations planned, substantial knowledge of both the general concepts and their specific application is required. Knowledge of the general can be gained from the literature and from theoretical notions; knowledge of the particular application, however, must come

Patricia A. Prescott, RN, PhD, is professor and chair, Graduate Department of Psychophysiological Nursing, School of Nursing, University of Maryland, Baltimore.

Karen L. Soeken, PhD, is an associate professor in the Center for Research, School of Nursing, University of Maryland, Baltimore.

From *Nursing Research,* January/February 1989, *38,* 60–62.

from the researcher's involvement in the setting with the subjects, operations, and measures.

It is primarily through empirical data that the researcher can come to understand the important issues related to construct validity in the planned study. Inadequate explication of constructs and related problems such as mono-operations bias (single exemplars of cause and effect), monomethods bias (single method of presentation of treatments or measurement of effects), and confounding constructs and levels of constructs (using operational manipulations at discrete levels when the variables actually are continuous) are potentially serious problems in research (Cook & Campbell, 1979). These problems can be addressed in pilot studies by asking methodological questions such as, "Do the treatments as delivered by the caregiving nurses actually represent the theoretical construct as intended?," "Did the treatment as delivered in practice contain all the elements it theoretically should and none of the elements of comparison or control treatments?," or "Are alternative measures of important variables available in the setting that could be used to avoid mono-operations bias?"

Design

The general outline of a study design can be established based on the researcher's purpose and the nature of the research question or hypothesis. Beyond this general level, however, the researcher is faced with many decisions that have a potential impact on the internal validity of the study. Some of the internal validity threats are controllable through use of random assignment. Pilot work relevant to these threats, then, centers on an assessment of whether random assignment actually can be implemented. In the event that random assignment to groups cannot be done, the researcher can use a fallback quasi-experimental design, provided the problem has been anticipated in sufficient time for design modifications to occur. A pilot study that implements the treatment protocol under the controlled conditions planned for the study can be helpful in this regard.

Other threats not controllable by random assignment to groups are more problematic, as often their effects are subtle and not evidenced until a study is under way. Of particular importance are internal validity threats related to application of the independent variable (diffusion of treatments and compensatory equalization of treatments) and the compensatory rivalry and resentful demoralization of respondents that can occur when treatments are perceived to have different value by subjects. A trial run of the treatment protocol helps identify the likelihood of these threats, as they cannot be statistically removed ex post facto.

To illustrate, think about a situation in which a nurse researcher plans an experimental study in which patients are to be randomly assigned to a health teaching group or to a group in which brief psychotherapy is provided to facilitate coping. The researcher plans to hold the simultaneous group sessions in different places to guard against the diffusion of treatments problem. While conducting a pilot study, however, the researcher learns that the subjects' (patients receiving radiation for oncological problems) radiation treatments are scheduled in such a way that patients in different treatment groups are in the waiting area at the same time. Further, in the course of the pilot study the researcher learns that the patients, who all know one another because of repeated visits for radiation therapy, are discussing the content of their experimental treatments. Clearly, the researcher has discovered a diffusion of treatment problem, and because it was discovered at the level of prestudy pilot work, corrective action such as changing the scheduling of radiation treatments or using separate waiting rooms can be taken.

Sampling

Pilot work is of critical importance to carefully conceived sampling designs, especially when there is not a substantial body of published research on the variables of interest. First, the relative variance of the dependent variable can be estimated; second, the appropriateness and feasibility of the sampling plan can be evaluated; and third, information needed to determine group size for a given level of power can be obtained.

Relative variance of the dependent variable, that is, the mean of the variable relative to its standard deviation, is critical for determining the sample size needed to represent the population of interest accurately and within known limits of sampling error. This is important to the external validity or generalizability of a study and is of particular importance when probability sampling designs are used. Representativeness of samples is of concern to survey researchers and those interested in describing the characteristics of patient populations.

Sampling designs differ in their efficiency and requirements. Most but not all probability sampling designs require that population size be known. Often it is not known in advance of entering the setting with a proposed study whether this condition can be met. In many clinical studies, for example, the researcher must know how client records and appointments are recorded before a sampling plan can be finalized. Systematic sampling often is chosen by clinical researchers specifically because the population size does not have to be known in advance of conducting the study. However, there are limitations to this sampling design as there are for all designs. Of particular importance is the requirement that there not be a periodicity in the sampling frame that corresponds to the chosen sampling interval and is related to the dependent variable. Failure to investigate this limitation could lead to a seriously biased sampling plan, which would produce nongeneralizable findings. For example, if one were interested in how long nurse practitioners spend with clients, and if one used a systematic sampling plan that called for selection of every third patient, and if every third patient scheduled were a new patient to the system in need of a complete workup, it is clear that the time nurse practitioners spend with patients would be overestimated and produce nongeneralizable findings.

Conducting a power analysis to establish the group sizes needed to detect a significant difference, if one exists, is an established principle of experimental and quasi-experimental research. Too often, however, researchers seem to establish group sizes based on convenience rather than plan. This is unfortunate, for many studies are de facto incapable of showing a treatment effect simply because the information needed for a power analysis prior to conducting the study was not collected. Such information, including the expected variability of the dependent variable, is available from a pilot study, which provides a data-based approach to establishing sampling parameters.

Measures

Among the steps required in the initial process of instrument construction is a preliminary trial of items so that revisions can be made as necessary. Subsequent steps include field testing of the items on a large sample representative of those for whom the test or measure is intended, item analysis and revisions, if necessary, and reliability and validity studies for the final form of the test. These steps are generally considered "... the minimum effort required to ensure that test scores ... serve as useful measurements" (Crocker & Algina, 1986). Even prior to initial item tryouts, however, decisions must be made regarding the test format (i.e., open-ended vs. closed-ended questions) or the number of response options on a Likert scale (i.e., odd vs. even). These decisions, too, should involve empirical assessment. Thus, it is not surprising that the discussion of a pilot study occurs most commonly in the context of assessing the proposed instrumentation. It seems, however, that what many authors refer to as a pilot study is the test construction process.

Assessment of an instrument during a pilot study can be viewed as examining the proposed instrumentation in light of the specific sample of interest. For example, reliability coefficients often are reported in the literature or a test manual for other samples. Because reliability is both sample- and situation-specific, though, it is necessary to determine whether the reliability estimates reported are based on samples similar in composition to the group for whom the test will be used. If not, a pilot study can be used to estimate reliability before implementing the study itself.

Similarly, it may be necessary to assess the respondent burden for the intended sample: What is the time required to complete the instrument? Do any items contain terminology that would be unfamiliar to the intended subjects? Are items written at an appropriate reading level? Can the instructions be clearly understood? Pilot testing with a sample similar to those who will be included in the intended study allow the researcher to answer such questions and make revisions as indicated.

A pilot test might reveal unexpected difficulties with the items themselves. For example, responses to an option such as "other, please specify" may indicate the need to create a new and specific response option category. Or the researcher may discover that a question does not elicit the type of response expected. For example, subjects are asked to "give a couple of terms you would use to describe yourself." The terms "easy-going" and "friendly" are provided as examples of the type of response expected. In a pilot testing, over half the respondents choose one or both of the terms provided as examples! Obviously, the question needs to be revised prior to the study.

Pilot studies also can be helpful for evaluating whether observational approaches to measurement can be implemented as planned. A researcher, for example, may find during pilot work that specific categories emerge from the general behaviors to be observed or that the proposed time sampling interval is insufficient. One researcher used a pilot study to determine where to position herself to best observe both the verbal and the nonverbal communication that occurred between the nurse and patient in a trauma setting.

Still another use of pilot work related to instrumentation is assessing the data collection form itself. A researcher may discover that the order in which the data are to be recorded on a form does not correspond to the order in which it appears on the monitor or in the patient's chart. A change in the form itself would make data collection more efficient and less error-prone. Extra room or so-called "white space" may need to be added to an interview guide where unexpected probing was necessary during an interview or where notes were needed to describe more fully what was observed.

Data Analysis

Not to be overlooked in the process of conducting pilot work is the opportunity to try out the proposed data analysis techniques to uncover potential problems with the proposed analysis. The result may be a tremendous savings in time later in the project.

Developing the code book, for example, and using it to code pilot data may reveal that more codes are needed for an item or that more columns are required for computer input. If the sample size is sufficient to enable data analysis, the researcher may determine if computer programs are correctly written to provide the expected output. Occasionally, analysis of the results of a pilot study may alert the researcher that instrumentation must be modified or that data as coded or entered into the computer will not permit the analysis envisioned. In one project, pilot data helped researchers determine whether the most efficient computer analysis of the data would be with the nurse or the patient as the person of record. In this instance, waiting until the final study data had been collected and possibly coded would have been a very time-consuming error.

Conclusion

More attention to pilot work may increase the time spent in preparation for a study, but we believe the time is well spent, as the data can provide the opportunity for the researcher to correct defects that cannot be removed or remedied after the study plan has been executed.

References

Cook, R., & Campbell, D. (1979). *Quasi experimentation design and analysis issues for field setting.* New York: Rand McNally.

Crocker, L., & Algina, J. (1986). *Introduction to classical and modern test theory.* New York: Holt, Rinehart and Winston.

Yaremko, R. M., Harari, H., Harrison, R. C., & Lynn, E. (1982). *Reference handbook of research and statistical methods in psychology: For students and professionals.* New York: Harper & Row, Publishers.

APPENDIX

List of Research Texts Reviewed

Ackerman, W. B., & Lohnes, P. R. (1981). *Research methods for nurses.* New York: McGraw-Hill Book Company.

Brink, P. J., & Wood, M. J. (1983). *Basic steps in planning nursing research.* Monterey, CA: Wadsworth.

Burns, N., & Grove, S. K. (1987). *The practice of nursing research conduct, critique and utilization.* Philadelphia: W. B. Saunders Company.

Lieswiadomy, R. M. (1987). *Foundations of nursing research.* Norwalk, CT: Appleton & Lange.

Polit, D. F., & Hungler, B. P. (1987). *Essentials of nursing research* (3rd ed.). Philadelphia: J. B. Lippincott.

Shelley, S. I. (1984). *Research methods in nursing and health.* Boston: Little, Brown and Company.

Treece, E. W., & Treece, J. W. (1986). *Elements of research in nursing* (4th ed.). St. Louis: The C. V. Mosby Company.

Williamson, Y. M., (Ed.). (1981). *Research methodology and its application to nursing.* New York: John Wiley & Sons.

Wilson, H. S. (1985). *Research in nursing.* Menlo Park, CA: Addison-Wesley Publishing Company.

The Consumer Approach to Recruitment of Elder Subjects

J. Elaine Souder

Successful completion of a research project is contingent on an adequate number of subjects. Despite resources and funding for such projects, recruiting older subjects for research remains a difficult and, at times, frustrating task. The purpose of this article is to present a personalized, "consumer" approach to recruitment of elderly subjects for research.

The varied factors that hinder successful recruitment of the aged for research have been documented. Many elderly individuals have diseases, limitations, or other disqualifying conditions. Several reports have noted that 9–12 interested elders have been required to yield one subject who met the necessary criteria and was successfully enrolled in a study. (Levy, Mohns, Rosen, & Davis, 1982; Williams, Vitiello, Ries, Bokan, & Prinz, 1988). Age itself has been negatively correlated with willingness to participate in research, and overall participation has been reported at less than 60% in the elderly (Zimmer et al., 1985). Studies are becoming increasingly more complex, and may involve invasive procedures, repeated assessment and data collection, and drug intervention. Fears of radiation, infection, and pain may hinder otherwise healthy older individuals who wish to contribute to research. Lipsitz, Pluchino, and Wright (1987) found that physiologic studies that involved discomfort and offered no direct benefit to subjects had the lowest recruitment rates (14–28%). Additionally, attrition due to morbidity and mortality means that more elderly must be recruited in order to assure adequate sample size in longitudinal projects. Other barriers to elderly individuals' participation in research include complex consent forms, safety concerns, cost of transportation, and distrust of the medical system (Leader & Neuwirth, 1987; Zimmer et al., 1985).

J. Elaine Souder, PhD, RN, is assistant professor, College of Nursing, and Department of Psychiatry, University of Arkansas for Medical Sciences, Little Rock, AR. At the time of the study, the author was a research associate, School of Nursing & Division of Nuclear Medicine, Department of Radiology, University of Pennsylvania, Philadelphia, PA.

From *Nursing Research,* September/October 1992, *41,* 314–316.

The personality of the recruiter affects the success of recruiting (Kaye, Lawton, & Kaye, 1990), as well as the recruiting approach, but have been only briefly noted in the literature. Zimmer et al. (1985) point out that it may be necessary to work with an older person over time to get beyond suspicion and hostility. Use of the same staff person in all contacts with potential subjects and their family members will also convey continuity in interest and approach and facilitate personalized interactions (Williams et al., 1988). Ideally, this individual will have sensitivity and clinical skills in dealing with older adults.

The Consumer Approach

A client-centered approach in dealing with the expressed needs of individuals using a psychiatric clinic has been described in the clinical literature (Burgess & Lazare, 1975). This approach also has implications for recruitment of research subjects. Elderly individuals cannot be considered a homogeneous group. They may be interested from a scientific perspective, prompted by concern about their health status, or altruistically motivated by the presence of a health condition in a friend. Although the research protocol must be maintained, recognizing and responding to the needs and motivation of potential subjects is prudent. A researcher can facilitate recruitment by observing clues that suggest an individual's motivation and strategically addressing these needs. This approach is "consumer" oriented. It assumes that subject willingness and satisfaction are tightly linked to the fulfillment of expectations.

The following classification is based on careful observations of questions, comments, and behaviors of potential and enlisted subjects during four years of recruitment of middle-aged and elderly subjects for aging and dementia studies. Eight descriptions of motivators are presented, along with suggestions for approaches by the recruiter.

Prototypes of Needs

Altruism

The opportunity to help others has been cited as a motivator for research participation (Hoffman, Marron, Fillit, & Libow, 1983; Lipsitz et al., 1987). Volunteers in this group verbalize satisfaction with their lives, and the desire to give something meaningful back to society. Individuals prompted by altruism tend to have few concerns about the protocol itself, trustful that the experts are competent and in control. They may brush off the consent form without reading it carefully, stating that since it is funded and being carried out by a major institution, it must be "okay." This group needs direction to read the consent form carefully before signing. Acknowledgment of their participation through verbal or written means or special certificates serves to recognize their contribution. They may also be ideal candidates (with consent) for publicity photographs.

Interpersonal Contact

Some individuals view research participation as a means of gaining additional interpersonal involvement in their lives. The contacts with professionals during the research process promote feelings of being special and increase self-esteem. The purpose and outcome of the research is not of primary concern to individuals in this group, since the research simply serves as a legitimate avenue by which to gain access to a person who is interested in them. This has been mentioned as a motivator in recruiting nursing home patients (Lipsitz et al., 1987), but may also be useful with those living independently in the community. Recruiters play an important role for these individuals as they care, nurture, and facilitate contacts with other members of the research team.

Documentation

Interest in obtaining baseline data about their health status may prompt some elderly to pursue research opportunities. Their first questions may focus on the availability of examination, laboratory, or test reports during their participation. Potential subjects carefully explain that they maintain a set of all their medical records and wish to add whatever is available to the current collection. Some potential recruits stipulate that participation is contingent on written agreement to receive a copy of chest X-rays, MRI films, and lab reports. These individuals are currently satisfied with the state of their health but seek baseline data upon which future deterioration can be measured. Since abnormal findings may be problematic, results should be sent only to the physician of their choice rather than to the individual. Success and satisfaction are directly correlated with the speed with which reports are made available to their physicians.

Novel Experiences

Individuals may be looking for an experience to break up the routine of retired life and frequently have a background of unusual endeavors. At times they may proudly refer to past intriguing activities, such as sailing alone for long periods, or relate personal knowledge and contact with a variety of well-known public figures. Participation in research is perceived as another chapter in their biography of "living the full life." The researcher can respond to this mind-set by emphasizing that research participation probably is different than anything encountered in the past, and by emphasizing novel aspects of the study.

Hope

Responders to research opportunities may be looking for hope through drug trials or other forms of treatment not yet available to the general public. While the motivation may be hope, recruiters should realize that guilt or desperation may also motivate this group. Feelings of having failed in some way (not seeking medical attention earlier, or ignoring previous medical advice) may cause such individuals to continually try to modify the course of a disease by experimental intervention. Researchers should emphasize that research participation is primarily useful to science and future victims of the disease, and that it may possibly have some benefit for the individual now. In a comparison of research studies, Lipsitz et al. (1987) found the highest rate (81%) of participation in a study of incontinence that offered potential direct benefit to subjects. For those responding from feelings of guilt or desperation, it may be helpful to indicate that each person has to make a decision as to the extent treatment of an incurable condition should be pursued. The humane response may be to give them permission not to push themselves into yet another study. Their choice regarding participation must take into consideration the demands of the study, disease status, and the availability of personal resources.

Scientific Involvement

Individuals seeking repeated research enrollment may be retired professionals who have prior experience with the research process or an interest in science. Kaye et al. (1990) found that those who participated in research felt very positively about research in general. Individuals in this group ask technical questions of the recruiter early in the interview process. They may pose specific questions only to the principal investigator. They may request prior publications by the research group. They may also take copious notes about the intended project and will usually seek an outside opinion from a lawyer, doctor, or trusted family member with expertise in the research area. Working with individuals with this need requires provision of detailed answers to all questions. They may become obsessed with particular details or concerns about the study, which are best handled with direct and open answers. Minimizing risk and profuse reassurance are not useful. If the potential recruit decides not to enroll and needs a way to save face after much discussion and effort to satisfy questions, it may be helpful to point out to them that the study under consideration is not for everyone.

Second Opinion

In research focused on the study of specific medical conditions, individuals may respond who are seeking a second opinion on an established health problem. In fact, they may consider a research avenue when prior medical contacts have been unable to provide a definitive diagnosis. Since dissatisfaction with previous diagnostic and therapeutic attempts may prompt their current interest, it is important to clarify expectations and limitations of participation. In particular, if the proposed protocol may not lead to a definite diagnosis or desired outcome at conclusion, that fact should be made clear in advance.

Reassurance

Elders who are anxious about some undiagnosed health concern may volunteer as healthy control subjects. They may enter a physical fitness study to see if their heart is normal or a dementia study to learn if their recent memory problems are, in fact, normative changes in aging. Their anxiety may be overt or covert and, in fact, may not surface until completion of the study when numerous phone calls convey their anxiety about test reports. Unlike those seeking written reports of their health, these individuals are seeking reassurance that will often be relieved by a verbal report. Abnormal results should be sent to their personal physician for further discussion and evaluation within the context of an ongoing relationship.

A variety of idiosyncratic factors may also be motivators for some individuals. For example, a subject may enroll to gain a specific service, such as completion of a medical form. Occasionally, someone may be interested in the financial incentive, although remuneration is typically modest for the required time and effort.

As with other endeavors and services, a satisfied consumer is an effective advertisement. A follow-up telephone call or survey can be used to determine overall level of satisfaction and to seek specific information and suggestions for improvements. Subjects who felt they were treated with respect and gained a sense of satisfaction through being part of a scientific endeavor will be more inclined to participate again and to refer friends.

References

Burgess, A. W., & Lazare, A. (1975). The customer approach to patienthood. *Community Mental Health.* Englewood Cliffs, NJ: Prentice-Hall.

Crosby, F., Ventura, M. R., Finnick, M., Lohr, G., & Feldman, M. J. (1991). Enhancing subject recruitment for nursing research. *Clinical Nurse Specialist, 5*(10), 25–30.

Hoffman, P. B., Marron, K. R., Fillit, H., & Libow, L. (1983). Obtaining informed consent in the Teaching Nursing Home. *Journal of the American Geriatrics Society, 31,* 565–569.

Kaye, J. M., Lawton, P., & Kaye, D. (1990). Attitudes of elderly people about clinical research on aging. *The Gerontologist, 30,* 100–106.

Leader, M. A., & Neuwirth, E. (1978). Clinical research and the noninstitutional elderly: A model for subject recruitment. *Journal of the American Geriatrics Society, 24,* 27–31.

Levy, M., Mohns, R., Rosen, W., & Davis, K. (1982). Research subject recruitment of gerontological studies of pharmacological agents. *Neurobiology of Aging, 3,* 77–79.

Lipsitz, L. A., Pluchino, F. C., & Wright, S. M. (1987). Biomedical research in the nursing home: Methodological issues and subject recruitment results. *Journal of American Geriatrics Society, 35,* 629–634.

Williams, D. E., Vitiello, M. V., Ries, R. K., Bokan, J., & Prinz, P. N. (1988). Successful recruitment of elderly community-dwelling subjects for Alzheimer's disease research. *Journal of Gerontology, 43*(3), 69–74.

Zimmer, A., Calkins, E., Hadley, E., Ostfield, A., Kaye, J., & Kaye, D. (1985). Conducting clinical research in geriatric populations. *Annals of Internal Medicine, 103,* 276–283.

The Overemphasis on Power Analysis

Thomas R. Knapp

It has been said that the question most often asked of statisticians is: What size sample should I use in my study? (See, for example, Hinkle & Oliver, 1983.) The statistician invariably answers that question with another question: How far wrong can you afford to be when you make an inference from your sample to the population from which the sample has been drawn?

Concern for appropriate sample sizes (not too small, not too large, but just right) in research investigations has led Jacob Cohen (1965, 1988, and elsewhere) and many others (e.g., Goodwin, 1984, Kraemer & Thiemann, 1987; Polit & Sherman, 1990; Yarandi, 1994) to recommend that statistical power analysis be used to determine optimal sample sizes. Given a hypothesized effect size, a desired power, a chosen significance level, and the requisite number of "tails" (a one-tailed test for a directional alternative hypothesis and a two-tailed test for a nondirectional alternative hypothesis), the appropriate sample size can be specified. Power analysis has caught on in a wide variety of disciplines (including nursing), so much so that in the preface to the latest edition of his text, Cohen (1988) says: "I am told that some major funding entities require power analyses in grant applications" (p. xiv).

The thesis of this commentary is that the emphasis on power analysis has gone too far, especially in nursing. The logic behind power analysis is impeccable: No study should be carried out if it has a very small probability of finding an "effect" that may be "there"; and nobody wants to fund such a study. (Several years ago, I co-authored a monograph on power that proclaimed that same logic—see Miller & Knapp, 1972.) But many researchers have been forced into using power analysis for determining sample size when that procedure does not fit their research design, and in the process, they have made all sorts of technical errors. My arguments now follow.

Thomas R. Knapp, EdD, is a professor of nursing and education, College of Nursing, Ohio State University, OH.

From *Nursing Research,* November/December 1996, *45,* 379–380.

Hidden Assumptions Underlying Power-Based Formulas and Tables

It is not widely known, or at least not widely acknowledged, that in addition to the traditional assumptions of normality and homoscedasticity, all of the readily available power-based formulas and tables for determining sample size assume *simple random* sampling from *infinite* populations. I know of no nursing research investigations that satisfy such assumptions. Most studies are carried out on "convenience" (nonrandom) samples or entire small populations (Barhyte, Redman, & Neill, 1990). (There are occasional studies that employ stratified random sampling or multistage cluster sampling, for which the usual power-based formulas and tables need to be adjusted.) It strikes me as improper for an investigator to "regard" his or her sample as a simple random sample from an infinite population (or even a population that is alleged to be much larger than the sample itself) when he or she knows full well that it is not.

Using the Wrong Formulas or Tables

As a person who does a great deal of methodological consulting, I am constantly amazed by the number of times I have encountered a sample size that is appropriate for a simple analysis (such as a one X, one Y regression) but is claimed to be appropriate for a more complicated analysis (such as multiple regression). For example, an *N* of 85 is fine for testing the null hypothesis of no relationship between two variables against an alternative hypothesis of .30 (a "medium effect"), at the .05 significance level (two-tailed) and a power of .80 (Cohen, 1988, p. 100 and Table 3.4.1). But for an alternative hypothesis of a .30 *multiple* correlation coefficient (α .09 R^2) with three independent variables, using the same alpha and power values, an *N* of approximately 110 is required (Cohen, 1988, p. 445 and Table 9.4.2). If a number of different analyses are carried out on the data collected in a particular study, the sample size must be large enough to test the smallest hypothesized effect for the most complicated analysis.

Post Hoc Use of Power Analysis

Some researchers report the results of a power analysis for determining sample size after they have completed their studies and have not been able to reject the null hypothesis. Typical statements read something like this: (a) "I did not get statistical significance, and the size of my sample probably was to blame, since the *N* that I used didn't give me much power"; or (b) "I did not get statistical significance, but the size of my sample probably was not to blame, since I had rather high power." As Darlington (1990) points out, that is not a proper use of power analysis, and confidence bands around the nonsignificant statistic are much more informative (see below).

A related problem is the calculation of power on the basis of an obtained effect size after the study has been completed. (See, for example, Rudy et al., 1995, and the section on power in Polit, 1996, pp. 139–142.) It is the power going into a study for a *hypothesized* effect size that is the important consideration. (The term *effect size* really should not be used to indicate an obtained result, but since that term is so ingrained in the meta-analysis literature, I am afraid we shall have to live with such ambiguity.)

An interesting example of the use of post hoc power analysis where a small sample (of 18 subjects) did unexpectedly reject the null hypothesis is a study by Redeker, Mason, Wykpisz, Glica, and Miner (1994). That is not an appropriate use either. If a small sample size can lead to the rejection of the null hypothesis (assuming that the chosen significance level is defensible), the researcher can be reasonably assured that the effect is "there." Contrary to some widely held beliefs, a statistically significant effect based on a small sample is more impressive than a statistically significant effect based on a large sample, since large-sample sizes can "buy" effects that are not scientifically important.

Hypothesis Testing versus Interval Estimation

It has been argued in several methodological articles and textbooks that hypothesis testing is inferior to interval estimation, as far as inferential statistics is concerned, and that one often gets hypothesis testing "for free" when using interval estimation. (See, for example, Cobb, 1985; Munro & Page, 1993.) There are formulas and tables for determining sample size that are based on desired amounts of confidence and interval widths, rather than desired powers and hypothesized effects. (See, for example, Darlington, 1990, chapter 15.) Many researchers find it difficult to hypothesize a specific effect size and a power value in any event and too often rely on Cohen's (1988) "defaults" of medium effect size and .80 power.

Cobb (1985) gives the example of a researcher who would like to estimate a population correlation coefficient to within .10 of its true value, with 95% confidence. With the appropriate formula, a sample size of 400 is required if it is believed that the population correlation is small, but smaller sample sizes (100 to 200) are sufficient for large-population correlations. Nice—simple, straightforward, and to the point.

Other Ways of Determining Sample Size

Mention was just made of the confidence-interval-based approach to sample size determination, which should be at least as equally highly regarded a method for sample size determination as any power-based procedure, particularly in the absence of any hypothesis to test. But there are several other ways of determining sample size.

One approach is to use an "*N* vs. *V*" (number of observations vs. number of variables) rule. Such rules abound in the research literature, with the 10 : 1 rule the most well known. (See, for example, Knapp & Campbell-Heider, 1989; Munro & Page, 1993.)

Another method is to base sample size determination on strictly practical considerations. If you have enough time, money, and effort to study only one person, then *N* is 1; if you have enough time, money, and effort to study only 25 persons, then *N* is 25; etc.

Perhaps the best way of all is to use sequential analysis (either sequential hypothesis testing or sequential estimation). This technique is particularly appropriate for clinical nursing research in which subjects are "run" one at a time. After each subject has been studied, the researcher takes a "look" at the data accumulated thus far and decides either to stop data collection and make the appropriate statistical inference or to continue sampling. It therefore permits the researcher to have a variable, rather than fixed, sample size, and it has been shown that the required sample size is less, on the average. (See Brown, Porter, & Knapp, 1993, for details regarding sequential hypothesis testing.)

Sample Size Determination in Qualitative Research

There is a vast qualitative research literature that provides excellent guidelines for sample size determination, none of which ever refers to power. A recent article by Sandelowski (1995) is particularly noteworthy in this regard. I know of a doctoral student in another discipline who was proposing a qualitative study and who was told by her committee that she would have to do a power analysis to determine the appropriate sample size, even if there was no way she could come close to that sample size.

Power Politics

The thing about the current emphasis on power-based techniques that I find most objectionable is that almost all nursing researchers who submit an R01, an R29, or other grant proposal are *required* to use power analysis to determine sample size and to justify the number that they come up with. I recently came across a "pink sheet" evaluation of a grant proposal in which the researchers were chastized for not using power analysis and for proposing a "sample" size that was too small, when, in fact, that was the size of the entire population. Not even in his wildest dreams did Jacob Cohen ever visualize a research world in which power-based techniques for sample size determination would be preferable to studying an entire population.

References

Barhyte, D. Y., Redman, B. K., & Neill, K. M. (1990). Population or sample: Design decision. *Nursing Research, 39,* 309–310.

Brown, J. K., Porter, L. A., & Knapp, T. R. (1993). The applicability of sequential analysis to nursing research. *Nursing Research, 42,* 280–282.

Cobb, E. B. (1985). Planning research studies: An alternative to power analysis. *Nursing Research, 34,* 386–388.

Cohen, J. (1965). Some statistical issues in psychological research. In B. B. Wolman (Ed.), *Handbook of clinical psychology* (pp. 95–121). New York: McGraw-Hill.

Cohen, J. (1988). *Statistical power analysis for the behavioral sciences* (2nd ed.). Hillsdale, NJ: Erlbaum.

Darlington, R. B. (1990). *Regression and linear models.* New York: McGraw-Hill.

Goodwin, L. D. (1984). The use of power estimation in nursing research. *Nursing Research, 33,* 118–120.

Hinkle, D. E., & Oliver, J. D. (1983). How large should the sample be? A question with no answer? Or . . . . *Educational and Psychological Measurement, 43,* 1051–1060.

Knapp, T. R., & Campbell-Heider, N. (1989). Numbers of observations and variables in multivariate analyses. *Western Journal of Nursing Research, 11,* 634–641.

Kraemer, H. C., & Thiemann, S. (1987). *How many subjects?* Newbury Park, CA: Sage.

Miller, J. K., & Knapp, T. R. (1972). *The importance of statistical power in educational research* (Occasional Paper No. 13). Bloomington, IN: Phi Delta Kappa Research Service Center.

Munro, B. H., & Page, E. B. (1993). *Statistical methods for health care research* (2nd ed.). Philadelphia: Lippincott.

Polit, D. F. (1996). *Data analysis and statistics for nursing research.* Stamford, CT: Appleton & Lange.

Polit, D. F., & Sherman, R. E. (1990). Statistical power in nursing research. *Nursing Research, 39,* 365–369.

Redeker, N. S., Mason, D. J., Wykpisz, E., Glica, B., & Miner, C. (1994). First postoperative week activity patterns and recovery in women after coronary artery bypass surgery. *Nursing Research, 43,* 168–173.

Rudy, E. B., Daly, B. J., Douglas, S., Montenegro, H. D., Song, R., & Dyer, M. A. (1995). Patient-outcomes for the chronically critically ill: Special care unit versus intensive care unit. *Nursing Research, 44,* 324–331.

Sandelowski, M. (1995). Sample size in qualitative research. *Research in Nursing & Health, 18,* 179–183.

Yarandi, H. N. (1994). Using the SAS system to estimate sample size and power for comparing two binomial proportions. *Nursing Research, 43,* 124–125.

Statistical Power in Nursing Research

Denise F. Polit ▪ Robert E. Sherman

A power analysis was performed on 62 articles that were published in *Nursing Research* and *Research in Nursing and Health* during 1989. The analysis revealed that when effects were small, the mean power of the statistical tests being performed to test research hypotheses was .26, indicating a very high risk of committing a Type II error. When effects were moderate, the mean power increased to .71, which is still below the conventionally acceptable power of .80. Only when a study involved large effects was the power adequate (mean of .95). Of the 583 power estimates calculated, 53% were for small effects. These analyses indicate that a substantial number of published nursing studies, and presumably even more of unpublished studies, have insufficient power to detect real effects, primarily because the samples used are too small.

Nursing research has experienced dramatic transformations over the past few decades, in terms of substance (a greater emphasis on problems of a clinical nature), theory (a higher degree of theoretical orientation), and methodology. Analyses of methodological trends in studies published in nursing journals have documented such changes as (a) an increase in research designs aimed at explanation compared to ones aimed at pure description; (b) the increased use of measuring instruments with established psychometric properties; and (c) greater reliance on multivariate statistical analyses to test research hypotheses (Brown et al., 1984; Moody et al., 1988).

With such increased sophistication in the design and execution of nursing studies, it is noteworthy that little change has been observed with respect to sampling plans. The majority of nursing studies continue to rely on small samples of convenience. Brown and her colleagues (1984), who analyzed research that was published in four journals in 1952, 1960, 1970, and 1980, noted that "there did not appear to be any trend toward the use of larger samples over the 30-year period" (p.30). The median sample size in 1952 was 84, and in 1980, it was 80. In a more recent analysis, Moody and associates (1988) noted that nursing studies still typically use samples of well under 100 subjects.

Denise F. Polit, PhD, is the president of Humanalysis, Inc in Saratoga Springs, NY.

Robert E. Sherman was a student in the Department of Sociology at Skidmore College at the time of this study.

From *Nursing Research,* November/December 1990, *39,* 365–369.

The clinical nature of much of nursing research undoubtedly makes it difficult to obtain large samples or to use probability sampling plans. Nevertheless, it must be understood that a price must be paid for relying on small samples. That price is known as statistical power.

Statistical Power

Standard statistical texts pay considerable attention to the problem of Type I errors. A Type I error occurs when the researcher wrongly rejects a true null hypothesis—that is, wrongly accepts as true the research hypothesis that a relationship exists between variables. The probability of committing a Type I error is established by the investigator as the level of significance, which is often referred to as alpha.

However, considerably less attention is paid to Type II errors, which occur when the researcher wrongly accepts a false null hypothesis—that is, wrongly rejects the research hypothesis that a relationship between variables exists. The probability of a Type II error is referred to as (β). The complement of beta (that is, $1 - \beta$) is the probability of obtaining a significant result, and is referred to as the power of a statistical test. When studies are designed with insufficient power, the risk of committing a Type II error is high.

Statistical power is a function of three other parameters: (a) the significance level, or alpha; (b) sample size; and (c) effect size. Each of these can be determined or estimated by the researcher prior to conducting a study, thus making power subject to the control of the researcher.

Power increases with higher Type I error rates. The conventionally accepted level for a Type I error is .05, meaning that the investigator is willing to assume the risk of committing such an error 5 times out of 100. If a stricter alpha criterion were established—say, an alpha of .01—power would decrease. Similarly, statistical power can also be increased by using directional hypothesis tests, since an alpha of .05 for a one-tailed test is analogous to an alpha of .10 for a two-tailed test.

The second parameter affecting power is the sample size. Larger samples increase the power of a test and reduce the risk of committing a Type II error. Thus, the researcher can directly affect power by increasing sample size, by using a directional hypothesis test, and/or by relaxing the alpha criterion of the test.

The third parameter that affects power is the effect size (ES). The ES is a measure of how "wrong" the null hypothesis is. In other words, it is an index of how strong the effect of the independent variable is on the dependent variable. With everything else equal, as the value of the ES increases, power also increases and the needed sample size decreases. Generally, the ES is the parameter over which the researcher has the least control, especially in nonexperimental research in which the independent variable is not manipulated or controlled by the investigator. Although ES is not easily controlled, its value can nevertheless be estimated.

A procedure known as statistical power analysis can, once an estimate of the ES is made, be used to solve for the sample size that would be needed to achieve a certain degree of power. Just as .05 has been adopted as the standard for the alpha criterion, a conventional standard for power ($1 - \beta$) is .80. This means that the risk of committing a Type II error is .20. While this risk may seem high, achieving greater power would mean using extremely large samples for most studies, since effect sizes are typically moderate.

The difficult part of doing a power analysis is to estimate before beginning a study what the ES will be. After all, the purpose of most research is to determine whether and to what extent variables are interrelated. There are four basic strategies. First, ES can be calculated on the basis of prior studies that have examined similar phenomena. These other investigations generally provide a sufficient basis for estimating whether the relationships being studied are likely to be strong or relatively modest, that is, for estimating the value of the ES. When several relevant studies have been conducted, a more reliable ES value can be determined, using meta-analytic procedures. A second approach that can be used when a study is on a groundbreaking topic is to conduct a small pilot study or pretest; the results from the pilot can then be used to calculate an ES that would be used as an estimate for the main study.

When no prior information is available and pretests are not feasible, a third strategy is to develop a "dummy table" analysis to calculate the smallest ES that would still be considered sufficiently large to have either practical or theoretical value. For example, if a smoking cessation intervention would be considered cost-effective and worthwhile only if it resulted in a 10% reduction in smoking among participants in the program, then an ES estimate could be developed on this basis. A fourth strategy, and one that is considered a last resort, is to estimate (based on prior research and clinical experience) whether the effects can be considered small, medium, or large. These qualitative labels can then be attached to quantitative ES values to conduct a power analysis. It should be emphasized that, as Cohen (1977) has noted, effect sizes are likely to be small in new areas of research inquiry. A medium ES should be estimated only when the effect is so substantial that it can be detected by the naked eye (i.e., without formal research procedures).

The value of ES is arrived at differently depending on the nature of the statistical test performed. For example, when the statistical test is the Pearson product moment correlation, the estimated value of ES is ρ, the expected population correlation coefficient. Table 1 presents Cohen's (1977) formulas for calculating effect size for five frequently used statistical tests and his definition of small, medium, and large effects for these tests.

Statistical power analysis is generally used in one of two ways. First, a researcher about to embark on a study can conduct a power analysis to determine how large the sample should be to reduce the risk of committing a Type II error. If the researcher has some constraints in recruiting a sample—let us say that a researcher knows in advance that obtaining a sample larger than 100 subjects would be impossible—then a power analysis should still be performed. In this situation, the researcher uses the sample size constraints and estimates of ES to calculate power, which indicates the risk of committing a Type II error. It is wasteful and unproductive to embark on a time-consuming study if it can be determined in advance that the power is, say, .50. This would mean that there would only be a 50–50 chance of obtaining significant results.

A second application of statistical power analysis is to calculate power *after* the study is completed and the data are analyzed. Power calculations provide readers of research reports with considerable information about the validity of the findings. Such an application of power analysis is especially important when nonsignificant results are obtained, since in such situations the findings seem inconclusive. When the researcher's real hypothesis

TABLE 1 **Formulas for Effect Size and Definitions of Levels of Effect Size for Five Statistical Tests**

Test	Effect Size Population Parameter	Effect Size Values		
		Small	*Medium*	*Large*
t-test for 2 group means	$d = \frac{\lvert \bar{X}_1 - \bar{X}_2 \rvert}{\sigma}$	.20	.50	.80
F-test for *k* independent means	$f = \frac{\sigma_{mi}}{\sigma}$	.10	.25	.40
$r\ (r \neq 0)$	r	.10	.30	.50
Difference between 2 proportions	$\phi_i = 2 \text{ arscine} \sqrt{P_i}$ $h = \lvert \phi_1 - \phi_2 \rvert$	.20	.50	.80
$F\ (R^2 \neq 0)$ (Multiple Regression)	$f^2 = \frac{R^2}{1 - R^2}$	.02	.15	.35

NOTE. The definitions of effect size values are based on Cohen (1977).

(not just the null) is that a relationship among the variables under study does not exist, power analysis should always be performed to corroborate the conclusions. Since our hypothesis-testing procedures are geared toward the disconfirmation of the null, power analysis can be an indispensable adjunct procedure in studies designed to demonstrate the absence of relationships.

Power in Nursing and Other Fields

As stated earlier, nursing studies generally are based on relatively small samples of subjects. This suggests that, unless nurse researchers have focused predominantly on problems in which effect sizes are large, these studies are likely to be underpowered, and the risk of committing a Type II error is likely to be great. Therefore, this study was undertaken to examine the statistical power of research published in prominent nursing journals.

Similar studies have been undertaken based on research published in journals in other disciplines. The results of studies from other disciplines are included here to illustrate that the problem of underpowered research is not unique to a single field of inquiry. Table 2 presents selected results from these studies. This table indicates that, regardless of the discipline, when the effects under study are small, power tends to be very low. In most disciplines, the probability of the researchers committing a

TABLE 2 **Comparison of Statistical Power Analyses in Other Disciplines**

Publications	Number of Studies	Mean Statistical Power for Different Effects		
		Small	*Medium*	*Large*
J. of Abnormal & Social Psych (1960)[a]	70	.18	.48	.83
American Ed. Research Journal (1969–70)[b]	47	.14	.58	.78
Nine communications journals (1975)[c]	46	.18	.52	.79
J. of Applied Psychology (1974)[d]	121	.25	.67	.86
Three management publications (1984)[e]	84	.31	.77	.91
American Journal of Medicine (1977)[f]	36	.12	.36	.60
New England Journal of Medicine (1977)[f]	66	.15	.44	.62
Journal of Pediatrics (1977)[f]	71	.16	.40	.64

NOTE. The studies analyzing the power in these publications are: (a) Cohen, 1962; (b) Brewer, 1972; (c) Chase and Tucker, 1975; (d) Chase and Chase, 1976; (e) Mazen et al., 1987; and (f) Reed and Slaichert, 1981. The power analysis based on medical studies by Reed and Slaichert (1981), unlike others in this table, were calculated only on studies that contained at least one nonsignificant result; therefore, the mean power values reported for these studies are likely to be depressed to a certain degree.

Type II error for their tests of significance is about 75% to 85% when the ES is small. Even when effects are moderate, the average power of the statistical tests being performed in every discipline is under the conventionally acceptable level of .80. Only when a study is examining very strong relationships among variables, as when the effects are large, does the power approach or exceed .80.

The purpose of the present study, therefore, is not to evaluate whether current nursing studies are better or worse than studies in other disciplines with respect to the issue of power, but rather to determine if, like researchers in other disciplines, nurse researchers are at high risk of finding nonsignificant results even when their research hypotheses are correct.

Method

The sample for this study consisted of articles from the 1989 volumes of *Nursing Research* and *Research in Nursing and Health*. Of the 124 articles that were published in the twelve 1989 issues of these journals, 62 (50% of the total) were found to yield data on which effect sizes and power could be calculated. Articles were omitted for the following reasons: the article was nonempirical (N = 28); the study was either qualitative or purely descriptive (N = 7); the study was primarily a psychometric analysis of an instrument (N = 16); the study yielded insufficient data for the computation of effect sizes (N = 5); the study was itself a meta-analysis (N = 2); or the study used a statistical test other than the five on which this analysis concentrated (N = 4).

As in previous research on power analyses, such as the studies cited in Table 2, each article rather than the individual test was used as the unit of analysis to avoid giving undue weight to those studies with a disproportionately large number of statistical tests. Within the 62 studies, an ES was calculated for each statistical test of the researchers' hypotheses, for the five tests shown in Table 1. No ES was computed for peripheral tests, such as an examination of demographic differences among subjects.

The method used to calculate the ES follows the formulas shown in Table 1. In instances where there were unequal groups, a weighted mean was used. After calculating the ES, the power of the test was estimated using the power tables presented in Cohen (1977). In calculating power for each ES, the .05 level of significance for a two-tailed test was used uniformly. On average, 9.4 effect sizes were calculated for each article included in the sample, for a total of 583 individual tests.

Once all calculations were made for each article, the effect sizes were grouped into three categories of small, medium, and large, based on Cohen's (1977) conventions of values in those ranges. For example, the convention for correlation coefficients is .10, .30, and .50 for small, medium, and large effects, respectively. The midpoint between these values was used for classification purposes. Thus, a correlation coefficient was considered a small effect if its absolute value was between .01 and .20; medium if its absolute value was between .21 and .40; and large if its absolute value was greater than .40. After classifying each effect according to these criteria, the average power per ES category per article was calculated.

In addition to these analyses, which follow the procedures used in other studies of statistical power, additional analyses were undertaken to consider the adequacy of the sample sizes. Here, the ES was used to obtain the number of subjects needed to detect significant findings for the average effect and the smallest effect in the study, with $\alpha = .05$ and $\beta = .20$.

Results

Table 3 presents the mean power values for the 62 nursing studies, according to ES category. The results are shown separately for studies in which the dependent variable was physiological or social-psychological. For both types of study, the average power for small effects was under .30. This means that when nurse researchers tested hypotheses involving small effects, there was less than a 30% probability of correctly rejecting the null hypothesis. Moreover, a very high percentage (52.7%) of

TABLE 3 Mean Power of Tests, by Effect Size and Type of Dependent Variable

Type of Dependent Variable	Small	Medium	Large	Number
Physiological	.25	.66	.98	18
Social-Psychological	.27	.73	.94	45
Total	.26	.71	.95	63[a]

[a] The total number does not add to 62 (the number of studies in the sample) because one study involved some physiological and some social-psychological dependent measures.

the effect sizes computed were small. Only 12 of the 62 studies in the sample (19%) had no effect sizes that were small. By contrast, 32 of the studies (52%) performed statistical tests where at least half of the effects were small, and one fifth of the studies involved tests for which 75% or more of the effects were small.

When the effects were medium in size, the analyses had substantially better power, as one might expect. However, even when effects were moderate, the average power was only about .70. Thus, the typical study with moderate effects was still at an unacceptably high risk of committing a Type II error. When the effects were large, the power in the studies surveyed was very high. However, only 3 of the 62 studies had effects that were exclusively large. Nearly one third of the studies (29%) had no effects classified as large. Overall, only 9 of the studies (15%) had adequate power for all of their analyses, regardless of ES. In only one of the studies included in the sample was power analysis used to determine sample size requirements. However, other researchers might have performed a power analysis without mentioning it in the article.

Table 4 presents the results in a somewhat different format. This table presents a frequency distribution for the mean power of the tests within the three ES groupings. Thus, there were 50 studies with small effects; of these, 50% had a mean power less than .20 (i.e., greater than an 80% probability of incorrectly retaining the null hypothesis). When effects were small, only 4% of the studies ($N = 2$) had an average power that was acceptable using Cohen's convention of .80. Of the 46 studies with effects in the medium range, the majority (54%) had an average power below .80. Surprisingly, even with large effects, 11% of the studies were underpowered.

These analyses indicate that many nurse researchers are undertaking inadequately powered investigations in which their hypotheses will fail to be supported, even when the hypotheses are correct. One underlying cause of low power is that the majority of hypotheses tested by nurse researchers involve effects that are small or small-to-moderate. This is not because nurse researchers are interested in unimportant or impractical problems. Rather, the phenomena under investigation are typically so complex and difficult to measure that no single study can hope to explain a substantial portion of their variance. In the present study, for example, the average correlation coefficient was .21, corresponding to less than 5% of explained variance.

The other major determinant of inadequate power is the tendency of nurse researchers to use small samples. The mean actual sample size (per group for tests in which groups were compared) was 115. (When the three studies with $N > 500$ are excluded, the mean N drops to 83). Two thirds of the studies had *N*s under 100. Based on the magnitude of the effects under study, these investigators would have needed an average of 218 subjects (per group, except for correlational tests) to detect the *average* effect with a power of .80 and an alpha of .05. Even if the investigators had had 218 subjects per group, effects below average would not, of course, have been detected. To have adequate power for *all* the statistical tests (i.e., even for the smallest effect), the researchers would have needed an average of 1,097 subjects per group. These numbers mask the fact that some studies are actually overpowered. For the 9 studies that had adequate power for all of their statistical tests, the average N was 187, and the average N needed to detect the smallest effect was 32.

Discussion

This study suggests that the majority of nursing studies do not have sufficient power to adequately test the investigators' research hypotheses at statistically significant levels. For several reasons, we believe that our analyses yielded

TABLE 4 **Frequency and Percentages of the Mean Power of the Nursing Studies to Detect Small, Medium, and Large Population Effects**

	Small Effect		Medium Effect		Large Effect	
Power	*f*	%	*f*	%	*f*	%
<.20	25	50	1	2	0	0
.20–.39	11	22	5	11	0	0
.40–.59	11	22	7	15	0	0
.60–.79	1	2	12	26	5	11
.80–.89	1	2	6	13	1	2
≥.90	1	2	15	33	38	86
Total	50	100	46	100	44	99

fairly generous estimates of the power of nursing studies. First, the sample consisted of only published reports.

A second reason for believing that the power estimates in these analyses were liberal is that they were based on studies published in two nursing journals where the methodological standards are especially rigorous. Many studies published in specialty journals are based on samples of 50 or fewer subjects.

Finally, even in the studies included in this study, there was a bias in the reporting of the results that led to further overestimates of power. When the results of analyses were statistically significant, the reports most often provided sufficient information for the computation of the ES. When the results were nonsignificant, however, the authors often stated this fact in narrative fashion, rather than giving quantitative details. For example, when correlation coefficients were significant, the value of *r* was reported; when the correlations were nonsignificant, the value of *r* was often not reported. Whenever possible, we estimated the ES in such situations, always using the most generous assumptions. For example, if the value of *r* was unreported but the text indicated a nonsignificant result, we estimated *r* as the highest possible value for a nonsignificant correlation, given the study's sample size. In some situations, it was not possible to estimate the ES for results that were reported to be nonsignificant, and these tests were omitted completely from our analyses. In both of these situations (that is, when estimates were or were not possible), the result would be to inflate the mean power estimates. Thus, we conclude that our analyses are unlikely to have yielded underestimates of the power of the statistical tests in contemporary nursing studies.

Several implications of the findings from this study bear mentioning. First, the results suggest that nurse researchers ought to undertake a power analysis prior to embarking on a study. Even modest studies are demanding of time and resources, and it is pointless to engage in such an activity when it can be shown in advance to have a high probability of failure; that is, failure to reject a false null hypothesis. The findings here also suggest that when the researcher is forced to use the convention of small, medium, and large to estimate ES, the researcher should generally assume small effects (or, at best, an effect midway between small and medium) unless there are specific theoretical or experiential reasons for expecting larger effects.

A related point is that when a proposal is being prepared for funding a quantitative study, power calculations should be included in the proposal. Review panels are often reluctant to invest in a project if they have no assurance at the outset that the endeavor has good prospects for success. Moreover, review panels do not want to waste resources by paying for more subjects than are needed to detect effects. In other words, researchers submitting a proposal for funding should provide evidence that their study will be neither underpowered (and hence lead to nonsignificant results) or overpowered (and hence use more resources than are necessary).

Given the increased emphasis on utilization of research results in nursing, it may also be important to calculate effect sizes and power estimates after the completion of a study. If the results of nursing studies are to be applied to nursing practice, then the nursing community needs assurance that the effects are substantial enough to warrant change (if there are significant effects) or that the absence of effects is not merely an artifact of an inadequate design. Given our inability to "prove the null hypothesis" using standard statistical procedures, any conclusion in favor of the null hypothesis needs to be bolstered by corroborating evidence, such as the calculation of an ES and power estimate.

The findings of this study indicate that nurse researchers need to pay greater attention to issues of power in designing their studies. Power can be enhanced by increasing ES through a number of methodological decisions. For example, the use of reliable instruments and powerful designs such as analysis of covariance can have positive effects on the ES. However, the most obvious and straightforward method of increasing power is to increase sample size.

References

Brewer, J. (1972). On the power of statistical tests in the American Educational Research Journal. *American Educational Research Journal, 9,* 391–401.

Brown, J. S., Tanner, C. A., and Padrick, K. P. (1984). Nursing's search for scientific knowledge. *Nursing Research, 33,* 26–32.

Chase, J., and Chase, B. (1976). A statistical power analysis of applied psychological research. *Journal of Applied Psychology, 61,* 234–237.

Chase, L., and Tucker, R. (1975). A power analytic examination of contemporary communication research. *Speech Monographs, 42,* 29–41.

Cohen, J. (1962). The statistical power of abnormal-social psychological research: A review. *Journal of Abnormal and Social Psychology, 65,* 145–153.

Cohen, J. (1977). *Statistical power analysis for the behavioral sciences.* New York: Academic Press.

Mazen, A. M., Graf, L. E., Kellogg, C. E., and Hemmasi, M. (1987). Statistical power in contemporary management research. *Academy of Management Journal, 30,* 369–380.

Lipsey, M. W. (1990). *Design sensitivity.* Newbury Park, CA: Sage.

Moody, L. E., Wilson, M. E., Smyth, K., Tittle, M., and Vancott, M. L. (1988). Analysis of a decade of nursing practice research: 1977–1986. *Nursing Research, 37,* 374–379.

Reed, J. F., and Slaichert, W. (1981). Statistical proof in inconclusive "negative" trials. *Archives of Internal Medicine, 141,* 1307–1310.

The Applicability of Sequential Analysis to Nursing Research

Jean K. Brown ■ **Laura A. Porter** ■ **Thomas R. Knapp**

Most statistical techniques have been developed to summarize data collected simultaneously from a group of subjects using traditional fixed-sample, power-based techniques. Inference is made from what is known about a sample at one point in time to what is unknown about a population at that same point in time. In contrast, most clinical nursing research involves the collection of data from subjects who enter the study at various points in time, yet the data are typically treated by traditional techniques.

A modification of inferential statistics, sequential analysis, includes both sequential estimation and sequential hypothesis testing (Wald, 1947; Wetherill, 1966). This paper is focused on sequential hypothesis testing, which seems tailor-made for much of nursing research. It incorporates two special features: a variable, rather than fixed, sample size; and three decisions, rather than two, with respect to the null hypothesis — accept it, reject it, or keep sampling.

Sequential hypothesis testing has been used extensively in manufacturing quality control situations and also in some medical randomized clinical trials (see Armitage & Berry, 1987; Gail, 1979; Pocock, 1983; Whitehead, 1992). The technique was introduced to psychological researchers (Fiske & Jones, 1954) but has had limited application in psychology. Rarely, if ever, has it been used in nursing research.

A major advantage of sequential hypothesis testing in clinical nursing research is the methodological fit, that is, subjects are often entered into studies one at a time. In addition, the sample size required is, on average, smaller than that required for traditional, power-based hypothesis testing (Dixon & Massey, 1983). The sample data analysis may converge toward a decision to accept or reject the null hypothesis after a relatively small number of subjects have been studied. This is very important in research where the cost of obtaining subjects is high or the number of subjects needed for traditional approaches is simply not available. It is also more ethical to terminate a study whenever the evidence is clear, rather than imposing further burdens on additional subjects and continuing to administer potentially harmful or ineffective experimental treatments to meet a predetermined, fixed sample size.

The basic principles of sequential hypothesis testing are summarized in this paper. Examples are given of applications to two existing datasets, and the technique is compared with the standard fixed-sample, power-based approach.

Basic Principles

In sequential hypothesis testing, a null hypothesis (H_0) is tested against an alternative hypothesis (H_1). As in traditional power-based hypothesis testing, H_1 must be explicit, and the researcher must set both alpha and beta. Randomly sampled observations are taken one at a time or in small groups. After each observation or group of observations is taken, a test statistic is calculated and compared to determine cutting points. Then the decision is made to accept H_0, to reject H_0 in favor of H_1, or to keep sampling. Formulas for these test statistics are functions of alpha, beta, the values specified in the H_0 and H_1, and the number of subjects tested thus far (Cox, 1952; Dixon & Massey, 1983; Ostle & Mensing, 1975).

Sequential hypothesis testing is applicable whenever most or all of the following conditions are present (Dixon & Massey, 1983). In most clinical nursing research these conditions are almost always the rule, not the exception:

1. Each test is expensive, thus the smallest sample size possible is preferable.

2. Response time is short, that is, outcomes can be evaluated soon enough to influence further sampling.

3. Test conditions permit testing only one subject at a time.

Jean K. Brown, PhD, RN, is an assistant professor, State University of New York at Buffalo, School of Nursing, Buffalo, NY.

Laura A. Porter, PhD, RN, is an assistant professor, Emory University, Nell Hodgson Woodruff School of Nursing, Atlanta, GA.

Thomas R. Knapp, EdD, is a professor of nursing and education, The Ohio State University College of Nursing, Columbus, OH.

From *Nursing Research,* September/October 1993, *42,* 280–282.

4. Test cases are available at infrequent intervals in time, for example, rare clinical conditions.

Applications

To determine the extent to which sequential hypothesis testing might have been appropriate, the technique was used to test hypotheses concerning proportions and correlations for two datasets. The fast dataset (Brown, 1991) included 60 lung cancer patients in a study of predictors of cancer-related weight loss. The second dataset (Porter, 1992) included 59 patients undergoing coronary angioplasty in a study of stress, cognitive appraisal, and life disruption. Both studies were approved by the Human Subjects Review Board.

Proportions

Because both studies were concerned with change in certain variables such as weight and the threat of heart disease, the proportion of subjects who had negative slopes across time was of interest (Kraemer & Thiemann, 1989; Suter, Wilson & Naqvi, 1991). For the Brown study, subject weights were recorded over time, and the slope of weight change for each subject was calculated. The following hypotheses were tested:

H_0: $\pi_0 = .50$ (50% of subjects have negative slopes indicating weight loss over time.)

H_1: $\pi_1 = .70$ (70% of subjects have negative slopes — a large effect.)

The results for the sequential test of H_0 against H_1 for the Brown data, with the usual defaults of $\alpha = .05$ and $\beta = .20$, are provided in Table 1. As can be seen, the decision to stop sampling and reject H_0 in favor of H_1 would have been made after sampling only 21 subjects. The proportion of the sample with negative slopes starts out high and stays high, never falling below .70 after the first three observations, so the test statistic cutting point for the alternative hypothesis is reached quickly. The fixed-sample approach would have required 37 subjects (Cohen, 1988; Kraemer & Thiemann, 1987).

For the Porter study, subjects were asked how threatened they were by heart disease prior to and following a coronary angioplasty, and the slope of change in heart disease threat was calculated for each subject. The hypotheses were as follows:

H_0: $\pi_0 = .50$ (50% of subjects have negative slopes or decreasing heart disease threat.)

H_1: $\pi_1 = .60$ (60% of subjects have negative slopes— a small effect.)

Again the usual defaults of $\alpha = .05$ and $\beta = .20$ were set. The results for the Porter data were quite different. After 59 subjects the decision would be to keep sampling, but there were no more subjects. As shown in Figure 1, the reason for the "keep sampling" decision was the lack of convergence toward either hypothesis because the sample proportions of negative slopes kept fluctuating around .55, halfway between the two values stipulated in the competing hypotheses. This can often happen for small effect sizes. The need for large sample sizes in order to differentiate between zero effects and very small effects is as necessary with sequential hypothesis testing as it is with traditional techniques. For this example, Cohen's (1988) table yields an n of 152.

TABLE 1 Sequential Hypothesis Testing for Proportions—Brown Data[a,b]

n	p	Test statistic
1	1.000	.336
2	.500	−.175
3	.667	.162
4	.750	.497
5	.800	.833
6	.833	1.167
7	.857	1.504
8	.875	1.841
9	.889	2.178
10	.900	2.513
11	.818	2.000
12	.833	2.335
13	.846	2.672
14	.786	2.166
15	.733	1.652
16	.750	1.988
17	.706	1.479
18	.722	1.809
19	.737	2.152
20	.750	2.485
21	.762	2.821

Decision: Reject H_0 in favor of H_1

[a] H_0:$\pi_0 = .50$, H_1: $\pi_1 = .70$ ($\alpha = .05$: $\beta = .20$).
H_0 cutting point: test statistic < -1.558.
H_1 cutting point: test statistic > 2.773.
[b] Test statistic: $n(.847\ p - .511)$, where n is the number of observations and p is the sample proportion based on n observations.

Correlations

The hypotheses concerning Pearson product-moment correlations for the Brown data dealt with the variables of height and weight:

H_0: $\rho_0 = 0$ (There is no relationship between height and weight.)

H_1: $\rho_1 = .50$ (A large effect)

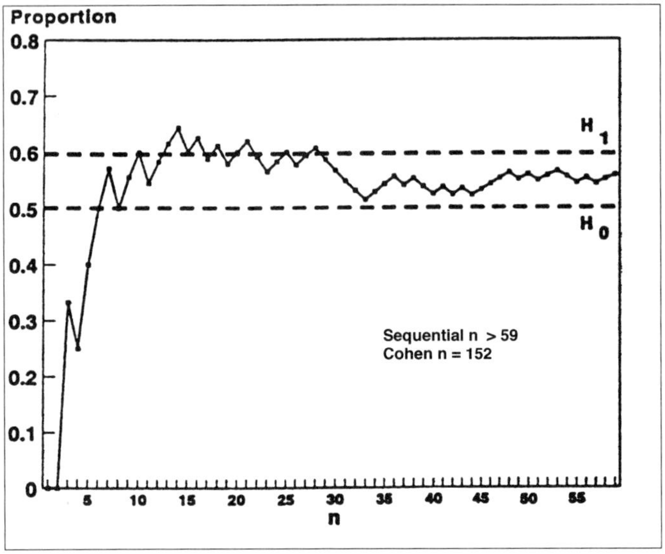

FIGURE 1 The Sequential Sample Proportions for the Porter Data

The first few observations in the Brown data (for $\alpha = .05$ and $\beta = .20$) resulted in negative correlations, taking longer for convergence to occur. The decision could have been made to *accept* H_0 after only 7 subjects because the test statistic cutting point was reached. Several more subjects were entered, however, because the *n* was so small. Moreover, a negative correlation was not commensurate with either H_0 or H_1. (The O'Brien and Fleming [1979] approach to sequential hypothesis testing would have avoided this problem because it is more difficult to cross the cutting points early in the analysis.) The decision to *reject* H_0 in favor of H_1 would have been made after 25 observations. The fixed-sample approach (Cohen, 1988) would have required only 22 observations.

For the Porter data, the relationship between optimism and heart disease threat was examined. In this analysis more stringent specifications were set ($\alpha = .01$. $\beta = .01$) than in previous examples. The hypotheses were as follows:

H_0: $\rho_0 = 0$ (There is no relationship between optimism and heart disease threat.)

H_1: $\rho_1 = -.30$ (A small, inverse effect)

The sample correlations started converging rapidly toward −.60 after the first few observations, and the decision to reject H_0 in favor of H_1 would have been made after only 34 observations, despite the stringent alpha and beta levels. Cohen's (1988) table would require an *n* of 229. This is an example of an apparent underestimation of the true effect size. Optimism and heart disease threat seem to have a strong inverse relationship, a much larger effect than that proposed in H_1.

Discussion

Sequential hypothesis testing resulted in a smaller sample size than traditional hypothesis testing for the Brown data proportions. Sequential analysis required 21 subjects, while traditional analysis would have required 37 subjects. Thus, 16 subjects were saved. An even greater savings was obtained for the Porter data correlations. The null hypothesis was rejected after 34 subjects were tested, whereas the fixed-sample, power-based approach would have required 229 observations.

Sequential hypothesis testing was not effective for either the Porter proportions or the Brown correlations. For the Porter proportions, convergence toward neither the null nor alternative hypotheses occurred. For the Brown correlations, three additional subjects were required to reject the null hypothesis. These two examples illustrate that sequential hypothesis testing has at least two disadvantages: (a) Convergence may never occur, and (b) more subjects may occasionally be required than for traditional approaches.

Another important point is that wrong decisions are just as likely in sequential hypothesis testing as in traditional statistical inference. Type I and Type II errors are always possible. In addition, both approaches assume random sampling, an assumption that is frequently violated by scientific researchers.

TABLE 2 Some Formulas for Sequential Hypothesis Testing

Parameter & Hypothesized Values	Test Statistic	Acceptance Value	Rejection Value
Proportion:[a] π_0 vs. π_1	$n\{[ln(\pi_1/\pi_0)] - ln[(1-\pi_1)/(1-\pi_0)]p - ln[(1-\pi_1)/(1-\pi_0)]\}$	$ln[\beta/(1-\alpha)]$	$ln[(1-\beta)/\alpha]$
Correlation:[a,b] ρ_0 vs. ρ_1	$(n-3)[2z - (\zeta_1 - \zeta_0)]$	$\frac{2ln[\beta/(1-\alpha)]}{(\zeta_1 - \zeta_0)}$	$\frac{2ln[(1-\beta)/\alpha]}{(\zeta_1 - \zeta_0)}$
Variance:[a] σ^2_0 vs. σ^2_1	$.5(n-1)(1/\sigma_0^2 - 1/\sigma_1^2)s^2 - (n-1)ln(\sigma_1/\sigma_0)$	$ln[\beta/(1-\alpha)]$	$ln[(1-\beta)/\alpha]$
Differences among means (ANOVA):[c] all μ's are equal vs. $var(\mu) = \lambda\sigma^2$	$(1+n\lambda)^{-.5(k-1)}\{c\}^{.5(nk-1)}$ where $c = \frac{(1+n\lambda)[k(n-1)+(k-1)F]}{k(n-1)(1+n\lambda)+(k-1)F}$	$\beta/(1-\alpha)$	$(1-\beta)/\alpha$

NOTE. Whitehead (1992) has developed PEST 2 software for many of these tests.
[a] *ln* is the natural logarithm (to the base *e*).
[b] The *z*'s and the ζ's are Fisher's *z* transformations of the Pearson *r*'s and ρ's.
[c] For the sequential ANOVA, $\lambda\sigma^2$ is the difference among the means postulated in the alternative hypothesis, i.e., a difference that is λ times as great as the within-population variance: *k* is the number of populations (and samples); *n* is the number of observations in *each* sample (since one observation must be taken from each of the *k* populations at each step); and *F* is the ratio of the mean square between samples to the mean square within samples.

Summary

The authors have described sequential analysis, specifically sequential hypothesis testing, pointed out some of its advantages and disadvantages, and applied it to a few examples involving proportions and correlations. Formulas for sequential analogues for more advanced statistical techniques are shown in Table 2. The sequential model provides an attractive option to traditional fixed-sample, power-based analyses because it is very appropriate for the methods and procedures used in clinical nursing research.

References

Armitage, P., & Berry, G. (1987). *Sequential methods in medical research.* London: Blackwell.

Brown, J. K. (1991). Precancer factors and outcomes of weight loss in adults with lung cancer. *Dissertation Abstracts International, 52,* 2989B.

Cohen, J. (1988). *Statistical power analysis for the behavioral sciences* (2nd. ed.). Hillsdale, NJ: Erlbaum.

Cox, D. R. (1952). Sequential tests for composite hypotheses. *Proceedings of the Cambridge Philosophical Society, 48,* 290–299.

Dixon, W. J., & Massey, F. J. (1983). *Introduction to statistical analysis* (4th ed.). New York: McGraw-Hill.

Fiske, D. W., & Jones, L. V. (1954). Sequential analysis in psychological research. *Psychological Bulletin, 51,* 264–275.

Gail, M. H. (1979). Monitoring and stopping clinical trials. In H. J. Tagnon & M. J. Staquet (Eds.), *Controversies in cancer* (pp. 455–484). New York: Masson.

Kraemer, H. C., & Thiemann, S. (1987). *How many subjects?* Newbury Park, CA: Sage.

Kraemer, H. C., & Thiemann, S. (1989). A strategy to use soft data effectively in randomized controlled clinical trials. *Journal of Consulting and Clinical Psychology, 57,* 148–154.

O'Brien, P. C., & Fleming, T. R. (1979). A multiple testing procedure for clinical trials. *Biometrics, 35,* 549–556.

Ostle, R., & Mensing, R. W. (1975). *Statistics in research* (3rd. ed.). Ames, IA: Iowa State University Press.

Pocock, S. J. (1983). *Clinical trials: A practical approach.* New York: Wiley.

Porter, L A. (1992). *Sources of psychological stress, cognitive appraisal, and life disruption.* Unpublished doctoral dissertation, University of Rochester.

Suter, W. N., Wilson, D., & Naqvi, A. (1991). Using slopes to measure directional change. *Nursing Research, 40,* 250–252.

Wald, A. (1947). *Sequential analysis.* New York: Wiley.

Wetherill, G. B. (1966). *Sequential methods in statistics.* London: Methuen.

Whitehead, J. (1992). *The design and analysis of sequential clinical trials* (2nd ed.). New York: Ellis Howard.

Planning Research Studies: An Alternative to Power Analysis

E. Benton Cobb

As evidenced by Goodwin's (1984) article, there is a growing awareness among nurse researchers of the importance of power calculations in the design of research studies. Cohen (1977) discussed applications for some commonly used statistical tests. Although the theory of hypothesis testing, as developed some 50 years ago by Neyman and Pearson (1933), has been discussed in many modern statistics textbooks, the concept of power has apparently not been fully understood or appreciated by researchers who use statistics. On the other hand, standard statistical tests such as *t* and *F* are widely used in all areas of research and have been for many years. The application of these tests has become so standardized that the rejection of a null hypothesis at the 5% level of significance has become a criterion by which a researcher's results are judged. This overly simplistic standard can lead to the publication of results that are statistically significant, but of no scientific importance. Since null hypotheses of equality are almost never true, sufficiently large sample sizes will lead to rejection of a null hypothesis of equality. In short, any such null hypothesis can be rejected, provided the researcher has enough time and money to spend on the study.

The choice of a minimum effective size (ES) in the design of a study is a statement about what constitutes an important scientific or clinical difference and should not be confused with a statistically significant difference. Choosing sample sizes to make the power sufficiently large at the ES allows the researcher to make a probabilistic statement about a difference being larger than ES if the null hypothesis is accepted; i.e., acceptance of the null hypothesis is statistical "proof" that the population difference is not more than ES. However, even with all this clarification, researchers are justified in thinking that the whole process is overly complicated. For example, the computation of power, as discussed in Goodwin (1984) for the ANOVA example, is based on a noncentrality parameter ϕ, which is a population measure of the amount of variance between groups relative to the amount of variance within groups. For three or more treatment groups, this parameter is not the most natural quantity for a researcher to consider.

E. Benton Cobb, PhD, is an associate professor in the Department of Mathematics, University of Kansas, Lawrence, KS.

From *Nursing Research,* November/December 1985, *34,* 386–388.

Confidence Intervals Instead of Tests

An alternative approach to the ANOVA and other statistical problems is to ignore testing and to concentrate on estimating treatment effects (or other parameters of interest) to a prespecified level of precision. That is, plan the study to yield confidence intervals of prescribed length for treatment effects. For many studies, estimation of treatment effects or other parameters is of more importance than the test of a hypothesis of equality. Confidence intervals provide not only information about where the differences occur, but also estimates of their magnitude. For orthogonal designs, ANOVA tables provide information about the relative importance of the various effects and interactions; *F* values are helpful as quantitative measures in this regard, but an *F* test, in effect, converts a measurement on a continuous scale to a binary measurement, thereby reducing the information contained in the data. The formulation of an acceptable minimal level of precision within the estimation framework is analogous to the formulation of ES within the hypothesis-testing framework. But, within the estimation framework, studies can be designed in a more natural way, and results can be presented in a more informative and understandable way.

One-way ANOVA

A one-way ANOVA with $k-1$ treatment groups and one control group can be used to illustrate the procedure. Let $\mu_1, \mu_2, \ldots \mu_k$ be the k population means, with μ_k the control mean, and let σ_e denote the population standard deviation. (As usual, we assume σ_e to be the same for each of the k populations.) Suppose the researcher wishes to compare each of the $k-1$ treatments with the control and has determined that a difference less than ξ between a treatment and a control mean is not important, but considers a difference greater than ξ to be important. Then, it is possible to determine a sample size n so that an interval estimate for a treatment-control difference, say $\mu_j - \mu_k$, will estimate population differences to within $\pm\xi$. This is accomplished by choosing the sample size n in each population large enough so that twice the standard error of the difference of the two sample means ($2\sigma_d$) is less than ξ. This is so because the 95% confidence interval for the difference $\mu_j - \mu_k$ is the interval of values between the confidence limits given by

$$(\bar{x}_j - \bar{x}_k) \pm 2\sigma_d \quad (1)$$

if σ_d is known. Because $\sigma_d = \sigma_e\,(2/n)^{1/2}$, the required sample size can be obtained by solving $2(2/n)^{1/2}\sigma_e = \xi$ for n, using an initial estimate for σ_e (it can be crude). This yields $n = 8\sigma_e^2/\xi^2$ which is the required sample size for each of the k groups.

For example, consider a one-way ANOVA based on the values:

$$\sigma_e = 10 \text{ (initial estimate)}$$
$$\xi = 5 \text{ (required precision).}$$

Then the required sample size for each group is given by

$$n = 8(10^2)/5^2 = 32$$

After data collection, σ_e is estimated in the usual way by s_e, the square root of the sample mean square for error; confidence intervals can be computed for all treatments and the individual treatment-control differences will be accurate to within an approximate tolerance ξ with 95% confidence (provided the initial estimate of σ_e used to determine n was not too small). That is, the intervals will be correct 19 times out of 20; a population difference will lie outside the interval only 1 time in 20, and the length of the intervals will be approximately 2ξ. The confidence limits are given by

$$(\bar{x}_j - \bar{x}_k) \pm t_{.025}(2/n)^{1/2} s_e, \quad (2)$$

where $t_{.025}$ is the upper 2.5% point of the t distribution with $k(n-1)$ degrees of freedom. Note that this is not the same as the usual two-sample t interval: The standard deviation s_e is computed from all k samples, not just samples j and k. This provides more degrees of freedom for error and a better confidence interval, provided the usual ANOVA assumptions are valid.

An initial estimate for σ_e can be based on a pilot study, the results of previous studies, or an educated guess. In the planning stage, it is better to overestimate σ_e as this will result in a sample size that is more than adequate for the goals of the study. When an initial estimate does not seem possible, the researcher must formulate precision in terms of standard units: i.e., instead of determining ξ as a raw difference, determine it as a fractional standard deviation, say $.25\sigma_e$ or $.50\sigma_e$. This is equivalent to setting $\sigma_e = 1$ in the calculations for n previously discussed, and setting $\xi = .25$ or $.50$.

The preceding example is a special case of a *contrast* among means: that is, a linear combination $\Sigma c_i\mu_i$ where the coefficients c_i sum to zero. Confidence limits for individual contrasts are easily calculated for one-way layouts, and sample sizes can be calculated to provide estimates of contrasts with prespecified precision. The contrast $\Sigma c_i\mu_i$ is estimated by $\Sigma c_i\bar{x}_i$ and its standard error is $\sigma_e(\Sigma c_i^2/n)^{1/2}$, which is a generalization of the quantity σ_d in the preceding example.

Correlation Coefficients

Another example in which estimation is often more appropriate than testing is correlation analysis. Studies designed to show correlation (or lack thereof) between variables can be designed to prespecified levels of precision. A confidence interval for a population correlation coefficient ρ provides the researcher with more information than a test of a null hypothesis. For example, suppose a study is designed to estimate ρ to within $\pm.10$ with 95% confidence. Assuming a bivariate normal population, the normal theory standard error for the sample correlation r is $\sigma_r = (1 - \rho^2)/(n-3)^{1/2}$ (cf., Johnson & Kotz, 1970, p. 229). Using an initial estimate for ρ, the required sample size can be determined by solving

$$2(1 - \rho^2)/(n-3)^{1/2} = .10$$

for n. For example, if ρ is close to zero, $n = 400$ is required. If $\rho = .55$, $n = 200$ will suffice, and if $\rho = .71$, then $n = 100$ is enough. If the researcher has no information about the magnitude of ρ, then the conservative solution is $n = 400$. After data collection, Fisher's z transformation (cf., Morrison, 1976, pp. 104–105) can be used to construct the actual confidence limits. This is preferred to the simpler normal theory limits because of the skewness of the distribution for r if ρ is not close to zero. Computational details are omitted.

If $n = 400$ is used in a study, the following reasoning applies: If the absolute value of ρ is larger than .10, then the confidence limits are not likely to bracket zero, in which case the researcher has statistical proof of a nonzero correlation in addition to an estimate of ρ with limits on the amount of error in estimation. On the other hand, if the confidence limits bracket zero, the researcher has statistical proof of negligible correlation. There is no need to explicitly state all this; the interpretation is for illustration only and is in accordance with the logic of hypothesis tests. It is much easier and more understandable to simply report the confidence interval and confidence coefficient.

Simultaneous Confidence Intervals

The discussion so far has centered on confidence intervals for individual contrasts. Many researchers prefer the simultaneous approach to testing and estimation; modifications are required for this approach. Miller (1966) discussed many methods for simultaneous estimation. An example of one of the simplest of these is the Bonferroni method, which is particularly easy to apply to the preceding ANOVA example. There are $k - 1$ comparisons in that example, and the overall confidence coefficient for the set of the $k - 1$ differences will be .95 provided that $t_{.025}$ is replaced by t_b in (2), where $b = .025/(k - 1)$. This makes the intervals wider, which means less precision for the individual contrasts if n remains fixed. Now, to determine n so that the *simultaneous* precision is ξ, substitute the upper $2.5/(k - 1)$ normal percentage point, z_b, for the number 2 in (1), and solve $z_b(2/n)^{1/2}\sigma_e = \xi$ for n. For example, if $k = 6$, then $b = .025/5$, and $z_{.005} = 2.6$. This, of course, will cause an increase in n over that required for ξ precision for individual intervals. Using $\sigma_e = 10$ and $\xi = 5$ as in the preceding example,

$$n = 2(2.6)^2(10)^2/5^2 = 54.08,$$

and so 54 or 55 subjects are required for each of the six groups.

Bonferroni's method can be applied to obtain simultaneous intervals for a set of parameters in any study in which confidence intervals for the individual parameters are available. Important examples include regression coefficients in a regression analysis and correlations among a set of variables in a multivariate study. Details can be found in Miller (1966) and Morrison (1976).

Modifications are possible with other methods of simultaneous estimation in ANOVA, such as Scheffé's method and Tukey's method. In many cases the modifications are straightforward, but will not be discussed here.

Improving the Precision

Most of the comments in Goodwin (1984) concerning ways to increase power translate to analogous methods of improving precision of estimates. For example, if only a single confidence limit is required, either upper or lower, for a parameter, then precision can be improved for a given sample size in the same way power is improved by a directional hypothesis. The choice of design to minimize σ_e improves precision in estimation just as it improves power.

Summary

Hypothesis testing is a cumbersome method of statistical analysis and sometimes leads to misinterpretation of results. Whenever possible, it is preferable to design studies and analyze data using estimation procedures. For ANOVA, correlation analysis, regression, and other standard statistical methods, it is possible, and no more difficult, to use estimation procedures.

References

Cohen, J. (1977). *Statistical power analysis for the behavioral sciences* (rev. ed.). New York: Academic Press.

Goodwin, L. D. (1984). The use of power estimation in nursing research. *Nursing Research. 33,* 118–120.

Johnson, N., & Kotz, S. (1970). *Continuous univariate distributions* (vol. 2). Boston: Houghton-Mifflin.

Miller, R. G., Jr. (1966). *Simultaneous statistical inference.* New York: McGraw-Hill Book Co., Inc.

Morrison, D. F. (1976). *Multivariate statistical methods* (2nd ed.). New York: McGraw-Hill Book Co., Inc.

Neyman, J., & Pearson, E. S. (1933). On the problem of the most efficient tests of statistical hypotheses. *Philosophical Transactions of the Royal Society of London, Series A, 231,* 289–337.

Systematic Sampling: Theory and Clinical Methods

Judith A. Floyd

Systematic sampling is a nonrandom probability sampling method. It is considered a type of probability sampling because each unit of the population has a known, nonzero probability of selection. However, the systematic process of taking every *k*th sampling unit after a random start sets this sampling method apart from random forms of probability sampling. This article is focused on systematically selecting *n* of *N* elements: however, the issues discussed here in terms of element sampling also apply when *a* of *A* clusters are systematically sampled.

The Systematic Sampling Procedure

Suppose a list of all adult patients admitted to the surgical suite of a hospital during the past calendar year is available to a researcher. Assume the researcher has determined that a sample size of 84 is needed to detect medium bivariate correlational effect sizes (Cohen, 1988). For ease of computation, let the list contain 840 patients. Then the systematic sampling interval *k* will equal *N* (840) divided by *n* (84), or 10. The interval *k* divides the population *N* into *n* segments or zones. The researcher will select every *k*th element, one from each zone, after a random start.

The purpose of a random start is to choose the first sampling unit in a manner that assures that all units on the list have a chance to be included in the sample. The first unit may be randomly selected from the entire list. Under most circumstances it is equally appropriate, and often more convenient, to select the first unit from the first *k* units randomly, or, in the case of the example, the first 10 patients. If the researcher does not randomly select the first unit, the procedure no longer qualifies as probability sampling. Regardless of how the random start *r* is obtained, if it were, for instance, number 7, then patients listed as numbers 7, 17, 27, 37 . . . 837 would be selected, for a total of 84 subjects.

Judith A. Floyd, PhD, RN, is an associate professor of nursing, Wayne State University, Detroit, MI.

From *Nursing Research,* September/October 1993, *42,* 290–293.

Systematic sampling can be done as a list is formed. If the researcher wishes to select every *k*th individual as they are admitted for surgery, the first subject must be identified using a random procedure to select *r*. The population list begins with the first potential subject, but it is the *r*th patient who becomes the first subject. After patient *r*, every *k*th patient is selected as a subject. After the final subject has been selected, consider the next *k* minus *r* patients as part of the population list.

Advantages of Systematic Sampling

The major reason to use systematic sampling instead of other forms of probability sampling is its relative simplicity. The use of systematic sampling as a list is formed can be especially useful in complex settings, such as health care facilities, where random types of probability sampling procedures may be too burdensome. It is easier for clinicians to collect data or implement an experimental treatment if subjects are selected on a regular schedule, rather than randomly.

Whatever sampling approach is chosen for a study, the researcher needs to make sure that it is implemented properly. Although it is difficult to check if a random procedure is implemented as planned, one can often review a list of population elements or clusters to see whether every *k*th unit was selected. With care, even the random start can be verified, or, if necessary, the researcher can determine the random start rather than leave it to others.

Another advantage of systematic sampling is that it generates a roughly proportionate sample whenever the population list has strata. A systematically drawn sample from the hypothetical list of 840 patients admitted over the calendar year will yield the same proportion of patients from each month as occured in the listing. Whatever stratification exists in the ordering of the population list, the systematic sample will reflect it with an absolute error of less than one element for any stratum (Kish, 1965). Under these same circumstances, simple random sampling is less likely to represent each stratum. Therefore, systematic sampling may be preferable to simple random sampling when a list is stratified (Babbie, 1973).

However, systematic sampling is limited in its ability to represent strata precisely, and when a stratum is smaller than k, it may be completely excluded. Therefore, both simple random sampling and systematic sampling should be bypassed in favor of stratified sampling methods when it is important to represent strata smaller than k and/or have strata represented precisely.

Issues in Systematic Sampling

The problem of intervals arises when the population list is not an integral multiple of k. In the example, 840 is evenly divisible by 84, yielding a zone length of 10. If one had a listing of 848 patients, and kept k equal to 10, the sample size would still be 84 if the random start fell at 9 or 10, but would be 85 if the random start fell between 1 and 8. One approach is to allow the sample to be of size n or of size $n + 1$, depending on where the random start falls (Kish, 1965). According to Cochran (1977), the disturbance is negligible when n exceeds 50 and unlikely to be large even when n is small. This approach to handling the problem of intervals yields an equal probability of selection for each element, which is equal to $1/k$. It also yields a close approximation to a proportionate sample when the population list is stratified.

A second approach is to consider the list as circular. The last unit is followed by the first. In the example, the 85th zone would be composed of patients 841, 842, 843, 844, 845, 846, 847, 848, 1, and 2. This approach guarantees a specific sample size a priori, but leads to unequal probabilities of selection since patients 1 and 2 have two chances of being included while the others have only one. As long as each element from the population list has a calculable nonzero probability of selection, the sampling method remains a type of probability sampling. Even when the population list is considered circular, systematic sampling with a random start from 1 to k has all the advantages of probability sampling. However, it lacks the additional potential benefit of equal probability selection methods. These benefits are related to the precision of population parameters estimated from sample statistics. If the situation allows a random start from 1 to N, equal probability of selection can be retained and will equal 84 divided by 848 (n/N).

A third approach is to use a random process to reduce the list to exactly the right length to achieve an integral multiple of k prior to the beginning of the systematic sampling procedure. In the example, the researcher would randomly select 8 of the 848 patients to be eliminated prior to selecting the random start. The probability of selection for each element is equal and has a value of n/N. However, if stratification exists in the ordering of the population list, random elimination of subjects will decrease the accuracy of a proportionate sample.

A fourth approach is to use fractional intervals. For example, if the researcher wants a sample size of 84 to be systematically sampled from a listing of 848 patients, k can be calculated by dividing 848 by 84. In this case, k rounds to 10.1. The researcher then chooses a random start between 1 and $10k$. In this case, $10k$ equals 101. The researcher adds the interval 101 successively until 84 numbers are obtained. These numbers are rounded down by eliminating the last digits, thus obtaining 84 numbers between 1 and 848. For a random start of 59, the first 12 numbers would be 59, then 59 + 101 = 160, then 160 + 101 = 261, and so on, to identify numbers 362, 463, 564, 665, 766, 867, 968, 1069, and 1170. Dropping the last digit to round down, the first 12 patients to be selected would be patients 5, 16, 26, 36, 46, 56, 66, 76, 86, 96, 106, and 117. Continuing in this manner, the 84th subject would be patient number 844. It can be shown that the probability of selection for each patient is equal and is n (84) divided by N (848), or 1 divided by k. This approach sets the sample size a priori. It does not interfere with the accuracy of a proportionate sample when stratification exists in the order of elements on the population list. The only disadvantage is its relative lack of simplicity compared to stating, "We will start with patient number 7 and then continue with every 10th patient."

If the primary purpose of a clinical study is exploratory, much work regarding measurement issues is likely to remain. In this case, sampling error due to unequal probability of selection methods is negligible in comparison to measurement error, and the researcher's choice of how to manage the problem of intervals is best guided by practical considerations.

In clinical experiments the researcher assigns subjects to groups following selection. Cost and accuracy may make it desirable to preset the sample size as well as to have equal probability of selection. If the problem of intervals arises, randomly deleting subjects to obtain the desired number of elements on the population list prior to systematic sampling is the most straightforward approach. However, if representation of strata from an ordered list is also important, the use of fractional intervals will be necessary.

Departures from randomness in the ordering of elements on the population list is the second major problem for the researcher who wishes to use systematic sampling. One type of departure, called a monotonic trend, exists when the list is ordered in such a manner that the values for some variable of interest slowly, but more or less steadily, rise or fall. Rapid and/or steady increases or decreases of values are of equal concern. However, they are more easily noticed and are thus less of a threat (Kish, 1965).

Assume a new surgical technique was developed for a condition that first develops in young adulthood but remains surgically correctable across the lifespan. The surgeons are eager to help those who have suffered the longest. A monotonic trend in age might appear because age is likely to be high initially, but will gradually show a downward trend as the backlog of long-suffering patients have surgery. Under these circumstances, the mean age of a systematic sample of every 10th element would depend on the value of the random start: A sample consisting of the first element from each zone, patients 1, 11, 21, would very likely have a higher mean age than a sample composed of the last element from each zone, patients 9, 19, 29. Based on the sample statistics, the population mean would be underestimated in the first case and overestimated in the second.

Another type of departure from randomness in the ordering of elements on a population list is periodic variation. A periodic variation exists whenever units are placed on a list in a manner that results in a recurring cycle. Such cyclical fluctuations are considered potentially more biasing than monotonic trends, but easier to find and avoid (Kish, 1965; Sudman, 1976).

In the example of 840 patients, suppose a cycle corresponds with the researcher's plan to select every 10th patient. The hospital tends to admit 2–4 emergency medical cases and then admit up to 10 elective surgery patients before repeating the cycle. Under these conditions, a random start of 1 or 2 would yield a very different sample (mostly, or all, emergency admissions) than a random start of 9 or 10, which would yield a sample of mostly, or all, elective surgery patients.

As the example shows, it is not the presence of cyclical patterns that creates the problem. The difficulty results from the synchronization of the periodic fluctuation with the sampling interval length. Generally, whenever fluctuations of period k are present in the population list, a sampling interval of k or any multiple of k—or even simple fractions such as $k/2$ or $k/3$—should not be used (Cochran, 1977; Kish, 1965). The problems created by either a monotonic trend or a periodic variation are clarified by a consideration of the third major issue regarding systematic sampling, which is the estimation of variance for systematic samples.

The Problem with Variances

Variance computations require at least two random selections per stratum to be considered valid, but systematic samples are composed of a single selection from each zone, which is an implicit stratum. Furthermore, these selections are not independent between strata. In fact, a systematic sample can be regarded as the result of choosing a single sample from a population of k samples; the interval k divides the population into k "clusters" of n elements each, and the random start from 1 to k selects one of these clusters as the sample. Each of the n elements in a systematic sample is considered to have both a random error component and a deviation from the population mean that is constant for all the elements in the sample. The random components tend to cancel out for large n, but the deviation from the population mean is a systematic deviation. This resembles a systematic bias of measurement, but is not formally called a bias because it cancels over all k possible samples (Cochran, 1977; Kish, 1965).

Because the deviation from the population mean remains unmeasured and therefore excluded from the variance computations, a systematic sample, although a probability sample, is not strictly "measurable" as it does not provide all the information for computing the variance. Therefore, the researcher must provide a model for the nature of variation over the listing order. Because the researcher must work from an assumed model of the nature of variation, the one-stage systematic sampling process described in this article is not recommended when the primary purpose of a study is to estimate population parameters (Cochran, 1977; Hansen, Hurwitz, & Madow, 1953; Kish, 1965).

Often the researcher can provide theoretical and empirical evidence to support the assumption of a simple random model for the nature of variation over the listing order. The argument usually is that if the population elements were thoroughly shuffled before they were ordered on the list, a systematic sample would be equivalent to a simple random sample. Although short of this ideal, in many population lists most of the variance in the variables of interest is irregular and haphazard, and the result of systematic selection can be accepted as a good approximation for random choice (Madow, 1949; 1953; Madow & Madow, 1944).

When a population list has divisions, the sample variance may be lower than the simple random model would indicate because of the proportionate stratification effect induced by systematic sampling. Under these circumstances, there is a tendency for nearby elements of the population list to resemble each other, that is, to deviate similarly from the population mean. In this case, the assumption of a stratified random model can more easily be defended (Cochran, 1977; Kish, 1965). Another choice of model is the paired selections model. It can be adopted when it is reasonable to assume that the $2k$ elements comprising every two consecutive zones are in random order (Kish, 1965).

A final model, the successive difference model, sometimes seems the most reasonable. It is a modified version of the paired selections model. It uses all the successive differences to form pairs, that is, the elements from zones 1 and 2, then the elements from zones 2 and 3, and so on. Although more tedious to determine if a computer program is not available, the precision of the computed sample variance using this model is somewhat increased over the paired selections model (Kish, 1965).

Detection and Management of Departures from Randomness

When there is a monotonic trend or periodic variation, none of the four models can be assumed. Thus, attention needs to be given to detecting and avoiding departures from randomness. In many situations, a researcher familiar with the clinical setting and clinical phenomenon under study may be able to dismiss the possibility of a monotonic trend or periodic fluctuation by simple scrutiny of the list.

Sometimes statistical analyses involving part or all of the population list can be helpful to rule out monotonic trends and periodic variations. One approach is to compare the means and variances of all k-possible samples from a subset of zones. Zones separated maximally from each other should be chosen. In the case of the original example of surgical patients, one could compare the 10 samples ($n = 8$) generated when patients from zones 1, 12, 24, 36, 48, 60, 72, and 84 are selected for r from 1 to k, respectively. If monotonic trends or periodic fluctuations exist in the list, significant linear, cubic, or quadratic trends should be found over the 10 sample means ordered from 1 to k (Weiner, 1971).

A second statistical approach is to use time series analysis to examine the data from the entire population list. Using the example, data from all 840 cases would be entered for computerized time series analysis. Any variable suspected of producing a monotonic trend or periodic variation over the length of the list would be analyzed (Cook & Campbell, 1979).

If the researcher is not confident that monotonic trends and periodic fluctuations have been avoided, it may be possible to shuffle the listing before using the systematic sampling procedure. If this is done, the opportunity to sample proportionately is lost. The practice of changing the random start many times may be more feasible. For example, in selecting 84 subjects from the list of 840 patients, one random start could be used to select the first 25% (21) of the subjects. Then a second random start could be chosen and used for the next 25%, and so forth (Kish, 1965; Madow & Madow, 1944; Madow, 1949; 1953). Unlike shuffling the list, changing the random start is feasible for studies where systematic sampling is used as the list forms. However, this procedure will interfere with selecting a proportionate sample.

Two other approaches can be used to manage monotonic trends. The first is to follow standard systematic sampling procedures and then weight the values obtained depending upon the subjects' place in the zone. If the subjects are from the first half of each zone, their scores on variables of interest are increased by the calculated weight; if they are from the latter half of each zone, their scores are decreased by the calculated weight. Bellhouse and Rao (1975) provide formulas for calculating weights.

The second approach is to use purposive procedures based on the researcher's knowledge of the distribution of sampling units on the population list. A typical purposive approach is the selection of a centrally located sample. Instead of using a random start, the researcher deliberately chooses the middle element of each zone, which is k divided by 2 if k is even or $k + 1$ divided by 2 if k is odd (Madow, 1953). In the example of 840 patients where k equals 10, k is even and k divided by 2 equals 5. Thus, the 5th patient on the list would be chosen, followed by every 10th patient. The rationale is intuitively clear: If some value is increasing or decreasing over the length of the list, selecting the middle unit from each zone will be more precise than a randomly located unit (Cochran, 1977). Variations on selecting a centrally located sample exist. All attempt to select the most representative elements based on knowledge of the monotonic trend (Murthy, 1967; Singh, Jindal, & Garg, 1968).

Although systematic sampling has much to recommend it, it is not problem-free. The greatest threats are undetected monotonic trends or periodic fluctuations in the order of the population list. However, if investigators carefully rule out these problems and use theoretical and empirical knowledge to select models of population distribution, systematic sampling may be the method of choice in many clinical research situations.

References

Babbie, E. R. (1973). *Survey research methods.* Belmont, C.A. Wadsworth.

Bellhouse, D. R., & Rao, J. N. K. (1975). Systematic sampling in the presence of a trend. *Biometrika, 62,* 694–697.

Cochran, W. G. (1977). *Sampling techniques* (3rd ed.). New York: Wiley.

Cohen, J. (1988). *Statistical power analysis for the social sciences* (2nd ed.). Hillside, NJ: Earlbaum.

Cook, T. D., & Campbell, D. T. (1979). *Quasi-experimentation: Design & analysis for field settings.* Chicago: Rand McNally College Publishing.

Hansen, M. H., Hurwitz, W. N., & Madow, W. G. (1953). *Sample survey methods and theory.* (Vols. 1–2). New York: Wiley.

Kish, L. (1965). *Survey sampling.* New York: Wiley.

Madow, W. G. (1949). On the theory of systematic sampling. II. *Annals of Mathematical Statistics, 20,* 333–354.

Madow, W. G. (1953). On the theory of systematic sampling, III: Comparison of centered and random start systematic sampling. *Annals of Mathematical Statistics. 24,* 101–106.

Madow, W. G., & Madow, L. H. (1944). On the theory of systematic sampling. *Annals of Mathematical Statistics, 15,* 1–24.

Murthy, M. N. (1967). *Sampling theory and methods.* Calcutta, India: Statistical Publishing Society.

Singh, D., Jindal, K. K., & Garg, J. N. (1968). On modified systematic sampling. *Biometrika, 55,* 541–546.

Sudman, S. (1976). *Applied sampling.* New York: Academic Press.

Weiner, B. J. (1971). *Statistical principles in experimental design* (2nd ed.). New York: McGraw-Hill.

Incorporating Auxiliary Variables into Probability Sampling Designs

Alison M. Trinkoff ■ Carla L. Storr

When data are collected using probability sampling methods, the credibility of conclusions are substantially increased. A sound sampling strategy provides the basis for making inferences and generalizing results beyond a single sample to a target population. Although probability sampling requires more effort than convenience sampling, for nonexperimental designs the effort is well worth it, and many descriptions of sampling using probability techniques are now available (e.g., Kish, 1965; Levy & Lemeshow, 1991).

Probability sampling is used to ensure unbiased estimates of a population (Royall, 1976; Smith, 1984). A major function is to achieve comparability on all variables, whether measured or unknown. However, the assumptions of random sampling are based on all possible samples. Therefore, they do not take into account the possibility that the sample selected may not be representative of the population (Royall, 1992). For example, when sampling a large geographic area, it is possible to wind up with more subjects from urban areas, underrepresenting the population in rural areas.

This report describes balanced stratified sampling, a strategy that incorporates the use of an auxiliary variable in selecting a probability sample. How this sampling strategy was used is illustrated by the Nurses Worklife and Health Study, the main purpose of which was to investigate factors that place a nurse at increased risk of substance use (Trinkoff & Storr, 1997). The goal of the sampling plan was to select a nationally representative sample of the registered nurse (RN) population for which there was no available nationwide sampling frame. The quality of the sampling scheme is evaluated and the efforts to achieve representativeness are discussed.

Alison M. Trinkoff, RN, ScD, is an associate professor, Department of Psychiatric, Community and Adult Primary Care Nursing, School of Nursing, University of Maryland, Baltimore, MD.

Carla L. Storr, MPH, is a research associate, Department of Psychiatric, Community and Adult Primary Care Nursing, School of Nursing, University of Maryland, Baltimore, MD.

From *Nursing Research,* May/June 1997, *46,* 182–185.

Theory and Mechanics of Balanced Stratified Sampling

Balanced stratified sampling, a model-based sampling method, can be used in concert with traditional probability sampling methods to increase the likelihood that a sample will be representative (Thompson, 1992). In balanced stratified sampling, the concept of a representative sample is given quantitative meaning by balancing on numerical properties of the population. This is consistent with the notion that inference is most secure when the sample is "like" the population.

The theoretical basis for model-based sampling comes from work by Royall and Cumberland (1981a, 1981b), who advanced the concept that observed units included in a sample are used to predict the values for the unobserved units in the population. This is performed using information available on an auxiliary variable (x) that is related to the study outcome (y). Auxiliary variables are of interest to the study only for the assistance they can provide in improving the sample. They are usually selected from census data or other information reflecting population size. For example, an auxiliary variable could be hospital bed size, school enrollment, number of cases of a particular surgery performed, or birth rates.

The basic steps for executing balanced stratified sampling are as follows: (a) Sampling units (e.g., schools, counties) are assigned their corresponding value for the auxiliary variable and are ordered on that variable. (b) Strata are formed, such that as much variation as possible exists among the means for the auxiliary variable for each of the strata. The object is to maximize heterogeneity between strata and minimize variability within a stratum. (c) Units within each stratum are selected whose moments are equal to the stratum moments on the auxiliary variable. This achieves balance and results in a sample of units that represents the population on the auxiliary variable; therefore it should also represent the population on the outcome of interest (Royall & Cumberland, 1981a, 1981b). Balance on an auxiliary variable (x) reduces the likelihood of nonrepresentativeness by ensuring that a particular sample resembles the population on variable (x). Moments are mathematical terms for describing the distribution of a variable, with the first moment representing the arithmetic mean and the second moment representing the population variance or sum of means squared. (d) Individual subjects within the chosen sampling units are selected, using traditional probability sampling methods, such as simple random or systematic random sampling.

By combining probability methods with balancing, one improves on both methods by addressing potential limitations of each (Thompson, 1992). Whereas in theory, over all possible samples, probability methods will result in a representative sample, each study is based on one particular sample in which adequate distribution of population characteristics may fail to occur. The advantage of including a probability sampling scheme to select individual sample elements along with balancing is to protect against the chance that while the selected sample will be balanced on (x), it may not be balanced on an unobserved variable (z). This protection is especially strong as the sample size increases, as the likelihood of balance on any other unobserved variables will be increased as well.

Application

Because no single, unduplicated list of licensed RNs existed in the United States (U.S.), lists of nurses needed to be obtained through individual State Boards of Nursing. If we selected nurses from all 50 states, if even one state declined to provide a list, we would have introduced noncoverage biases. Noncoverage biases are systematic errors that are introduced when one cannot contact a portion of the target population. An assumption of probability samples is that all elements of the population have a known and nonzero chance to participate. Therefore, a state-level strategy was devised, using a 20% sample of states. To maximize the chance of selecting a representative sample that would produce estimates that were generalizable to the U.S. RN population as a whole, balanced stratified sampling was used to select the states.

The first step was to choose an appropriate auxiliary variable. As substance use tends to increase with population density, the RN population per state was chosen as the auxiliary variable. Data for this variable were obtained from the most recent survey of RNs licensed in each state and the District of Columbia, produced by the Division of Nursing, Bureau of the Health Professions, Department of Health and Human Services (preliminary report of Moses, 1994). States were then listed in ascending order by size of the RN population. Fortunately, the boundaries of the strata were relatively easy to assign. Grouping 10 to 11 states into five approximately equal-sized strata resulted in strata containing states with similar values on the auxiliary variable (Table 1). This achieved the goal of minimizing within-stratum variability and maximizing between-strata variability.

TABLE 1 Calculation for Balance on First and Second Moments: Nurses Worklife and Health Study 1994

	Stratum 1	Stratum 2	Stratum 3	Stratum 4	Stratum 5
Population					
No. of states (including District of Columbia)	10	10	10	11	10
Range of RNs/state[a] (1,000s)	3.5–9.2	11.1–17.0	20.0–33.0	42.2–56.9	78.3–207.6
Total no. of RNs (1,000s)	68.7	133.1	276.1	525.0	1236.6
Mean [First moment]	6.9	13.3	27.6	47.7	123.7
Mean sum of squares [Second moment]	50.2	180.8	1779.2	2302.7	17043.4
Sample					
No. of states	1	1	2	2	4
Mean [First moment]	6.7	12.7	27.6	47.8	123.7
Percent deviation (population-sample/population × 100)	2.9	4.5	0	0	0
Mean sum of squares [Second moment]	44.9	161.3	793.0	2291.2	6966.0
Percent deviation (population-sample/population × 100)	10.5	10.8	1.8	1.8	0.4

[a]March 1992 National Sample Survey of Registered Nurses preliminary estimates, Division of Nursing, Bureau of Health Professionals, United States Department of Health and Human Services (USDHHS).

The number of states selected per stratum was determined using an optimal allocation formula. Optimal allocation is a strategy for selection of stratum elements that is designed to generate estimates of population parameters with the lowest variance, given a fixed number of stratum elements (Levy & Lemeshow, 1991). In this study, the number of stratum elements was fixed at 10 states. To reflect the more diverse range of RNs per state in the stratum containing the largest states, the formula designated the selection of four states within this stratum. For the three strata in which more than one state was to be selected, all possible combinations of states were evaluated by calculating the moments for each combination and comparing them with the population moments for the respective strata. For strata in which more than one combination of states balanced on the moments, the geographical dispersion over the entire sample of states also was considered. This is appropriate when considering elements to be selected, as long as balance is maintained (Survey Sampling lecture notes, Department of Biostatistics, Johns Hopkins University).

Ten states were selected based on balance on the size measure on the first and second moments, although one state had to be replaced because it was not possible to draw a comparable probability sample from its list of nurses. Balancing data for the final set of states are included in Table 1. The moments for the sample design and the selected states were extremely similar. Deviation from the first moment was minimal, ranging from 0% to 4.5%. For the second moment, the level of balance achieved was within 10%. Simple random sampling was then used to randomly select 600 subjects per state, for a total of 6,000 RNs.

Sampling Frame

To obtain the sampling frame, a description of the project detailing the research purpose, goals, and procedures was sent to the Board of Nursing for each of the selected states. After meeting legal and monetary requirements, each licensing agency provided listings of all RNs with active or current licenses. Lists were checked for duplicate names. Because some nurses were licensed in more than one state, any RNs with out-of-state addresses were excluded from the original state listings. Accuracy of the mailing information varied because each state had its own process for updating lists, and license renewal dates ranged from annual to triennial. All 10 states were recontacted early in the data collection phase to obtain updated addresses on subjects to whom the postal service could not deliver or forward an introduction letter. Overall, the undeliverable rate was only 5%.

Findings

Usable data were obtained from 4,438 respondents out of 5,706 eligible addresses, for a response rate of 78%. This was based on a data collection scheme with up to six mailed contacts per subject. Comparison of respondent characteristics with estimates from the 1992 National Nurse Survey (Moses, 1994), the only RN population estimates available for the U.S. as a whole, indicates that this study's aim of obtaining a representative sample (Table 2) was accomplished. Overall, there was good agreement between the two. Both were predominantly white and female. The respondents in this study were slightly older, more educated, and somewhat less likely to be staff nurses than population estimates. The sample in this study differed slightly in the distribution of work characteristics, which may reflect the rapidly changing role of nurses over the 2-year period.

Discussion

Although balanced stratified sampling introduces additional requirements and expenditure of time, the chance of selecting a representative sample is greatly enhanced by using information on an auxiliary variable that is related to the outcome of interest. Aside from the statistical advantages, there are some practical advantages. Unlike cluster or multistage sampling, no design effects are introduced because this design is considered to be a stratified sample. As a result, this eliminates the need for complex techniques to calculate variance estimates such as Taylor series approximation. In addition, balanced stratified sampling limits the number of units from which one needs to obtain complete listings to construct the sampling frame. This is especially advantageous when listings are not available for the complete population, and therefore selection of a probability sample seems unachievable. For example, in this study, only the lists for the states that were selected as stratum elements had to be obtained; the entire sampling frame of all RNs in the U.S. did not need to be available. Furthermore, use is not limited to very large data sets. In small samples, the assumptions of probability sampling may be harder to meet because it is difficult to ensure a representative distribution of a large population in a small sample, as suggested by Hansen, Madow, & Tepping (1983).

Researchers interested in other populations could choose appropriate auxiliary variable data based on a hypothesized relation to the major study variable. For example, when studying data from patients discharged from hospitals, data may be available on number of procedures, deliveries, or bed size. Any of these figures could

TABLE 2 Registered Nurse Population by Sociodemographic and Work Characteristics (%)

	1992 DHHS[a] (*n* = 2,239,816)	NWHS[b] (*n* = 4,438)
White	90.1	93.5
Male	4.0	4.1
Marital status		
Married	72.2	74.0
Widow/divorced/separated	16.6	16.6
Never married	11.2	9.4
Highest education		
Diploma	33.7	27.9
Associate	28.3	25.1
Bachelors	30.0	36.6
Masters or above	8.0	10.4
Age (mean)	(43.1)	(44.3)
< 30	11.1	7.5
30–39	33.7	30.0
40–49	27.6	33.8
50–59	16.5	16.9
60–64	5.4	6.1
65+	5.7	5.7
Employment		
In nursing	82.7	84.4
Not in nursing	4.2	4.2
Work setting		
Hospitals	66.5	59.6
Ambulatory/physician offices/HMO	7.8	7.2
Nursing home/extended care/	7.0	8.4
Nursing education	2.0	2.1
Home health agency	3.1	7.6
Community/government/other	13.3	15.1
Position		
Staff general/charge	61.7	56.4
Private duty	0.6	0.7
Head nurse/supervisor/coordinator	12.3	13.8
Administration	6.2	6.0
Advanced practice	5.6	6.5
Educator/research/consultant	4.8	5.9
Other	8.9	10.7

[a]1992 National Sample Survey of Registered Nurses, USDHHS, 1994.
[b]Nurses Worklife and Health Study.

potentially serve as an auxiliary variable when measuring outcomes such as complication rates or readmissions.

Despite one's best efforts, the final sample may still not be representative because of faulty enumeration or sample selection. For example, surveys depend on complete and timely listings in order to avoid noncoverage biases. Therefore, attention needs to be paid to other aspects of the research design and implementation to ensure an optimal participation rate that will result in high-quality data.

To summarize, stratum elements were selected through balancing on the auxiliary variable. Then, individuals within the selected stratum elements were randomly selected. Thus, a combination of probability and model-based sampling methods was used. A well-designed sampling plan can allow one to make inferences and generalize results beyond a single sample. When additional information is available on a population, such as with an auxiliary variable, it is prudent to use this information in the sample selection phase (Hansen, et al., 1983).

References

Hansen, M.H., Madow, W.G., & Tepping, B.J. (1983). An evaluation of model-dependent and probability-sampling inferences in sample surveys. *Journal of the American Statistical Association, 78,* 776–793.

Kish, L. (1965). *Survey sampling.* New York: Wiley.

Levy, P.S., & Lemeshow, S. (1991). *Sampling of populations: Methods and applications* (2nd ed.). New York: Wiley.

Moses, E.B. (1994). The Registered Nurse Population: Findings from the National Sample Survey of Registered Nurses, March 1992 (USDHHS Publication No. [PHS]55-4872). Rockville, MD: Bureau of Health Professions.

Royall, R.M. (1976). Current advances in sampling theory: Implications for human observational studies. *American Journal of Epidemiology, 104,* 463–474.

Royall, R.M., & Cumberland, W.G. (1981a). An empirical study of the ratio estimator and estimators of its variance. *Journal of the American Statistical Association, 76,* 66–77.

Royall, R.M., & Cumberland, W.G. (1981b). The finite-population linear regression estimator and estimators of its variance—an empirical study. *Journal of the American Statistical Association, 76,* 924–930.

Royall R.M. (1992). Robustness and optimal design under prediction models for finite populations. *Survey Methodology, 18,* 179–185.

Smith, T.M.F. (1984). Present position and potential developments: Some personal views sample surveys. *Journal of the Royal Statistical Society, 147 part 2,* 208–221.

Thompson, S.K. (1992). *Sampling,* New York: Wiley.

Trinkoff, A.M., & Storr, C.L. (1997). *Substance use among nurses: Specialty differences.* Manuscript accepted for publication, University of Maryland, Baltimore.

Randomization by Cluster

Walter W. Hauck ■ Catherine L. Gilliss ■ Allan Donner ■ Susan Gortner

In traditional, simple randomization, each subject entered in the study is assigned to either the intervention or control group. In effect, a separate coin is flipped for each subject. In practice, this simplicity is complicated by stratification and blocking to ensure nearly equal allocation within each stratum. In cluster randomization, groups or clusters of subjects are formed or identified, and each group is separately assigned, as a whole, to either intervention or control. A coin is flipped once for the group and all members of the group receive the same assignment. However, the unit of analysis is still the individual subject. The key property of cluster randomization is that the unit of randomization, the group, is different from the unit of analysis, the individual subjects forming the group. If the group were randomized and the group retained as the unit of analysis, the design would be one of simple randomization, not of cluster randomization.

Given the accepted strength of individual randomization, why randomize by cluster? For nursing interventions, there are a number of potential reasons. (See Buck and Donner, 1982, for additional discussion.) The first is contamination. In some trials it may not be possible to keep experimental and control subjects separated. For instance, even when it is possible to randomize only one hospitalized patient per room, study staff seldom have control over whether patients are moved between rooms, or whether experimental patients and their family members discuss study interventions with control patients. The potential for contamination can be reduced with cluster randomization. The cluster can be formed by entering consecutive patients into the study as the group or cluster, and then randomizing the group. Once the full group is entered, study entry can be temporarily closed before reopening entry to the next group. This process eliminates contamination, as groups of subjects with different experimental conditions are never co-mingled.

A second reason for adopting a cluster randomization design is that using simple randomization may not be feasible. Some interventions may be difficult to implement except on the group in which they naturally occur. For example, if one wanted to implement hypertension screening as part of a patient contact that would not normally involve such screening, the simplest implementation would be by practice unit (i.e., everyone in a practice unit is either screened or not). When there is no way to introduce an intervention except to groups, randomization by cluster is not simply feasible, it is necessary. If an intervention is additional education for a nurse practitioner (NP) and the outcome is something that does or does not happen to the NP's patients, cluster randomization is a necessity—the NP is randomized to receive or not receive the education and the cluster is the NP's patients.

Improving feasibility may also enhance adherence. In interventions aimed at behavior modification such as reduction of dietary sodium, adherence will likely be aided if the patient's family is also recruited to the study. If data from the subject alone were analyzed the study would be a standard randomized trial. However, in this approach data are wasted since family members could be analyzed to assess the effect of the intervention. In the latter case, the family is a cluster, and the design could be cluster randomization.

Ethical considerations may also lead to the choice of cluster randomization. A practitioner may not be willing to treat some patients differently from others. This would dictate that the practitioner's patient group be considered the unit of randomization.

Walter W. Hauck, PhD, is professor and Head, Division of Biostatistics, Department of Epidemiology and Biostatistics, University of California, San Francisco, CA.

Catherine L. Gilliss, DNSc, RNC, FAAN, is associate professor, Department of Family Health Care Nursing, University of California, San Francisco, CA.

Allan Donner, PhD, is professor and Chairman, Department of Epidemiology and Biostatistics, The University of Western Ontario, London, Ontario, Canada.

Susan Gortner, PhD, MN, FAAN, is professor and Director, Cardiac Recovery Laboratory, Department of Family Health Care Nursing, University of California, San Francisco, CA.

From *Nursing Research,* November/December 1991, *40,* 356–358.

However, as desirable as cluster randomization may seem, there are prices to be paid. The most important of these costs is loss of efficiency, particularly in terms of effective sample size. In a simple randomized study of 100 subjects, the effective sample size is the number of randomized units, namely 100. If the 100 subjects fall into 10 groups and the 10 groups are randomized, the effective sample size will be dependent upon observed similarity of responses within clusters, that is, the intracluster correlation. In an extreme case, the members of each group all respond alike so that no additional information is gained by analyzing more than one subject per group. In this case, the effective sample size is 10. The other extreme occurs when members of the same group are as dissimilar in responses as members of different groups, in which case the effective sample size remains 100. Generally, given a positive intraclass correlation, the effective sample size would fall between 10 and 100. Therefore, the benefits of cluster randomization come at the price of reduced efficiency and loss of power. A cluster-randomized study will require more subjects to maintain desired power than a simple randomized study.

The magnitude of the reduction in effective sample size increases with the average number of individuals per cluster and with the value of the intracluster correlation. The intracluster correlation can be thought of as a measure of the extent to which subjects in a group are more or less like each other than to members of other groups. One way to identify intracluster correlations is to ask if the groups could be expected to differ in outcome even in the absence of an intervention. Practice units will demonstrate intracluster correlation because outcomes would be expected to vary depending on the training and experience of the care provider and the characteristics of the patients who selected those practices.

The notion of effective sample size can be quantified. If K clusters are randomized, each containing n subjects (Kn subjects total), the effective sample size (ESS) is:

$$ESS = (Kn)/[1 + (n - 1)\, \rho],$$

where ρ is the intraclass correlation (Donner, Birkett, & Buck, 1981). The two extremes referred to above correspond to $\rho = 1$ (ESS = K) and $\rho = 0$ (ESS = Kn). If the groups are not of equal size, the effective sample size can be approximated by substituting the average group size for n in this formula.

Unfortunately, given the importance of ρ in ESS, the range of intracluster correlations that one might expect to observe is not generally well known. What is known suggests that ρ will tend to be small, on the order of .01–.05 for nonfamilial clusters (Donner, 1982), as in randomized practice units, with larger clusters tending to have the smaller intracluster correlations. While such correlations may seem too small to have practical consequences, note that the ESS depends on $(n-1)\,\rho$, not just ρ. A small intracluster correlation in clusters that are at least moderately large can have a major impact on the ESS. For example, if $\rho = .01$ and $n = 11$, the effective sample size will be 10% less than the total number of subjects. When the family is the unit of randomization, much larger intracluster correlations should be expected.

Another price to be paid for the use of cluster randomization is that statistical analyses are more complicated. Standard methods, based on simple randomization, would treat the effective sample size as the total number of subjects (Kn). We know from the results above that this would overstate the effective sample size, with the consequence that standard errors and p-values would be inappropriately small and thus any observed statistical significance may be spurious.

One rationale for randomization is that it reduces the likelihood that the experimental and control groups will differ on an important prognostic factor. The effectiveness of this property increases with the number of units randomized and will therefore be impaired in studies randomizing a relatively small number of large clusters. For example, if only two clusters were to be randomized, there is no way that cluster randomization can eliminate differences between the two clusters. If the nature of the study requires that the number of clusters be small, the likelihood of imbalance can be reduced by first pairing clusters and then randomizing one of each pair to the intervention and one to control (Donner, 1987; Donner & Donald, 1987).

Analysis of Cluster Randomized Studies

Univariate

Standard Student's t and chi-square tests can be corrected for clustering. If the sample size is effectively reduced by the factor $f = 1 + (n - 1)\,\rho$, this suggests that the variances of our effect measures should be increased by the same factor. Since t statistics are ratios of differences of means to the standard errors (not variance) of these differences, t statistics are modified by dividing by f. For chi-square tests the variance is used, and chi square is divided by $\sqrt{f}$. This approach provides simple adjustments for these univariate tests. Additionally, if the statistic is not statistically significant before correcting for clustering, the correction will only make it less significant. For confidence intervals of the form ± a multiple of the standard error, the standard error is first multiplied by $\sqrt{f}$.

The major problem created by this simple correction is determining an estimate of ρ. Estimation procedures, with examples, are given by Donner, Birkett, and Buck (1981) for use with t-statistics and by Donner and Donald (1988) for chi squares. When results are very significant prior to correction for clustering, a first look at the effect of the correction can be obtained by setting $\rho = 1$ ($f = n$). If the statistic remains statistically significant even with this most extreme correction, it will remain significant for any value of ρ.

Multivariate

There are two statistical approaches that incorporate clustering into multivariate analyses. The first is derived from the survey sampling field where clustering is present whenever the survey unit is a group, such as household or census tract. Numerical survey data can be analyzed by the method of generalized least squares (Donner, 1985). Computer packages are available for the analysis of cluster samples, notably SUPERCARP (Hidiroglou, Fuller, & Hickman, 1980) and SURREGR (Research Triangle Institute, Research Triangle Park, NC). Use of either of these programs requires some familiarity with sample survey terminology.

The second multivariate approach is based on mixed-effects analysis of variance. The mixed-effects approach is essentially an extension of the univariate analysis of repeated-measures designs. In a repeated-measures design, each subject forms a cluster, and the "members" of the cluster are the various times at which the subject provides data. It is well known that repeated-measures data must be analyzed in a way that recognizes that each subject appears multiple times in the data. Statistical programs that recognize clusters with intraclass correlations can be used for the analysis of repeated-measures designs and, more generally, any clustered design.

The mixed-effects analysis of clustered designs uses the same assumptions as the univariate analysis of repeated-measures, namely, that the correlation between any pair within a cluster is the same. In cluster randomization designs with nonfamilial clusters, this is likely a reasonable assumption, more reasonable than for repeated measures where time ordering suggests that points close together in time may be more highly correlated than more distant pairs. The equal-correlation assumption may be less reasonable in familial clusters.

One complication in analyzing repeated-measures data and, more generally, clustered data is that many programs require equal group sizes (equivalently, complete cases for repeated-measures). Two programs which can be used to analyze clustered data with unequal cluster sizes are available in the BMDP package: BMDP-3V and BMDP-5V (Dixon et al., 1990). The recently distributed BMDP-5V also permits alternative correlation assumptions.

In recent years, multivariate methods based on these two approaches have been developed for dichotomous measures. Ware, Lipsitz, and Speizer (1988) and Neuhaus, Kalbfleisch, and Hauck (1991) provide a discussion to aid in choosing methods. These methods are not yet offered in widely available computer programs. Mixed-effects logistic models can be used on a personal computer with the new package EGRET (Statistical Epidemiology Research Corp., Seattle).

An Example of Randomization Cluster

Improving Recovery from Cardiac Surgery (NR01031; Gilliss et al., 1989) was a cluster-randomized clinical trial of nurse-managed instructional support intended to improve the health of individuals undergoing cardiac surgery and the functioning of their family group. The clusters consisted of consecutive consenting patients. With this essentially artificial grouping, we expected that clustering would lead to little loss of power. The results of the analysis incorporating clustering produced only a few variables with more than trivial differences as compared to when clustering was excluded.

Data were collected presurgery (baseline) and 4, 8, 12, and 24 weeks postsurgery. All analyses were run first ignoring the clustering; that is, treating the analyses as standard repeated-measures analyses. A clustered analysis was then run consisting of specified subjects as a random effect nested within cluster and clusters as a random effect nested within intervention groups. All analyses included time and group by-time effects and, as a covariate, the baseline value of the dependent variable.

A variable where the two analyses differed substantially was the general subscale of the self-reported activity measure. In part A of Table 1 the means at each time are presented, (a) unadjusted for missingness, then (b) adjusted first in the repeated-measures analysis (no clustering), and then (c) in the doubly-nested (with clustering), analysis. Part B of Table 1 shows p-values for the group, time and group-by-time effects, where the interaction effect is adjusted for the two main effects (and baseline) and the two main effects are adjusted only for the other main effect (and baseline). In Part B, the type of change expected is seen for the group variable, namely a larger p-value in the clustered analysis.

TABLE 1 Results of Analyses of Self-Reported General Activity Measure

A. MEANS (SE'S)

Group	Time (weeks)	Observed	Predicted from Analysis	
			Random Effects	*Clustered*
Experimental				
	4	13.62	13.54 (.34)	13.51 (.40)
	8	14.85	14.82 (.34)	14.79 (.40)
	12	15.32	15.27 (.33)	15.24 (.40)
	24	15.76	15.71 (.34)	15.69 (.40)
Control				
	4	12.63	12.63 (.34)	12.59 (.40)
	8	13.55	13.63 (.31)	13.65 (.37)
	12	14.39	14.42 (.32)	14.42 (.38)
	24	15.69	15.77 (.32)	15.77 (.38)

B. P-VALUES

Allowance for Clustering	Effect		
	Group	*Time*	*Group X Time*
No	.011	<.001	.178
Yes	.103	<.001	.181

References

Buck, C., & Donner, A. (1982). The design of controlled experiments in the evaluation of nontherapeutic interventions. *Journal of Chronic Diseases,* 35, 531–538.

Dixon, W. J., Brown, M. B., Engelman, L., & Jennrich, R. I. (1990). *BMDP statistical software manual,* volume 2. Los Angeles: University of California Press.

Donner, A., Birkett, N., & Buck, C. (1981). Randomization by cluster. Sample size requirements and analysis. *American Journal of Epidemiology, 114,* 906–914.

Donner, A. (1982). An empirical study of cluster randomization. *International Journal of Epidemiology, 11,* 283–286.

Donner, A. (1985). A regression approach to the analysis of data arising from cluster randomization. *International Journal of Epidemiology, 14,* 322–326.

Donner, A. (1987). Statistical methodology for paired-cluster designs. *American Journal of Epidemiology, 126,* 972–979.

Donner, A., & Donald, A. (1987). The analysis of data arising from a stratified design with the cluster as unit of randomization. *Statistics in Medicine, 6,* 43–52.

Donner, A., & Donald, A. (1988). The statistical analysis of multiple binary measurements. *Journal of Clinical Epidemiology, 41,* 899–905.

Gilliss, C., Gortner, S., Shinn, J., & Sparacino, P. (1989). Improving recovery from cardiac surgery: Final report (NIH, NCNR, 2R01-01031).

Hidiroglou, M. A., Fuller, W. A., & Hickman, R. D. (1980). *Supercarp* (6th ed.). Ames, IA: Statistical Laboratory, Iowa State University.

Neuhaus, J. M., Kalbfleisch, J. D., & Hauck, W. W. (1991). A comparison of cluster-specific and population-averaged approaches for analyzing correlated binary data. *International Statistical Review, 59,* 25–35.

Ware, J. H., Lipsitz, S., & Speizer, F. E. (1988). Issues in the analysis of repeated categorical outcomes. *Statistics in Medicine,* 7, 95–107.

Permuted Block Design for Randomization in a Nursing Clinical Trial

Ellen B. Rudy ■ Patricia L. Vaska ■ Barbara J. Daly ■ Mary Beth Happ ■ Pamela Shiao

The random assignment of subjects to treatment and control groups is a basic tenet of experimental design. Randomization attempts to balance treatment and control groups with respect to prognostic factors and attempts to alleviate bias. The randomized control trial is the most powerful way to ascribe results to experimental variables and represents the "gold standard" of research design. However, randomized assignment of subjects to experimental and control groups in health care research often presents problems. The following discussion describes some of these problems and details an approach successfully used to address the difficulties.

Selection bias can be avoided in blind experiments in which the treatment allocation is made by a third party and the researcher and subject are ignorant of the group to which the subject has been assigned (van der Linden, 1980). However, blind experiments are impractical for most clinical trials other than some drug studies. This is particularly true for testing specific nursing interventions that cannot be kept blind to either the investigators or the subjects. When blinded studies are not possible, the standard recommended procedure for complete randomization is to use a random number table or to flip an unbiased coin. But in many cases involving the realities of a clinical setting, neither of these procedures is feasible.

Our interest in randomization of subjects is the result of current experience with a research study of the long-term critically ill, and the application of random assignment procedure to compare patient outcomes for different interventions. The population of interest for this study are patients who are admitted to an intensive care unit (ICU) for an acute episode but who require extended stays in the ICU because of complications, comorbidities, or exacerbations of chronic conditions. Typical examples in this category might include a patient admitted with pneumonia who is in acute respiratory distress with underlying chronic obstructive pulmonary disease, or a patient requiring coronary bypass graft surgery for unstable angina who has advanced left ventricular failure. Such patients are admitted to ICUs and remain there even when the need for intensive medical therapies is past because they still require intensive nursing care, often in the form of ventilatory support. For the most part, such patients cannot be cared for in general or step-down nursing divisions because of their acuity (Daly, Rudy, Thompson, & Happ, 1991). We have labeled these long-term patients "chronically, critically ill." They make up a significant portion of patient days and place financial and personnel burdens on the hospital.

To test the effects of an alternative method of care for these long-term patients adequately, the investigators designed a unit with a specific physical layout, including private rooms and areas for family visits and overnight stays, a case management care delivery system, and a shared governance model of management for the nursing staff. We labeled this unit a Special Care Unit (SCU) for the chronically, critically ill and designed a research study to compare patient outcomes between patients cared for in the SCU, the experimental group, versus those cared for in the traditional ICU, the control group.

Eligibility for the SCU study is established by means of the Acute Physiology and Chronic Health Evaluation (APACHE II) (Knaus, Zimmerman, Wagner, Draper, & Lawrence, 1981) and the Therapeutic Intervention Severity Scale (TISS) (Cullen, Civetta, Briggs, & Ferrara, 1974) scoring systems. All ICU patients are scored after 7 days in the ICU. They are considered eligible if their APACHE II scores are less than 18 and their TISS scores are less than 39. The patients, their families, and their physicians are approached for informed consent, and the patients are transferred to the SCU if assigned to the ex-

Ellen B. Rudy, PhD, RN, FAAN, is dean and professor, University of Pittsburgh, School of Nursing, Pittsburgh, PA.

Patricia L. Vaska, MSN, RN, is a clinical nurse specialist, Sioux Valley Hospital, Sioux Falls, SD.

Barbara J. Daly, MSN, RN, FAAN, is an assistant professor, Case Western Reserve University, School of Nursing, Cleveland, OH.

Mary Beth Happ, MSN, RN, is a clinical nurse specialist, Riverside Hospital, Columbus, OH.

Pamela Shiao, MSN, RN, is a project director, Case Western Reserve University, School of Nursing, Cleveland, OH.

From *Nursing Research,* September/October 1993, *42,* 287–289.

perimental group. Permission to be in the study is obtained from all patients, regardless of placement.

In the initial stages of the study, a fair coin was tossed and patients were randomized to either the experimental or control group. This fair coin randomization became impractical almost immediately. The SCU is a seven-bed unit, and at least four beds must be filled at all times in order for it to be financially feasible for the hospital to keep the unit open. We recognized that unconstrained randomization may lead to imbalances in group assignment if there are, by chance, long unbroken runs of assignments to one group. A line of unbroken assignment either to the SCU or to the ICU could be disastrous in maintaining the new patient unit. We estimated that with the number of eligible patients available for the study, we needed approximately twice as many in the SCU as in the ICU to keep the census adequate in the SCU. Therefore, we adopted an alternative to complete randomization, using a permuted block design for randomization and assigning subjects by blocking patients into groups of three. Out of every three patients two were randomized to the experimental group (see Figure 1).

The literature on randomization for clinical trials confirms the need to balance the groups at some time during a study. A variety of mechanisms have been suggested, all under the rubric of a biased coin mechanism or adaptive randomization (Efron, 1971; Hjelm-Karlsson, 1992; Meinert & Tonascia, 1986). Some investigators suggest using a table of random numbers, where probability is altered as subjects are assigned to groups to keep the groups more equal. This means that once one group has a subject, the next subject assignment by the altered (biased) table of random members will have a higher probability of being assigned to a different group (Efron, 1971; Hjelm-Karlsson, 1991). However, this approach, while achieving the desired specific balance by the end of the study, still allows the possibility of a long run of assignment of subjects to one group.

In a permuted block design, the pure randomization process is constrained to ensure ongoing balance in the assignments made to the treatment and control groups. In our particular situation we wanted a 2:1 ratio. In the procedure suggested by Efron (1971), we randomized subjects in groups of three, with two out of three requiring SCU placement. Steps of the full assignment procedure are listed in Table 1. The randomization procedure is as follows:

Example 1 Flip a coin. If patient goes to ICU, next two automatically go to SCU with no coin flip.

OR

Example 2 Flip a coin. If patient goes to SCU, flip a coin for assignment of second patient. If second patient goes to SCU, third one automatically goes to ICU.

OR

Example 3 Flip a coin. If patient goes to SCU, flip a coin for assignment of second patient. If second patient goes to ICU, third one automatically goes to SCU.

In reviewing this assignment procedure, the reader can easily see that the permuted block design is effective in preventing grossly unbalanced subject assignments. However, the disadvantage is that at certain times the investigators know ahead of time the group assignment of the next subject. This, of course, can lead to the possibility of selection bias. In our study, we use the time a patient becomes eligible for the study to determine who is next in line for assignment. Since this is not under the direct control of the investigator, it tends to mitigate the selection bias. Furthermore, the nursing and medical

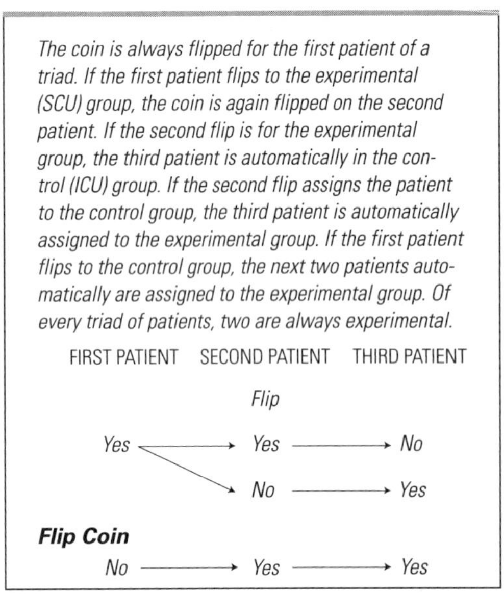

FIGURE 1 Assignments of Patients to SCU Study (Yes = experimental; No = control)

TABLE 1 Assignment Procedure for Special Care Unit

1. Assess all patients in the ICUs for eligibility
2. Randomly assign all eligible patients by coin toss or block assignment
3. Obtain physician permission to transfer for experimental subjects
4. Obtain patient/family consent
5. If experimental transfer to SCU

personnel in the SCU and the ICU are not involved in either determining patient eligibility or the assignment to the units.

While this assignment procedure is successful in achieving the benefits of randomization, problems still exist. Occasionally we have the dilemma of patients who qualify for inclusion in the study and randomize to a group; then their physical condition deteriorates and prevents or delays their entry to the study group. When this occurs, they are ineligible, and we move to the next eligible patient for assignment. If the original patient becomes eligible for the study at a later time, he is assigned at that later time according to the block procedure, irrespective of where he was originally assigned.

More troublesome problems are delays in obtaining family consent, physician consent, or an available SCU bed after the patient has been assigned to a group. To handle these delays, we have established a rule to guide our patient assignments. The rule states that we can hold patients for a maximum of 7 days after eligibility scoring before entering the study. Patients who exceed the 7-day limit are dropped from the study. For those patients who enter the study within 7 days, APACHE II and TISS are again scored immediately prior to entry; these scores are then compared to those of subjects who entered the study immediately to make sure their acuity level is comparable. These problems illustrate the importance of supplementing randomization procedures with specific rules to deal with the practical difficulties unique to clinical research.

Another issue unique to clinical research is the need to accommodate preferences of patients and others. Occasionally a family member or a physician will specifically request assignment to either the SCU or the traditional ICU. Because these patients meet eligibility criteria and give consent, we do not want to lose them from the study. Therefore, we have created separate groups of nonrandomly assigned patients in both the experimental and control group. When the SCU needs patients to keep the census at the minimum of four, eligible patients can be nonrandomly assigned to the experimental group. The randomization scheme skips these nonrandomly assigned subjects and resumes with the following patient. Statistical analysis will be conducted with the nonrandom patients both as part of the whole group and as separated from the randomly assigned patients. If significant differences are discovered by analysis with the nonrandomly assigned patients separated, we will report our findings as such.

To date, we have entered 122 subjects in the study. Of these, 103 (84%) have been randomized according to our block design, and only 19 (16%) are nonrandom subjects. Preliminary analysis shows no significant difference between the randomized subjects and the nonrandomized subjects by sex, age, or acuity. The principal reasons for nonrandom assignment have been physician preference, need to fill the SCU bed, and family preference.

When one considers the difficulties of randomization in clinical trials, it is surprising that there are any randomized nursing research studies at all. Nurses encounter the problems discussed every day in the blueprint stages of their research, as do researchers in many other fields.

References

Cullen, D. J., Civetta, J. M., Briggs, B. A., & Ferrara, L. C. (1974). Therapeutic intervention scoring system: A method for quantitative comparison of patient care. *Critical Care Medicine, 2,* 57–62.

Daly, B. J., Rudy, E. B., Thompson, K. S., & Happ, M. B. (1991). Development of a special care unit for chronically critically ill patients. *Heart and Lung, 20,* 45–51.

Efron, B. (1971). Forcing a sequential experiment to be balanced. *Biometrika, 58,* 403–417.

Hjelm-Karlsson, K. (1991). Using the biased coin design for randomization in health care research. *Western Journal of Nursing Research, 13,* 284–288.

Knaus, W. A., Zimmerman, J. E., Wagner, D. P., Draper, E. A., & Lawrence, D. E. (1981). APACHE-acute physiology and chronic health evaluation: A physiologically based classification system. *Critical Care Medicine, 9,* 591–597.

Meinert, C. L., & Tonascia, S. (1986). *Clinical trials. Design, conduct and analysis.* New York: Oxford University Press, pp. 90–112.

van der Linden, W. (1980). Pitfalls in randomized surgical trials. *Surgery, 87,* 258–262.

Three Methods of Random Assignment: Comparison of Balance Achieved on Potentially Confounding Variables

Michael Conlon ■ Gene C. Anderson

Random assignment of subjects to a nursing intervention has the primary benefit of removing selection bias by preventing the investigator from selecting "more suitable" subjects for a promising innovation and leaving "less suitable" subjects for the control (customary) treatment. When the assignment sequence is known, as in alternating assignment, in which every other subject is assigned to the control, the possibility of selection bias through subjective interpretation of entrance criteria is present. An extreme case of nonrandomization is assigning subjects on the basis of medical or subject judgment or choice, a method which creates such large possibilities for bias that Pocock (1983) writes "judgment is generally regarded as obviously unacceptable."

A second benefit of randomization is that it helps achieve balance between the intervention and control groups for factors (covariates) correlated with outcomes. This implies that repeated randomized studies with positive findings cannot be attributed to covariate differences. The same cannot be said of quasi-experimental studies. Note that randomization helps balance not only recorded covariates but also unknown, or as yet unsuspected, covariates. Randomization in the context of clinical trials is discussed in the review by Fetter et al. (1989).

Randomization only helps achieve balance—it does not guarantee it. Later in this article, our simulation experiment will show that small studies, which use randomization methods that do not consider covariate levels, are at considerable risk for producing samples in which the treatment assignment is strongly imbalanced in one or more levels of the covariates.

In simple random assignment, each eligible subject receives either treatment with equal probability. Simple random assignment is easy to implement since it requires no information concerning the subject to be randomized, nor any information regarding previous assignments (Polit & Hungler, 1987). However, simple random assignment may not be adequate to balance the total number of subjects assigned to each treatment and the number of subjects with various important prognostic (covariate) values assigned to each treatment. This is especially true for studies with less than 100 subjects. Several modifications of simple random assignment have been introduced to rectify imbalance in the total number of subjects assigned to each treatment. These modifications include re-randomization (Pocock, 1983), permuted block assignment (Zelen, 1974), biased coin techniques (Efron, 1971), and urn methods (Wei, 1978). However, none of these techniques address imbalance in covariate values.

Michael Conlon, PhD, is an assistant research scientist in the Division of Biostatistics, University of Florida, Gainesville, FL.

Gene C. Anderson, PhD, RN, FAAN, is a professor in the College of Nursing, University of Florida, Gainesville, FL.

From *Nursing Research,* November/December 1990, *39,* 376–379.

Stratification Techniques

The balance of assignment for important covariates can be improved by stratification techniques, which involve the random selection of subjects from two or more strata populations independently. One disadvantage of stratification is that far more planning and control are needed than for simple random assignment methods. For this reason, some authors have argued that stratification should be used only in smaller studies ($N < 100$) where balance on covariates is most difficult to achieve (Lachin, Matts, & Wei, 1988). However, stratification will improve assignment balance even when the sample size is over 100.

One simple technique for achieving balance for treatment assignment within strata is to use permuted blocks within each strata (Zelen, 1974). A separate randomization list, or set of envelopes, is prepared for every combination of strata levels. For example, with three stratifying factors, each with two levels, $2^3 = 8$ lists are required. Each list is created by randomly assigning innovation (I) and control (C) in fixed length blocks, usually of size four or six. A typical block might look like CCICII or ICIICC. Permuted blocks assure balance between treatments at every *b*th patient, where *b* is the size of the block. To randomize a subject we must know the levels of each of the stratifying variables, but we can still prepare all randomization materials in advance of the study. Unfortunately,

TABLE 1 Minimization Example

Stratifiers	Strata Levels	Control[a]	Intervention[a]	Current Imbalance
	Subjects in Each Stratifier			
Gestation age	≤30 wks	6	8	2
	>30 wks	5	5	0
Infant sex	Male	2	6	4
	Female	9	7	2
Mother's choice of feeding	Breast	8	11	3
	Bottle	3	2	1
				12

[a] Strata marginal total

preparing the many randomization lists required for this technique may not actually achieve the desired effect. When several of the strata level combinations occur infrequently, it is possible that substantial imbalance in assigned treatment can occur.

A second technique called minimization can also be used to achieve balance for treatment assignment within strata (Pocock & Simon, 1975). Minimization requires that the investigator maintain a collection of tables showing the number of subjects in each stratum and the number that have been assigned to each treatment. The first subject is assigned by a simple coin toss. Each following subject is assigned to whichever treatment will minimize the imbalance in the strata. To randomize a subject we must know the levels of each of the stratifying variables and maintain a history of the previous assignments.

For example, consider a study where newborn infants will receive either standard care (control) or a new individualized nursing care (intervention) designed to minimize crying. We wish to insure that the treatment groups are balanced for gestational age (≤ 30 weeks vs. > 30 weeks), sex of infant, and mother's choice of feeding (breast, bottle). Suppose we have assigned 24 infants with the current imbalance shown in Table 1. Suppose also that the next infant who meets the selection criteria and is to be randomized is a female under 30 weeks and has a mother who will bottle feed. Placing the subject in the control group results in an imbalance of $|7-8| + |5-5| + |2-6| + |10-7| + |8-11| + |4-2| = 1 + 0 + 4 + 3 + 3 + 2 = 13$. Note the vertical bars indicate that the signs of each difference are ignored. Placing the same subject in the intervention group results in an imbalance of $|6-9| + |5-5| + |2-6| + |9-8| + |8-11| + |3-3| = 3 + 0 + 4 + 1 + 3 + 0 = 11$. Thus, the subject should be assigned to the intervention group to reduce covariate imbalance (Table 2). The same decision can be reached by adding up the current number of subjects in each stratum level of the new subject, within each possible assignment. For control we have $6 + 9 + 3 = 18$, whereas for intervention we have $8 + 7 + 2 = 17$, so the subject should be assigned to the intervention. The tables are updated to reflect the new assignment (Table 2) and the next subject is handled in the same

TABLE 2 Imbalance Minimized by Adding New Subject to Intervention Group

Stratifiers	Strata Levels	Control[a]	Intervention[a]	Current Imbalance
	Subjects in Each Stratifier			
Gestational age	≤30 wks	6	9	3
	>30 wks	5	5	0
Infant sex	Male	2	6	4
	Female	9	8	1
Mother's choice of feeding	Breast	8	11	3
	Bottle	3	3	0
				11

[a] Strata marginal total

manner. When each assignment produces the same degree of imbalance, a coin toss is used.

Randomization lists cannot be prepared in advance, since the assignment depends on the order in which subjects are encountered in the study. Accurate records of all previous assignments are needed, as well as up-to-date tables showing the number of subjects randomized within each stratum level.

Experiment

To compare these three techniques, a simulation experiment was conducted in which clinical trials were randomly generated using a computer. Each trial consisted of 36 patients to be randomly assigned to either intervention or control. Each patient had three strata levels randomly selected with equal probability from each of two possible levels. There were eight possible combinations of strata levels and six strata marginal totals. Each patient was entered into three concurrent trials: one assigned by simple random assignment, one assigned by permuted blocks of size six within strata levels, and one assigned by minimization. When 36 patients had been assigned, total imbalance and maximum strata imbalance were computed and recorded.

Total imbalance is the sum of the differences in assigned counts within the strata marginal totals. Table 1 shows the results of such a trial after 24 patients have been entered, using the minimization method. The total imbalance is 12 in Table 1 and has been reduced to 11 in Table 2. Maximum strata imbalance is the largest discrepancy between control and intervention totals in any of the margins. In Tables 1 and 2 the maximum strata imbalance is for male infants with a value of 4. A total of 10,000 trials were conducted for each method.

Results

Percentiles for the imbalance measures are presented in Table 3. For simple random assignment, half the trials had a total imbalance of 20 or less. Half the trials assigned by simple random assignment had a maximum strata imbalance of 7 or less. This means that half the trials had a strata with imbalance of 8 or more. Ten percent of these trials had a strata with imbalance of 12 or more. Since each stratum value occurred with equal probability, each stratum should contain about 18 subjects. An imbalance of 12 would occur if 15 subjects were assigned to one treatment and 3 to the other. Ten percent of the trials conducted using simple random assignment contained a stratum level with this serious imbalance.

TABLE 3 Resulting Percentiles for Imbalance

	Method of Randomization		
Percent	*Simple Random*	*Permuted Blocks*	*Minimization*
	Total Imbalance		
50	20	10	2
75	26	14	6
90	34	18	6
95	38	18	6
99	48	24	8
	Maximum Strata Imbalance		
50	7	3	1
75	9	4	1
90	11	5	2
95	12	5	2
99	15	7	2

Permuted blocks within strata had half its trials resulting in total imbalance of 10 or less. Recall that permuted blocks of size six, as used in this simulation experiment, insure balance after every sixth subject within each stratum. But since subjects come to the study with random strata levels, there is no assurance that the number of subjects in each stratum level combination will be a multiple of six. Many of the blocks of six will be partially used, leading to the imbalance observed in Table 3. While achieving far better results than simple random assignment, 10% of the permuted blocks trials resulted in maximum strata imbalance of 6 or more. An imbalance of 6 in a group of 18 subjects results when 12 are assigned to one treatment and only 6 to the other.

Minimization is designed to minimize total imbalance each time a subject is entered into the study. It results in half its trials having a total imbalance of 2 or less. The results are similar for maximum strata imbalance. Half the trials have a maximum strata imbalance of 1 or zero. Ninety-nine percent of the trials have a maximum strata imbalance of 2 or less.

Figure 1 shows the distribution of total imbalance for each set of 10,000 trials. Figure 2 shows the resulting distributions of maximum strata imbalance for the three randomization methods. Each method was compared to the other two methods on both total imbalance and maximum strata imbalance. Minimization produced significantly lower total imbalance and maximum strata imbalance than permuted blocks within

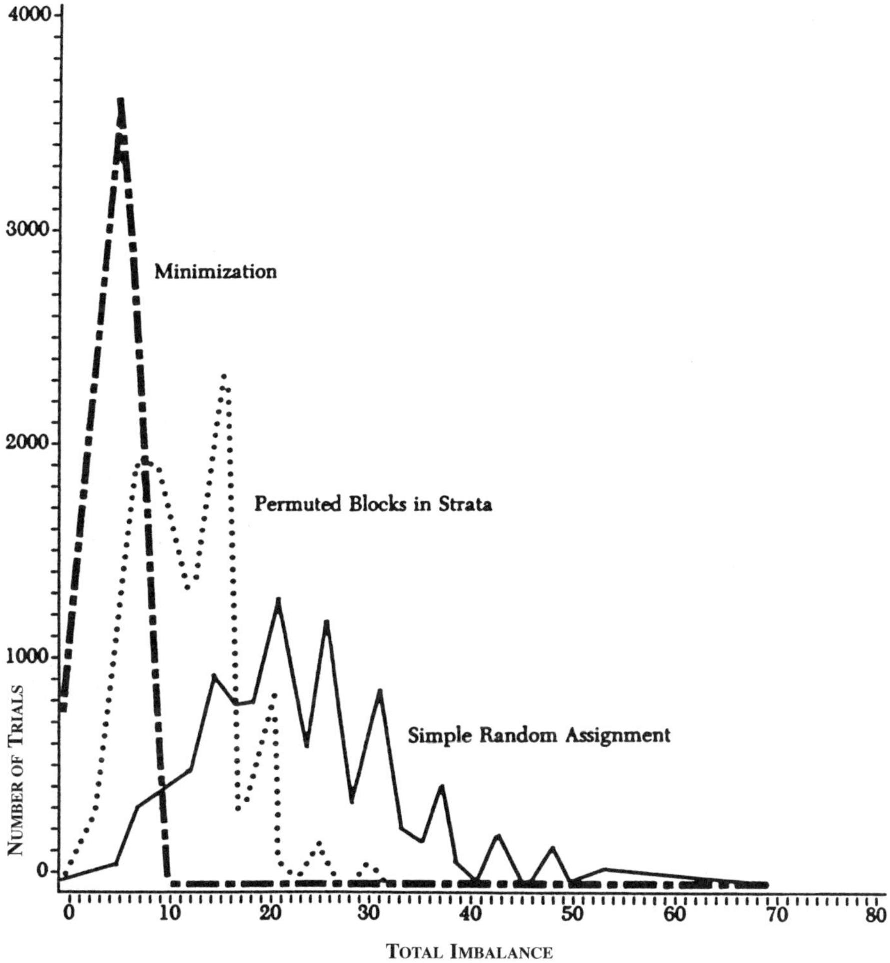

FIGURE 1 Total Imbalance for 30,000 Computerized Randomization Trials (10,000 per method)

strata or simple random assignment. Permuted blocks within strata produced significantly lower total imbalance and maximum strata imbalance than simple random assignment. All comparisions were significant at $\alpha = 0.0001$.

Discussion

Stratified random assignment is important in controlled clinical trials to overcome selection bias and the possibility of serious imbalance among covariates at study end. Stratified random assignment procedures are more complex to administer than simple random assignment. Permuted blocks within strata require separate randomization lists for each combination of strata levels. When the number of strata and levels is small, such lists may be feasible. The findings from our simulation experiment indicate that in small studies ($N = 36$) minimization achieves significantly better covariate balance than either simple random assignment or permuted blocks within strata. Minimization is also recommended for large samples with numerous strata and levels. Minimization can be easily administered with the aid of a computer program to record assignment of subjects already randomized.

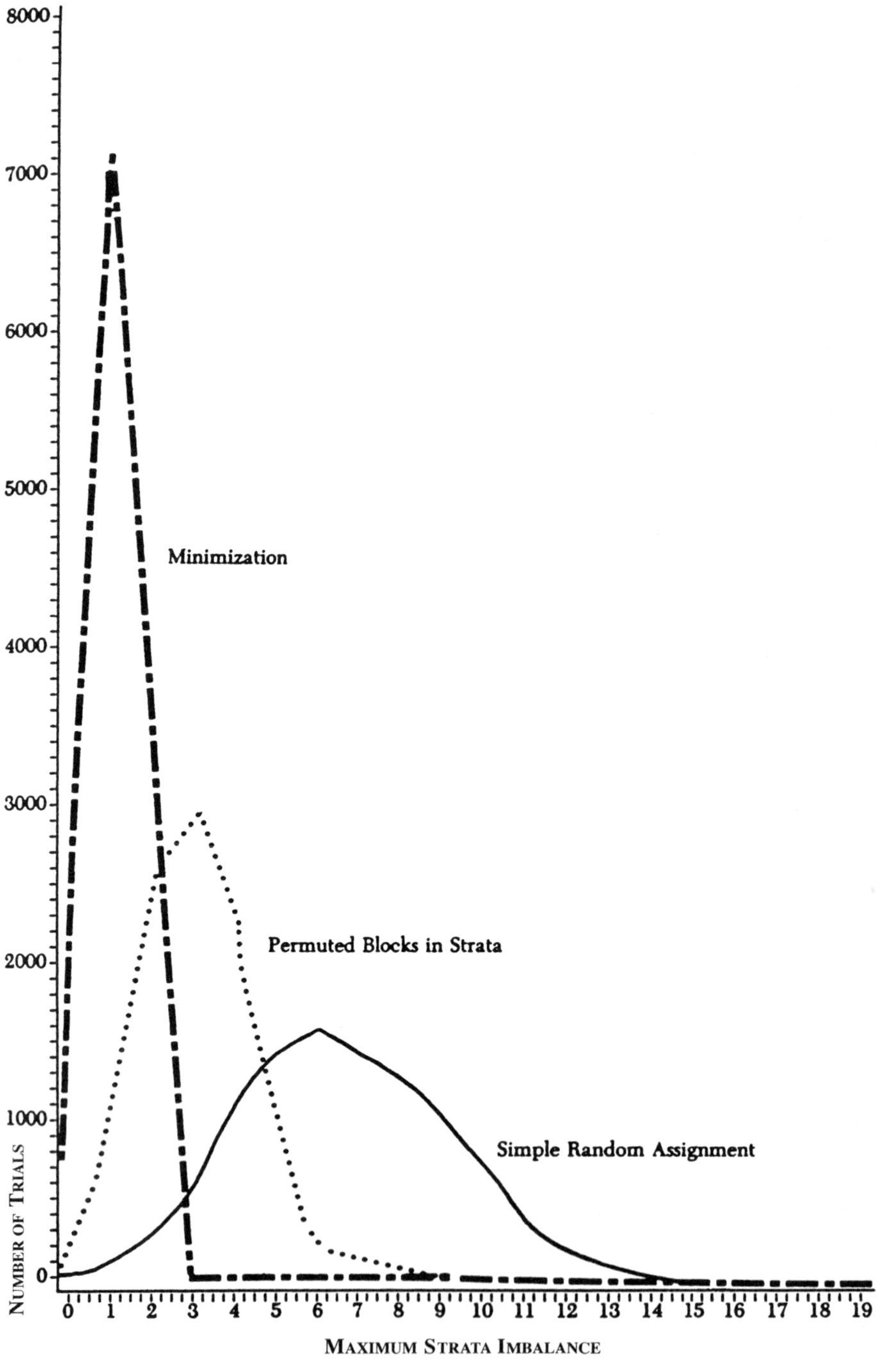

FIGURE 2 Maximum Strata Imbalance for 30,000 Computerized Randomization Trials (10,000 per method)

References

Efron, B. (1971). Forcing a sequential experiment to be balanced. *Biometrika, 58,* 403–417.

Fetter, M. S., Feetham, S. L., D'Apolito, K., Chaze, B., Fink, A., Frink, B. B., Hougart, M. K., & Rushton, C. (1989). Randomized clinical trials: Issues for researchers. *Nursing Research, 38,* 117–120.

Lachin, J. M., Matts, J. P., & Wei, L. J. (1988). Randomization in clinical trials: Conclusions and recommendations. *Controlled Clinical Trials, 9,* 365–374.

Pocock, S. J., & Simon, R. (1975). Sequential treatment assignment with balancing for prognostic factors in the controlled clinical trial. *Biometrics, 31,* 103–115.

Pocock, S. J. (1983). *Clinical trials: A practical approach.* Chichester, UK: Wiley.

Polit, D. F., & Hungler, B. P. (1987). *Nursing Research: Principles and methods.* Philadelphia, PA: Lippincott.

Wei, L. J. (1978). An application of the urn model to the design of sequential controlled clinical trials. *Journal of the American Statistical Association, 73,* 559–563.

Zelen, M. (1974). The randomization and stratification of patients to clinical trials. *Journal of Chronic Diseases, 27,* 365–375.

PART TWO

Qualitative Techniques

Qualitative vs. Quantitative Research or Qualitative and *Quantitative Research?*

Laura D. Goodwin ■ **William L. Goodwin**

In recent years there has been increased discussion about the relevance of *qualitative* versus *quantitative* methodological strategies used for research in nursing (Klenow, 1981; Knafl & Howard, 1984; Swanson & Chenitz, 1982), as well as in education and other social and behavioral fields. Although qualitative and quantitative are frequently used in supposedly lucid, precise, and unambiguous terms, a number of methodologists have pointed out that the qualitative-quantitative distinction is inexact and somewhat artificial (Downs, 1983; Lynch, 1983; Smith, 1978). Discussions about the relative merits of the two approaches often become heated debates, and "taking sides" seems to be especially popular. Once immersed in the discussions or debates, it is easy to forget that the focus of all this attention is directed on two different methods of data collection and analysis rather than two different philosophies of life! The purpose of this paper is to discuss several myths about the differences between the two approaches and to point out two advantages of using *both* strategies in a single study.

There are three popular myths about the differences between qualitative and quantitative research that are prevalent in qualitative-versus-quantitative discussions. For related and more detailed discussions of these and other myths, the reader is referred to Reichardt and Cook (1979) and Smith (1978).

Myth #1: Qualitative and quantitative research strategies represent clearly different, mutually exclusive paradigmatic perspectives. Those researchers who take this position usually adopt Kuhn's (1962) definition of *paradigm:* a world view or set of assumptions and perspectives that provides a conceptual framework for the organized study of the real world. A number of methodologists have argued that quantitative research methods are inherently linked to a logical-positivist paradigm and qualitative methods are inherently associated with a phenomenological paradigm (Rist, 1980; Smith, 1983; Watson, 1981). Others, however, have convincingly pointed out that a linkage between paradigm and method is neither an inherent nor necessarily consistent requirement (Reichardt & Cook, 1979; Lynch, 1983). The qualitative-quantitative distinction is primarily one of methods of data collection, analysis, and interpretation. As Reichardt and Cook said, it is possible to approach the study of a phenomenon with a certain paradigmatic orientation using *either* method:

> Is the researcher who uses quantitative procedures necessarily a logical positivist, and conversely, is the researcher who uses qualitative procedures necessarily a phenomenologist? Certainly not, for, on the one hand, many social researchers who use quantitative methods subscribe to a phenomenological stance. For example, social psychological theories of attribution are phenomenological in that they are aimed at understanding behaviors and beliefs from the perspective of the actors themselves. Yet most, if not all, of attribution research is conducted in the laboratory with quantitative methods. . . . On the other hand, it would be possible, though perhaps unlikely, for an ethnographer to conduct research from a logical-positivist stance. For example, imagine a researcher who believes that socioeconomic status is defined solely in terms of material possessions such as televisions, cars, houses, and clothes. Since these material goods can be observed and counted without reference to the meanings that they may have for their owners, such a measure of SES is clearly in the logical-positivist tradition. Then a researcher who uses this measure and who verifies an individual's possessions by ethnographic fieldwork would be subscribing to logical-positivism while using qualitative methods. [1979, p. 12]

Although certain methods are usually linked to certain paradigms, the association between paradigm and method is far from exclusive. The choice of research procedures—including design, sampling plan, instrumentation, data collection methods, and data analysis techniques—should match the research question and be optimally efficient,

Laura D. Goodwin, PhD, is an associate professor of education at the University of Colorado at Denver and adjunct associate professor of nursing at the University of Colorado Health Sciences Center, Denver.

William L. Goodwin, PhD, is a professor of education at the University of Colorado at Denver.

From *Nursing Research,* November/December 1984, *33,* 378–380.

powerful, valid, and reliable. Sometimes the methods of choice will be qualitative, sometimes quantitative, and sometimes they will be a combination of both procedures. Trying rigidly to link paradigm with method will inevitably lead to research that is conducted inappropriately and which, therefore, will produce findings that lack credibility. At a time when methodological advances (including substantial contributions from ethnographic and other qualitative approaches) have increased the options available to researchers, it seems unfortunate to artificially dichotomize quantitative and qualitative research procedures into two nonoverlapping sets with cross-use prohibited.

Myth #2: Qualitative methods are always "naturalistic," unobtrusive, and subjective, whereas quantitative methods are always controlled, obtrusive, and objective. The data-collection methods typically considered qualitative are observation, especially participant observation; in-depth or key-informant interviewing; document or record review; and other nonreactive measures such as physical-trace collection (Denzin, 1978). Although these types of measures tend to be highly subjective and to yield data in the form of narrative descriptions, they do not *necessarily* have those characteristics. Document-reviews, for example, can certainly be conducted in a very objective manner (using standardized formats and multiple recorders for reliability checks) and thus produce numerical data best termed quantitative. Interviews and observation can be quite obtrusive; in fact, the well-known Hawthorne effect is a formidable obstacle to the validity of many studies that employ such methods. Conversely, methods usually considered quantitative—randomized experiments, laboratory studies, paper-and-pencil tests, questionnaires, rating scales—are not inherently controlled, objective, or obtrusive. True or quasi-experimental studies conducted in field settings can be fairly unobtrusive. For example, consider the nurse practitioner-physician comparison studies of the last decade. Many involved nonrandom assignment of patients to providers and collection of data via record review. Most studies of this type would be classified as quantitative, yet they possessed several methodological features considered qualitative. They were conducted in a naturalistic environment, were generally unobtrusive to patients and providers, and involved indirect, nonreactive measurement techniques. Similarly, quality assessment research studies, frequently relying on record audits as the chief measurement strategy, have been viewed as quantitative by most reviewers (Bloch, 1980).

Myth #3: Measurement-related validity and reliability are irrelevant in qualitative research. Traditional notions of validity and reliability seem to have become associated with quantitative research methods and, at the same time, have been more or less ignored by qualitative researchers. This tendency is especially apparent if one looks at the more popular qualitative research textbooks or methodological source books (Glaser & Strauss, 1967; Lofland & Lofland, 1984; Spradley, 1979, 1980). Denzin (1978), a well-known sociologist who has written about qualitative methodology, specifically noted that little systematic attention has been given to validity and reliability. The reasons for this situation are difficult to discern. A partial explanation may lie in the attitude of some qualitative researchers, especially those with a strong anthropological/ethnographic orientation, who view the researcher as the instrument and therefore feel the instrument has no standing independent of the researcher. Traditional validity and reliability estimation techniques, devised for objective, quantitative measurement strategies, thus appear inappropriate to these researchers (e.g., Smith, 1983).

Although the traditional quantitative methods of estimating validity and reliability are problematic with some qualitative measurement strategies, it does not automatically follow that the concepts of validity and reliability are irrelevant. For research to produce credible findings, the data must be collected in a consistent, reliable way, and must be valid indications of reality. LeCompte and Goetz (1982) comprehensively analyzed the constructs of validity and reliability as defined by ethnographers. They noted that the treatment of these constructs has been haphazard and sporadic, but managed to synthesize and suggest an impressive number of strategies that qualitative researchers can use to estimate and enhance the validity and reliability of their investigations.

Similarly, Goodwin and Goodwin (in press) applied traditional notions of validity and reliability estimation to data collection methods and also to data analysis/interpretation techniques in qualitative research. They showed how inter-interviewer or inter-observer reliability, inter-analyst reliability, and internal consistency reliability are important issues that must be considered and can be empirically or logically estimated. They also demonstrated it was possible to estimate content, concurrent, and construct validity, which are even more critical concerns. For example, some qualitative researchers advocate a technique known as *triangulation* to achieve comprehensiveness in data collection (Denzin, 1978; Filstead, 1982; Reichardt & Cook, 1979). Triangulation refers to data collection via multiple methods (such as observation, interviewing, and record review), and subsequent examination of the data for congruence across methods. Thus, in actuality it is closely related to concurrent validation techniques long used by quantitative psychometricians. What is beginning to emerge in terms of validity and reliability issues is a realization that the positions and best interests of quantitative and qualitative researchers are not dramatically distinct.

Use of Both Strategies in a Single Study

Whether or not it is appropriate to use both strategies in the same study is an issue closely associated with the three myths, and especially the first one. That is, those researchers who believe that there is a paradigmatic distinction between qualitative and quantitative methods usually reject the notion that the two types of strategy can be used together (Rist, 1980; Smith, 1983). Curiously, however, other methodologists support the paradigmatic distinction and yet also acknowledge the advantages of a combined or integrated use of qualitative and quantitative methods in a single study (Bogdan & Biklen, 1982; Filstead, 1982). And, of course, there is an increasingly large number of methodologists who find the paradigm issue fairly irrelevant and strongly advocate the combined use of the two approaches (Gorenberg, 1983; Mullen & Iverson, 1982; Reichardt & Cook, 1979).

Although the advantages of an integrated or combined approach do not apply to every research study (i.e., for some research studies it is appropriate to use *only* qualitative or *only* quantitative strategies), many studies could be enhanced considerably if a combined approach were taken. Two examples are:

Achieving a Comprehensiveness That Neither Approach, If Used Alone, Could Achieve

This comprehensiveness refers to several aspects of the research. First, delineating the problem and specifying the exact research questions to be answered can be aided by considering both quantitative and qualitative types of questions in a single study. Many research studies have multiple purposes or attempt to answer several different questions. Some of the purposes or questions (e.g., those that deal with contextual, baseline, or process variables) are frequently best approached by qualitative strategies; others (e.g., those that focus on outcome variables) might optimally be answered with quantitative methods (Fetterman, 1982). Second, it is sometimes advantageous to add a qualitative component to what is basically a quantitative design to increase the meaning of the obtained data. For example, qualitative measurement techniques such as intensive observations or interviews can help the researcher identify the values and perspectives of subjects in ways that are often impossible with strictly quantitative strategies.

Relatedly, those qualitative techniques can help identify unanticipated program effects in quantitative program evaluation research studies (Mullen & Iverson, 1982). In general, use of qualitative techniques in true or quasi-experimental designs can enhance the validity and reliability of the study by (a) providing an enlarged contextual and procedural framework within which to analyze and interpret the data, thus increasing the understanding of the phenomenon being studied; and (b) helping to eliminate alternate explanations for findings in the weaker quasi-experimental designs.

Cross-validating the Findings

No single measurement strategy or method is perfectly reliable or valid; relatedly, every data collection technique has certain strengths and weaknesses. Use of multiple measures in a single study has long been advocated as a means of strengthening the study (e.g., Polit & Hungler, 1978). Increasingly, such advice to researchers about multiple measures includes using quantitative, objective measures in conjunction with qualitative, subjective measures (although, as noted in the discussion of Myth #2, there is no absolute objectivity-subjectivity distinction between these measures). Ianni and Orr (1979) and Sieber (1978), for example, suggested using field observations to validate survey results, and survey data to validate field observational data. Pelto and Pelto (1978) recommended the collection of both self-report and observational data within a single study as a way to enhance the generalizations or external validity of the research. Other methodologists have also noted the need to check for congruence in findings obtained via different methods (some qualitative and some quantitative), a type of triangulation mentioned in Myth #3. Most research studies can benefit from multiple measures of the process and/or outcome variables of interest; careful choice of a combination of qualitative and quantitative measurement strategies can increase the information yield and strengthen the external validity of the results.

A myriad of topics can be discussed in reference to qualitative and quantitative research. Only a few have been presented here. It is hoped that more methodological discussions of this type on key issues and concerns about the two types of methods will help clarify their relative advantages and disadvantages, and strengthen the quality of studies conducted by the research community.

References

Bogdan, R. C., & Biklen, S. K. (1982). *Qualitative research for education: An introduction to theory and methods.* Boston: Allyn & Bacon.

Bloch, D. (1980). Interrelated issues in evaluation and evaluation research. *Nursing Research, 29,* 69–73.

Denzin, N. K. (1978). *The research act* (2nd ed.). New York: McGraw-Hill.
Downs, F. S. (1983). One dark and stormy night. *Nursing Research, 32,* 259.
Fetterman, D. M. (1982). Ibsen's baths: Reactivity and insensitivity. *Educational Evaluation and Policy Analysis, 4,* 261–279.
Filstead, W. J. (1982). Qualitative and quantitative information in health policy decision making. In E. R. House & Associates (Eds.), *Evaluation studies review annual:* Vol. 7 (pp. 704–717). Beverly Hills, CA: Sage Publications.
Glaser, B. G., & Strauss, A. L. (1967). *The discovery of grounded theory: Strategies for qualitative research.* Chicago: Aldine.
Goodwin, L. D., & Goodwin, W. L. (1964). *The validity and reliability of data collection and data analysis/interpretation techniques in qualitative evaluation research.* Manuscript submitted for publication.
Gorenberg, B. (1983). The research tradition of nursing: An emerging issue. *Nursing Research, 32,* 347–349.
Ianni, F. A. J., & Orr, M. T. (1979). Toward a rapprochement of quantitative and qualitative methodologies. In T. D. Cook & C. S. Reichardt (Eds.), *Qualitative and quantitative methods in evaluation research* (pp. 67–98). Beverly Hills, CA: Sage Publications.
Klenow, D. J. (1981). Qualitative methodology: A neglected resource in nursing research. *Research in Nursing and Health, 4,* 281–282.
Knafl, K. A., & Howard, M. J. (1984). Interpreting and reporting qualitative research. *Research in Nursing and Health, 7,* 17–24.
Kuhn, T. S. (1962). *The structure of scientific revolutions.* Chicago: University of Chicago Press.
LeCompte, M. D., & Goetz, J. P. (1982). Problems of reliability and validity in ethnographic research. *Review of Educational Research, 52,* 31–60.
Lofland, J., & Lofland, L. H. (1984). *Analyzing social settings: A guide to qualitative observation and analysis* (2nd ed.). Belmont, CA: Wadsworth.
Lynch, K. B. (1983). Qualitative and quantitative evaluation: Two terms in search of meaning. *Educational Evaluation and Policy Analysis, 5,* 461–464.
Mullen, P. D., & Iverson, D. (1982, May-June). Qualitative methods for evaluation research in health education programs. *Health Education,* pp. 11–18.
Pelto, P. J., & Pelto, G. H. (1978). *Anthropological research: The structure of inquiry* (2nd ed.). Cambridge: Cambridge University Press.
Polit, D., & Hungler, B. (1978). *Nursing research: Principles and methods.* Philadelphia: J. B. Lippincott Co.
Reichardt, C. S., & Cook, T. D. (1979). Beyond qualitative versus quantitative methods. In T. D. Cook & C. S. Reichardt (Eds). *Qualitative and quantitative methods in evaluation research* (pp. 7–32). Beverly Hills, CA: Sage Publications.
Rist, R. C. (1980). Blitzkrieg ethnography: On the transformation of a method into a movement. *Educational Researcher, 9*(2), 8–10.
Sieber, S. D. (1978). The integration of fieldwork and survey methods. In N. K. Denzin (Ed.), *Sociological methods: A sourcebook* (2nd ed.) (pp. 358–380). New York: McGraw-Hill.
Smith, J. K. (1983). Quantitative versus qualitative research: An attempt to clarify the issue. *Educational Researcher, 12*(3), 6–13.
Smith, L. M. (1978). An evolving logic of participant observation, educational ethnography, and other case studies. *Review of Research in Education, 6,* 316–377.
Spradley, J. P. (1979). *The ethnographic interview.* New York: Holt, Rinehart & Winston.
Spradley, J. P. (1980). *Participant observation.* New York: Holt, Rinehart & Winston.
Swanson, J. M., & Chenitz, W. C. (1982). Why qualitative research in nursing? *Nursing Outlook, 30,* 241–245.
Watson, J. (1981). Nursing's scientific quest. *Nursing Outlook, 29,* 413–416.

Guidelines for Integration of Quantitative and Qualitative Approaches

Sheila Taylor Myers ■ **Joan E. Haase**

Integration of quantitative and qualitative research approaches is inevitable and essential in furthering nursing science. However, integration can be more easily accomplished when guidelines are used to make decisions about research programs and specific designs. Such guidelines for integration are proposed in this article.

The guidelines are based on three principles. First, nursing practice synchronizes integration of qualitative and quantitative approaches. Nurses in practice have long recognized the uniqueness of an individual's experiences and interactions (the qualitative approach) while simultaneously identifying commonalities from which to make predictions (the quantitative approach). Current thinking about nursing models provides further evidence of how nursing practice guides integration. To illustrate, in earlier years, Roy's Adaptation Model was consistent with the quantitative research approach. Roy recently added "health as a process" to the model (Roy, 1984) which indicates to some (Parse, 1987) that the model now includes ideas usually associated with the qualitative approach. To be congruent with the shift in approach, the type of research questions asked by those using Roy's model should also change to include qualitative questions and methods. Thus, questions arising from discussions of nursing models which define practice also serve to accommodate the integration of approaches to research.

A second principle used to develop the guidelines is that each approach must be equally valued. If both approaches are not valued, problems arise when decisions must be made about how and in what order specific qualitative and quantitative methods will be incorporated into a program of research. Therefore, in order to achieve a dynamic balance between qualitative and quantitative approaches, we considered the unique contributions of each.

The third principle is that the link between method and assumptions (Smith & Heshusius, 1986; Powers, 1987) demands simultaneous consideration. Such simultaneous consideration occurs on several levels by identifying commonalities in assumptions between the two approaches rather than emphasizing differences (Haase & Myers, 1988). Combined methods will be more than a conglomeration of strategies if investigators are sensitive to these commonalities and view the approaches as complementary.

Thus, the guidelines are proposed as an initial step toward explicating any decision making involved in integration. They are presented here as broad conditional statements and provide a framework to stimulate and redirect thought. New designs may be formulated and new phases of research may be developed for theories previously considered complete if the guidelines are used.

Guidelines for Integration of Research Approaches

The first guideline specifies that the world is viewed as a whole, an interactive system with patterns of information exchange between subsystems or levels of reality. This world view can be thought of as a multidimensional gameboard. In such a game one must visualize simultaneous moves both across levels and between levels on the board in order to plan successful game strategies. Levels exist within the whole and are interactive so that changes on one level reverberate between levels.

In the "world" where nurses practice, these levels can be viewed in various ways. A familiar stratification is seen in the levels proposed by Engle (1979) for the health sciences: cellular, organ system, person, family, community, culture and society. Specific clinical areas of nursing differ in the strength of their reliance on certain levels. For instance, medical and surgical nursing is strongly grounded in organ systems, the cellular level, while community nursing is focused on family systems and the social group or community. However, even though there is a central focus on a primary level for each clinical area,

Sheila Taylor Myers, MS, RN, is an assistant professor at the University of Oklahoma, Oklahoma City, OK.

Joan E. Haase, PhD, RN, is an assistant professor at the University of Oklahoma, Oklahoma City, OK.

From *Nursing Research,* September/October 1989, *38,* 299–301.

other levels are always considered and patterns emerge because of the strong interaction between levels and a general blurring of boundaries. Thus, nurses in all clinical areas recognize many levels in the interaction between themselves and a client, while drawing predominantly from a selected few levels.

Following the nursing practice model, at least two levels should be incorporated into research questions and represented in the data base. In studies of bonding, for example, nurse researchers consider various levels of data from physiological reactions, individual interaction patterns, statements of belief and experiences, and family function indicators are included in an investigation. Physiological response data alone would be inadequate for nursing because that explanation of bonding, by itself, is too limited to be useful. When only one level is represented, the understanding of reality is artificial and recognition of interrelationships across levels is not possible.

In addition to considering interactive levels, interdependence between levels should be anticipated in research plans. Information exchange between levels and consideration of the context within which that communication occurs allows flexibility in planning research so that interactive parts of the whole are considered. For example, in bonding research, data about beliefs and experiences may influence interpretation of data about physiological responses or family functioning. While strategies to isolate parts are an effective way to begin understanding the world, use of these strategies to establish control must be recognized as artificial, offering incomplete knowledge.

If the world is conceived as an interactive whole, one cannot justifiably negate the legitimacy of data based on its source. Hence, the second guideline: Both subjective and objective data are recognized as legitimate avenues for gaining understanding.

All data sources offer a reflection of the whole and are necessary to understand the phenomenon under investigation. Issues about the legitimacy of data sources have, in the past, limited understanding gained from either qualitative or quantitative approaches. Similarly, when either objective or subjective data is held as superior, an important source of information is eliminated. Although one may omit a particular source of data at specific phases of a research program, valuing both data sources increases the potential for information. Furthermore, some questions about legitimacy of data are more appropriately viewed as questions of validity or reliability.

To illustrate the importance of different data sources, consider two potential data sources for research on bonding: the subjective descriptions of mothers' progressive ability to anticipate their infants' needs contrasted with objective observations of the mother-infant interaction. When both data sets are valued, efforts are made to identify useful data from each. The task then becomes one of integrating the understanding of data from the various sources. Rather than assuming that one source is more important—or even negates the other when contradictions seem apparent—commitment to deal with both sources of data will ultimately enrich the findings.

The third guideline asserts that both atomistic and holistic thinking be used in design and analysis. Different people have different styles of thinking and approach problems in different ways. Atomistic thinkers tend to focus on the individual parts of a problem while holistic thinkers focus on the overview of the situation within which a problem is posed. The type of thinking used to conceive a problem influences the research design as well as the methods and analysis employed in the investigation. Different thinking styles can complement one another rather than create chaos. Research approaches negotiated by people using both atomistic and holistic thinking styles will expand the way problems are conceived. In so doing, the power as well as the efficiency of the research questions will be increased.

The fourth guideline is that the concept of research "participant" includes not only those who are the subjects of the methodology but also those who administer or operate the methodology. Traditionally, in quantitative research, the investigator attempts to maintain an observer neutral stance. This position reinforces a sense of false security. The impossibility of this stance is evident in the many methods developed to deal with investigator bias. Recognition of contributions from both the investigator and the subject are increased when the interaction between the two are acknowledged. Using the example of bonding once more, a mother's affirmation or modification of an investigator's description of bonding can strengthen the validity of that description as well as expand that knowledge.

To increase the effectiveness of the first four guidelines, the fifth provides that maximally conflicting points of view are sought with provision for systematic and controlled confrontation. Respectful, honest, open confrontation on points of view between investigators is essential. Here, conflict is seen as a positive value because it offers potential for expanding questioning and consequent understanding. Confrontation occurs between co-investigators with differing expertise who recognize that both approaches are equally valid and vulnerable. Ability to consider participants' views which may differ from the investigator's perspective is equally important.

Implications of Using Guidelines

When individuals with varied expertise are involved in the planning stages of a research project, greater flexibility and more creative solutions can be expected. More than direct causal relationships will be anticipated in the construction of the design. Design planning will be progressive with investigators using feedback from the data and from all participants in the research process. At the same time, through negotiation of conflicting positions, strategies to establish rigor and to ensure trustworthiness of the data will be available.

Recognition of consequences will be enhanced by the participation of several types of thinkers with differing perspectives, both investigators and subjects. It may be necessary to plan programmatic research with co-investigators whose thinking patterns complement one another. Oberst (1986) defined programmatic research as "A systematic line of investigation involving multimodal approaches over time" (p. 1). That definition could extend to the use of interdisciplinary teams as well. Mitchell (1986) has already described investigator triangulation for nursing research. Combinations of clinical nursing staff and faculty is yet another fruitful strategy. Successful efforts in such ventures have already been reported (Pettingill & Knafl, 1985). Including subjects as participants in the process and product of research also enhances efforts to obtain different perspectives.

Cooperation between people with varied orientations and areas of expertise is expected when the guidelines are instituted, and personal costs will be a major consideration for participants. Differences, from terminology to territory, from personality to conceptual orientation, must be recognized and reconciled. Acceptance and respect for these varied positions can be rewarded as an evolving, primary value that advances project goals rather than experienced as a personal loss of position or power. When differences are viewed positively, systematic and controlled confrontation is enhanced. The result is a mutuality which is initially costly in terms of time and energy, but which ultimately yields high dividends.

Project costs may need to be constructed differently when research is collaborative. Increased expenses may arise from the elaborate designs that will evolve. Funding sources will need to be identified as well as strategies for securing funds. However, phasing of projects and sequential planning can offer long-range budget forecasting and can increase strategies that offer flexibility in unit or departmental development.

Other implications of using the guidelines are the ethical issues of confidentiality and disciplinary boundaries. Protection of human rights through the mechanism of institutional review boards will be an interesting phenomenon to watch. Ethical principles may need to be redefined. For example, the right of a subject to anonymity has traditionally been valued to the exclusion of the right to identification. However, when participants share their experiences, as called for in the guidelines, they often consider this a contribution to others. The idea of anonymity may negate this contribution and will need to be addressed as a human right of major value. Therefore, the protection of an individual's right to privacy may need to be expanded to consider also the human right to the ownership of contribution.

The proposed guidelines are viewed as a step toward integrating qualitative and quantitative approaches in order to answer questions that confront the practice of nursing. The consequences may be reflected in more unified investigative approaches, broader questions, different team compositions, and costs and benefits at the personal and organizational levels.

References

Engle, G. L. (1979). The Biomedical model: A Procrustean bed? Man and medicine. *The Journal of Values and Ethics in Health Care, 4*(4), 257–275.

Hasse, J. E., & Myers, S. T. (1988). Reconciling paradigm assumptions of qualitative and quantitative research. *Western Journal of Nursing Research, 10*(2), 128–137.

Mitchell E. S. (1986). Multiple triangulation: A methodology for nursing science. *Advances in Nursing Science, 8*(3), 18–26.

Oberst, M. T. (1986). Establishment of a research office: Why now? *School of Nursing Research Newsletter University of Wisconsin-Madison, 6*(1), 1.

Parse, R. R. (1987). *Nursing science: Major paradigms, theories, and critiques.* Philadelphia: W. B. Saunders Company.

Pettingill, M., & Knafl, K. (1985, April). *Methodological considerations and future directions for studying clinical nurse researchers.* [Abstract]. Paper presented at the Ninth Annual Conference of the Midwest Nursing Research Society, Chicago, IL. (unpublished).

Powers, B. A. (1987). Taking sides: A Response to Goodwin and Goodwin, *Nursing Research, 36,* 122–126.

Roy, C. (1984). *Introduction to nursing: An adaptation model* (2nd ed.). Englewood Cliffs, NJ: Prentice-Hall.

Smith, J. K., & Heshusius, L. (1986). Closing down the conversation: The end of the quantitative-qualitative debate among educational inquirers. *Educational Researcher, 15*(1), 4–12.

Approaches to Qualitative-Quantitative Methodological Triangulation

Janice M. Morse

Recently, there has been discussion in nursing journals regarding the appropriateness, advantages, and disadvantages of methodological triangulation.[1] The issue that has prompted the most interest is combining qualitative and quantitative methods within the same project. Some authors have published examples on how this was accomplished within a particular project, identifying the issues involved with such strategies (Imle & Atwood, 1988; Knafl, Pettengill, Bevis, & Kirchhoff, 1988; Murphy, 1989; Tripp-Reimer, 1985). Others have identified unresolved issues (Clarke & Yaros, 1988; Duffy, 1987a, 1987b; Phillips, 1988a, 1988b) or noted that guidelines for the use of methodological triangulation are lacking (Mitchell, 1986). In particular Mitchell (1986) notes five areas of concern: the difficulty of merging numeric and textual data; the interpretation of divergent results obtained from the use of qualitative and quantitative methods; the lack of delineation of concepts and the merging of concepts; the weighing of information from different data sources; and the difficulty in ascertaining the contribution of each method when assimilating the results. The purpose of this article is to explore the principles underlying the use of methodological triangulation when combining qualitative and quantitative methods. These principles are related to consistency between the purpose of research, the research question, the method used, the selection of sample, and the interpretation of results.

Methodological Triangulation

Methodological triangulation is the use of at least two methods, usually qualitative and quantitative, to address the same research problem. When a single research method is inadequate, triangulation is used to ensure that the most comprehensive approach is taken to solve a research problem. A less common use of triangulation is to ensure validity of the instruments used (Knafl & Breitmayer, 1989). However, this approach should be used cautiously, since an instrument should be tested prior to implementation or its validity established during a pilot stage.

Methodological triangulation can be classified as simultaneous or sequential (Field & Morse, 1985). *Simultaneous triangulation* is the use of the qualitative and quantitative methods at the same time. In this case, there is limited interaction between the two datasets during the data collection, but the findings complement one another at the end of the study. *Sequential triangulation* is used if the results of one method are essential for planning the next method. The qualitative method is completed before the quantitative method is implemented or vice versa.

The first step in qualitative-quantitative triangulation is to determine if the research problem is primarily qualitative or quantitative. Characteristics of a qualitative research problem are: (a) the concept is "immature," due to a conspicuous lack of theory and previous research; (b) a notion that the available theory may be inaccurate, inappropriate, incorrect, or biased; (c) a need exists to explore and describe the phenomena and to develop theory; or (d) the nature of the phenomenon may not be suited to quantitative measures (Field & Morse, 1985).

If a research problem is primarily quantitative, the above characteristics are not applicable. The researcher can locate substantial and relevant literature on the topic, create a theoretical framework, and identify testable hypotheses. In this case, the research design is comparative or correlational (i.e., Level II) or experimental or quasi-experimental (i.e., Level III) (Brink & Wood, 1989).

Thus, in methodological triangulation, the key issue is whether the theory that drives the research (May,

Janice M. Morse, RN, PhD (Nursing), PhD (Anthropology), is a professor and MRC/NHRDP Research Scholar in the faculty of nursing and is adjunct professor in the Department of Family Studies at the University of Alberta. She is associate clinical nurse researcher at the University of Alberta Hospitals and is adjunct professor in the Department of Nursing at the University of Northern Arizona.

From *Nursing Research,* March/April 1991, *40,* 120–123.

[1] In addition to methodological triangulation, Knafl & Breitmayer (1989) discuss investigator, data source, unit of analysis, and theoretical triangulation, and the reader is referred to this source for a discussion on the role and purpose of other types of triangulation.

1989) is developed *inductively* from the research per se or used *deductively* as in quantitative inquiry.

This differentiation results in several types of methodological triangulation. If the research is driven by an inductive process and the theory developed qualitatively and complemented by quantitative methods, the notation *QUAL+ quan* is used to indicate simultaneous triangulation. If the project is deductive, driven by an a priori theoretical framework, quantitative methods take precedence and may be complemented by qualitative methods. In this case, the notation *QUAN+ qual* is used. Sequential triangulation is indicated by *QUAL→quan* with an inductive project, that is, when the theoretical drive is inductive and uses a qualitative foundation. When the notation *QUAN→qual* is used, it indicates a deductive approach. That is, when following the completion of the quantitative step, a qualitative method is used to examine outliers or to explore unexpected findings. Note that the theoretical drive does *not* refer to the valuing of the qualitative or quantitative paradigm (Myers & Haase, 1989), the amount of effort required nor the amount of time spent answering each qualitative or quantitative question.

The following cases are examples of simultaneous triangulation:

QUAL + quan

What is it like to be a relative of a patient in the ICU? This is clearly a qualitative problem, and the methods of ethnography or grounded theory may be used to describe the experience of anxious, waiting relatives. From the inception of the project, we can quite safely assume that the relative will be anxious. But how anxious? Clearly, it would strengthen our description of the sample if we could administer a standardized anxiety scale and include a description of the levels of anxiety that relatives may be experiencing.

QUAN + Qual

The conceptual framework of this study predicts that the sicker the child, the greater the spatial distance between the parents and the child; and the greater the spatial distance between the parents and the child, the greater the child's anxiety. How do we measure spatial distance in this situation? One way would be to do participant observation at randomly selected intervals; another way would be to use video cameras to observe the distance between the parents and their child. From these observations an ordinal scale is developed: close (touching range), midway (from arm's reach to the end of the bed), and distant (beyond the end of the bed). Hypotheses related to parental spatial distance and severity of illness of the child can then be tested.

The following cases are examples of sequential triangulation:

QUAL→quan

A qualitative study on the responses of adolescents to menarche provided many insights into adolescent behavior and their affective response to menstruation at this time. But what were the normative attitudes of adolescent girls towards menarche? The domains from the content analysis were used to construct a Likert scale, and the items were derived directly from the qualitative data. Quantitative methods of ensuring reliability and validity were used, and the Likert Scale was administered to a randomly selected sample.

QUAN→Qual

A large infant feeding survey of a Third World country produced the unexpected finding that there was no difference in the incidence of infantile diarrhea in infants from homes with or without refrigeration. Qualitative interviews with a sample of residents from homes with refrigerators revealed that infant formula bottles were not kept in the refrigerator. Refrigerators were used for making and storing ice, which was sold to supplement the family income.

From the above examples, it is obvious that the qualitative and quantitative aspects of a research project cannot be equally weighted; rather, a project must be either theoretically driven by the qualitative methods incorporating a complementary quantitative component, or theoretically driven by the quantitative method, incorporating a complementary qualitative component. The important point is that each method must be complete in itself; that is, all methods used must meet appropriate criteria for rigor. If qualitative interviews are conducted, then they must be conducted as if this method stands alone. The interviews should be continued until saturation is reached, and the content analysis conducted inductively, rather than forcing the data into some preconceived categories to fit the quantitative study or to prove a point. Further, this standard enables each component to be published independently. This may be particularly important to an investigator using sequential triangulation in a project extending over several years.

Implementing Methodological Triangulation

Given the fact that methods need to be used independently within a single project, the real issue in triangulation is not incompatibility between the different assumptions of the two paradigms as many researchers have argued (see Duffy, 1987b; Phillips, 1988a). It is not the incompatibility of contrasting philosophical issues from static and dynamic realities, objective and subjective perspectives, inductive and deductive approaches, or holistic and particular views. Nor is it the infeasible merging of textual and numerical data or of simultaneously considering the antagonistic approaches of acausality and causality. Blending or merging of the data does not occur in the process of analysis but in the fitting of the results from each study into a cohesive and coherent outcome or theory, or confirming or revising existing theory. This is achieved by being aware of and adhering to the rules and assumptions inherent in each method related to the selection of the sample, the purpose of the method, and the contribution of the results to the overall research plan.

Combining Samples

The greatest threat to validity is the use of inadequate or inappropriate samples. Perhaps for reasons of convenience, investigators are tempted to use the same subjects for both qualitative and quantitative methods, even though it is clearly inappropriate to interchange these samples. For instance, quantitative research is based on the assumption that large, randomly selected samples will be used so that the sample will be representative of the population. Adequacy of the sample is determined statistically (using *n* or sample size) and appropriateness is determined by the representativeness of the sample to the total population. In qualitative research, appropriateness is ascertained by how well the sample can represent the phenomena of interest (i.e., to what extent the participants have experienced the phenomena and can articulate their experiences), and the sample is deemed adequate when saturation of data is reached (Morse, 1987). Yet, in light of the overall purpose of the research, there is no reason (other than that of convenience) to use the same subjects for both samples. Clearly, when incorporating quantitative methods into a qualitative study, the qualitative sample is apt to be inadequate for quantitative purposes. The lack of representativeness of the purposefully selected qualitative sample is inappropriate and threatens validity. The sample selection for the qualitative and quantitative components of sequential (QUAL→quan) or simultaneous (QUAL+quan) triangulation must be independent. As the qualitative sample is inappropriate and inadequate, the investigator has no choice but to draw a quantitative sample from the population. However, when quantitative methods are being used to add further information about the qualitative sample (QUAL+quan), exceptions may be made if norms or a normal comparison group are available for interpreting the findings. In the example of the anxious relatives in the waiting room, the anxiety scale scores would be interpreted within the norms available for the anxiety scale (See Table 1).

A subsample of the larger quantitative sample may be used for the qualitative component of QUAN+qual or QUAL→quan triangulation, but those subjects included or incidents observed in the qualitative portion must be selected according to the criteria for "good" participants rather than randomly selected. That is, the subjects selected from the quantitative sample should be the most experienced and articulate, and the observations chosen should be considered the best examples of the situation.

Combining Results

Mitchell's (1986) problem of weighing the results of each component are resolved if findings are interpreted within the context of present knowledge. As such, each component should fit like pieces of a puzzle. This type of interpretation is not accomplished using a mathematical formula to weigh the findings from each method; rather, it is an informed thought process, involving judgment, wisdom, creativity, and insight, and includes the privilege of creating or modifying theory. It is an exciting part of every research project, and when triangulating different methods, it can be especially exciting. If contradictory results occur from triangulating qualitative and quantita-

TABLE 1 Limitations and Resolutions for Each Type of Methodological Triangulation

Approach	Type	Purpose	Limitations	Resolution
QUAL+quan	Simultaneous	enrich description of sample	Qualitative sample	Utilize normative data for comparison of results
QUAL→quan	Sequential	test emerging H_o; determine distribution of phenomena in population	Qualitative sample	Draw adequate random sample from same population
QUAN+qual	Simultaneous	to describe part of phenomena that cannot be quantified	Quantitative sample	Select appropriate theoretical sample from random sample
QUAN→qual	Sequential	to examine unexpected results	Quantitative sample	Select appropriate theoretical sample from random sample

tive methods, then one set of findings is invalid and/or the end result of the total study inadequate, incomplete, or inaccurate. If the study is deductively driven, the theoretical framework may be incorrect.

Methodological triangulation is not a term that is applied to ethnography, when the research method includes the use of semi-structured interviews, some level of participant observation, the use of records, and perhaps, the administration of questionnaires. It is the combination of such techniques that constitute ethnography and that make ethnography, ethnography. It is not a matter of blending or "integrating guidelines from both qualitative and quantitative texts" (Knafl et al., 1988), but rather, the use of appropriate strategies for maintaining validity for each method. QUAN+qual methodological triangulation is not merely the "addition of narrative and linguistic data" to an experimental design (Clarke & Yaros, 1988), unless interview data are collected and analyzed with adherence to the assumptions and principles of the qualitative method (see Haase & Myers, 1988; May, 1989, pp. 205–206). Similarly, incorporating one or two open-ended questions into a quantitative survey does not make the study qualitative.

Conversely, the use of quantitative data in a qualitative study, such as frequency data to enhance description, does not constitute a quantitative study. Methodological triangulation is not a technique to be used for reasons of researchers' speed and convenience (see Knafl et al., 1988, p.31). Properly done, it probably has the reverse short-term effect, greatly increasing the work involved in a project and increasing the duration of a project. But the long-term gains achieved from such thorough groundwork are immeasurable.

Simultaneous methodological triangulation is not a technique of concurrent validation. Although the same strategies may be used, they are implemented in a study for different reasons. The purpose of concurrent validation is to ascertain whether the results of two methods measuring the same concept are equivalent. The purpose of simultaneous triangulation is to obtain different but complementary data on the same topic, rather than to replicate results.

Methodological triangulation is not a matter of "maximizing the strengths and minimizing the weakness of each" (Knafl et al., 1988). If not approached cautiously, the end result may be to enhance the weakness of each method and invalidate the entire research project. Rather, methodological triangulation is a method of obtaining complementary findings that strengthen research results and contribute to theory and knowledge development.

Some of the controversy on methodological triangulation has focused on the issue of "qualitative versus quantitative research." This controversy advocates combining methods "as long as there is consistency with the 'theoretical researcher'" (Clarke & Yaros, 1988; Phillips, 1988b). Researchers who purport to subscribe to the philosophical underpinnings of only one research approach have lost sight of the fact that research methodologies are merely tools, instruments to be used to facilitate understanding. Smart researchers are versatile and have a balanced and extensive repertoire of methods at their disposal.

References

Brink, P. J., & Wood, M. J. (1989). *Advanced design in nursing research.* Newbury Park, CA: Sage.

Clarke, P. N., & Yaros, P. S. (1988). Transitions to new methodologies in nursing science [Commentary]. *Nursing Science Quarterly, 1*(4), 147–149.

Duffy, M. (1987a). Methodological triangulation: A vehicle for merging quantitative and qualitative research methods. *Image: Journal for Nursing Scholarship, 19,* 130–133.

Duffy, M. E. (1987b). Quantitative and qualitative research: Antagonistic or complementary? *Nursing and Health Care, 8,* 356–357.

Field, P. A., & Morse, J. M. (1985). *Qualitative nursing research: The application of qualitative approaches.* Rockville, MD: Aspen.

Haase, J. E., & Myers, S. T. (1988). Reconciling paradigm assumptions of qualitative and quantitative research. *Western Journal of Nursing Research, 10,* 128–137.

Imle, M. A., & Atwood, J. R. (1988). Retaining qualitative validity while gaining quantitative reliability and validity: Development of the Transition to Parenthood Concerns Scale. *Advances in Nursing Science, 11,* 61–75.

Knafl, K. A., & Breitmayer, B. J. (1989). Triangulation in qualitative research: Issues of conceptual clarity and purpose. In J. M. Morse (Ed.), *Qualitative nursing research: A contemporary dialogue* (pp.209–220). Rockville, MD: Aspen.

Knafl, K. A., Pettengill, M. M., Bevis, M. E., & Kirchhoff, K. (1988). Blending qualitative and quantitative approaches to instrument development and data collection. *Journal of Professional Nursing, 4,* 30–37.

May, K. A., (1989). Dialogue: On triangulation. In J. M. Morse (Ed.), *Qualitative nursing research: A contemporary dialogue* (pp. 205–206). Rockville, MD: Aspen.

Mitchell, E. S. (1986). Multiple triangulation: A methodology for nursing science. *Advances in Nursing Science, 8*(3), 18–26.

Morse, J. M. (1987). Qualitative and quantitative research: Strategies for sampling. In P. Chinn (Ed.), *Nursing Research: Methodological Issues* (pp. 181–193). Rockville, MD: Aspen.

Murphy, S. A. (1989). Multiple triangulation: Applications in a program of research. *Nursing Research, 38,* 294–298.

Myers, S. T., & Haase, J. E. (1989). Guidelines for integration of quantitative and qualitative approaches. *Nursing Research, 38,* 299–301.

Phillips, J. R. (1988a). Research blenders. *Nursing Science Quarterly, 1,* 4–5.

Phillips, J. R. (1988b). Diggers of deeper holes [Response]. *Nursing Science Quarterly, 1,* 147–151.

Tripp-Reimer, T. (1985). Combining qualitative and quantitative methodologies. In M. M. Leinenger (Ed.), *Qualitative research methods in nursing* (pp. 179–194). Orlando, FL: Grune & Stratton.

Triangulation: Operational Definitions

Judith Kimchi ■ **Barbara Polivka** ■ **Joanne Sabol Stevenson**

Triangulation in research has been defined as the combination of two or more theories, data sources, methods, or investigators in the study of a single phenomenon (Denzin, 1970). Although this definition is seemingly straightforward, closer scrutiny reveals that the word "combination" can be interpreted in many ways. Idiosyncratic interpretations could lead to difficulties for researchers attempting to triangulate and for research consumers questioning whether or not triangulation took place. The lack of specificity and step-by-step procedures for implementing triangulation merits attention. The purpose of this paper is to present operational definitions for the types of triangulation described by Denzin (1989) in an effort to make triangulation clearer and thus more appealing to larger numbers of nurse investigators.

Based on Denzin's (1989) theoretical definitions, a set of operational definitions for the types of triangulation was drafted. Definitions were intended to be clear, specific, and to provide indicators that research consumers could use to judge whether triangulation had occurred. The operational definitions were refined during a review of all data-based articles ($n = 319$) in six nursing research journals published during 1986 and 1987. The six journals were: *Advances in Nursing Science, Image, International Journal of Nursing Studies, Nursing Research, Research in Nursing and Health,* and *Western Journal of Nursing Research.* The operational definitions are presented below together with an example of each type.

Judith Kimchi, RN, MS, is a clinical nurse researcher at Columbus Children's Hospital and a doctoral candidate in nursing at The Ohio State University, Columbus, OH.

Barbara Polivka, PhD, RN, is adjunct assistant professor, The Ohio State University, Department of Family & Community, Columbus, OH.

Joanne Sabol Stevenson, PhD, RN, FAAN, is a professor, Department of Life Span Process, The Ohio State University, Columbus, OH.

From *Nursing Research,* November/December 1991, *40,* 364–366.

Theory Triangulation

Denzin (1989) defined theory triangulation as an assessment of the utility and power of competing theories or hypotheses. This definition involves testing through research, the competing theories, rival hypotheses, or alternative explanations of the same phenomenon. Campbell's (1989) study of women's responses to battering provides an example of theory triangulation. The *grief model* and the *learned helplessness model* were competitively tested on the same sample of women. Both models had previously been used to explain women's responses to battering. The objective was to pit them against each other in a single study to determine which provided the better explanatory model of the battering phenomenon. Data collection approaches were used to measure concepts (variables) specific to each model. The published report stated the *a priori* objective of testing the two competing theories—a necessary component of the operationalization of theory triangulation.

Data Triangulation

The use of multiple data sources with similar foci to obtain diverse views about a topic for the purpose of validation is considered data triangulation. Denzin (1989) listed three types of data triangulation: time, space, and person. Time triangulation represents data collection on the same phenomenon at different points in time (e.g., days, weeks, months). Time must be relevant to the study. Longitudinal studies are not time triangulation. The objective of a longitudinal study is to document changes over time; whereas, the purpose of time triangulation is to validate the congruence of the same phenomenon across points in time.

Space triangulation is the collection of data on the same phenomenon at different sites. Space must be the central variable. Studies in which data are collected at multiple sites but are not cross-validated, are not considered space triangulation. In space triangulation, data are collected in two or more settings and analyzed to test multisite consistency and rule out cross-site variation.

The following example illustrates use of both time and space triangulation. Browner (1987) investigated sources of work stress for psychiatric technicians who cared for mentally retarded long-term care residents. Participant observation was used to gather information on four residential treatment units (space triangulation) and on three shifts (time triangulation). If the investigator's purpose for using the three shifts and the four units had been to compare and contrast them as different environments, it would not have been triangulation. In triangulation, discovery of commonalities across time and space is the goal. In Browner's study, space and time triangulation were used to reflect essential components of work stress related to the care of these residents on any shift or unit.

Person triangulation is the collection of data from at least two of the three levels of persons: individuals, groups (dyads, families, or groups), or collectives (communities, organizations, or societies). The investigator could collect data from both individuals and groups; both dyads and groups; any other pair, or each of the three types. Data collected from one source is used to validate data from the other source(s). For example, Hutchinson (1987) studied the recovery process of chemically dependent nurses at two levels. Data were collected from weekly meetings of the recovering groups of nurses over one year (group level) and in-depth interviews of selected nurses (individual level). The phenomenon of interest was the recovery process; each data level was used to validate findings from the other data level. On the other hand, Tomlinson's (1987) study of marital satisfaction during transition to parenthood did not include person triangulation. In the Tomlinson study, each spouse completed questionnaires as an individual. No dyadic data were collected; hence there was no cross-validation of couple-level data with individual-level data.

Methods Triangulation

Methods triangulation is the use of two or more research methods in one study and may occur at the level of design or data collection. Denzin (1989) described two types of methods triangulation: within methods and between methods. Within-methods triangulation is defined as the combination of two or more similar data collection approaches in the same study to measure the same variable. The use of two or more quantitative measures of the same phenomenon in one study is one example. The inclusion of two or more qualitative approaches such as observation and an open-ended interview to assess the same phenomenon is also considered within-methods triangulation. The observational data and the interview data are coded and analyzed separately, then compared as a way to validate the findings. A project classified as within-methods triangulation consisted of a sample of infants who were studied for behavioral pain responses to heel sticks (Franck, 1986). The two quantitative data collection techniques used were (a) time and velocity of first leg movement and all leg movements after the stick, and (b) time to first cry and total number of cries. Both measurements were done to quantitatively assess infants' responses to painful stimuli and to compare each response with the other.

Between-methods triangulation is the use of a qualitative measurement approach and a qualitative data collection approach in one study to measure the same unit (Denzin, 1989). Dixon's (1986) study of help-seeking behaviors of black adolescents provides an example of between-methods triangulation. Quantitative data were obtained using The Family Environment Scales (FES) which measures relationships, personal development, and system maintenance/change. Interview data (qualitative data) were collected to explore the same concepts and to augment information obtained through the FES.

Investigator Triangulation

Investigator triangulation is considered present when two or more "research trained" investigators with divergent backgrounds explore the same phenomenon. Investigator triangulation is considered to have occurred when (a) each investigator has a prominent role in the study, (b) the expertise of each investigator is different, and (c) the expertise (disciplinary bias) of each investigator is evident in the study. This definition elaborates and extends Denzin's (1989) definition that investigator triangulation occurs when two or more skilled researchers examine the data. The salient concern for investigator triangulation is that different disciplines' biases are compared or neutralized throughout the study. Generally, it is not possible to discern from published research if co-authors have met the requirements of this definition. Investigator triangulation is difficult to validate unless authors explicitly claim it and describe how they achieved it. In the future, authors who engage in investigator triangulation could best serve their readership by indicating how a multidisciplinary mix resulted in investigator triangulation.

Investigator triangulation was judged to be present in a study in which the relationships between subjective stress, job satisfaction, and job performance of hospital nurses (Packard & Motowidlo, 1987) were examined. Packard was listed as an Associate Professor of Nursing and Motowidlo as being employed by the Personnel Decision Institute in Minneapolis. Motowidlo had previously published widely in the area of job satisfaction and occupational stress and was considered the expert in the general area of human resources. Packard's expertise was in nurse staffing. The influence of both investigators, who were from diverse backgrounds, was evident in the study. This example suffers somewhat from lack of evidence that the disciplinary biases of the two investigators, fields were neutralized through the collaboration effort.

Multiple Triangulation

Multiple triangulation occurs when more than one type of triangulation is used in the analysis of the same event (Denzin, 1989). The advantages of each of the individual types of triangulation are combined to further validate the findings and gather a more comprehensive and satisfactory sense of the phenomenon. Multiple triangulation is defined as the combination of any two or more types of triangulation in one study. The use of within-methods triangulation and investigator triangulation in one study, or the use of within-methods and between-methods triangulation in one study are two examples of multiple triangulation. Wallston et al. (1987) combined investigator and within-methods triangulation. The team represented a multidisciplinary mix of investigators and the study goals reflected the distinct values of the different disciplines. Within-methods triangulation was evidenced by the use of three measures of distress, each used to validate the others. One measure was physiological and two were paper and pencil instruments.

Analysis Triangulation

Analysis triangulation, a more recently developed type, is the use of two or more approaches to the analysis of the same set of data for the purpose of validation (Kimchi, Polivka, & Stevenson, 1990). Comparing results of data analyzed using different "families" of statistical tests or differing qualitative analyses techniques to assess similarity of findings enables researchers to note similar patterns and thus verify findings. The use of divergent methods of data analysis for the purposes of cross-validation offers yet another potential means of triangulation.

The major goal of triangulation is to circumvent the personal biases of investigators and overcome the deficiencies intrinsic to a single-investigator, single-theory, or single-method study, thus increasing the validity of the findings (Denzin, 1989). The purpose of this paper was to develop further the definitions of the types of triangulation put forth by Denzin (1989) in the hope that clearer, more specific explanations would stimulate nurse investigators to use triangulation more often. Once a mass of triangulated studies is published, critical reviews can then be used to evaluate the overall merit of the triangulation approach to improve the validity of nursing studies.

References

Browner, C. H. (1987). Job stress and health: The role of social support at work. *Research in Nursing and Health, 10,* 93–100.

Campbell, J. C. (1989). A test of two explanatory models of women's responses to battering. *Nursing Research,* 38, 18–24.

Denzin, N. K. (1970). *The research act: A theoretical introduction to sociological methods.* Chicago: Aldine Publishing Co.

Denzin, N. K. (1989). *The research act* (3rd ed.). New York: McGraw Hill.

Dixon, M. A. (1986). Families of adolescent clients and non-clients: Their environments and help-seeking behaviors. *Advances in Nursing Science, 8*(2), 75–88.

Franck, L. S. (1986). A new method to quantitatively describe pain behavior in infants. *Nursing Research, 35,* 28–31.

Hutchinson, S. A. (1987). Toward self-integration: The recovery process of chemically dependent nurses. *Nursing Research, 39,* 339–343.

Kimchi, J., Polivka, B., & Stevenson, J. S. (1990). Re: Multiple triangulation: Applications in a program of research [Letter to the editor]. *Nursing Research,* 217.

Packard, J. S., & Motowidlo, S. J. (1987). Subjective stress, job satisfaction, and job performance of hospital nurses. *Research in Nursing and Health, 10,* 253–261.

Tomlinson, P. A. (1987). Spousal differences in marital satisfaction during transition to parenthood. *Nursing Research, 36,* 239–243.

Wallston, B. A., Smith, R. A., Wallston, K. A., King, J. E., Rye, P. D., & Heim, C. R. (1987). Choice and predictability in the preparation for barium enemas: A person-by-situation approach. *Research in Nursing and Health, 10,* 13–22.

Multiple Triangulation: Applications in a Program of Nursing Research

Shirley A. Murphy

This article describes the research processes and outcomes of an eight-year disaster project using multiple triangulation. According to Campbell and Fiske (1959) and Denzin (1970), validity of research methods and theory construction is best established by the use of multiple triangulation–the use of multiple methods within a single research study. Four types of triangulation were outlined by Denzin.

Data triangulation involves collecting data from multiple sources for analyses within the same study. Multiple data sources provide the opportunity to test how an event is experienced by different groups at different points in time. Each data source is selected to meet a particular research goal. In this study example, specifically, how a stressful life event, a natural disaster, was experienced by diverse groups of subjects and how the event influenced their health and adjustment at different times in recovery was investigated.

Investigator triangulation includes multiple observers, interviewers, or analysts who pose specific research questions or bring specific methodological expertise to a project. Reliability in data collection, analysis, and interpretation of results is greater when numerous researchers are involved. For example, reliability is increased when multiple raters score an observation similarly. Investigator triangulation can also be a cost-effective means of doing research. That is, research questions can be asked that were not initially posed, such as differences by gender or age groups on outcome variables.

Theoretical triangulation considers rival hypotheses, tests existing theories, and proposes new theories. Testing rival hypotheses within the same data set increases knowledge of a specific phenomenon by lending support for a current theory or by providing evidence contrary to the theory and perhaps suggesting alternative hypotheses to be tested. For example, in the development and testing of a causal model, several alternative models can be tested which may support working hypotheses. If hypotheses are not supported, reconceptualization of a problem may be necessary or alternative measurement strategies may be recommended.

Methodological triangulation, the most complex type of triangulation, involves multiple procedures for data collection and analysis in a single study. In this study example, data were collected using multiple paper and pencil tests for quantitative analysis and interviews were conducted with stratified subsets of study group participants for qualitative analyses. The use of several types of statistical analyses on the same data set serves an important purpose. That is, if results of several analyses prove to be identical or similar, more confidence can be placed in the findings. Therefore, when studying a unique phenomenon or when samples are limited, it is important to show consistency across procedures.

The Longitudinal Disaster Study

The event that precipitated the research was the May 1980 volcanic eruption of Mt. St. Helens in southwestern Washington in the United States. Massive public and private property destruction occurred. Sixty persons died or were presumed dead, and several hundred persons lost their homes, farms, and employment associated with lumber and tourist industries. Although there were some warnings, the major eruption occurred suddenly and lasted only a few minutes.

As the consequences of the event unfolded, it seemed logical to assume that grief associated with the loss of loved ones would be more intense and prolonged than the loss of one's home because: (a) the deaths were unpredicted and sudden, (b) some families experienced the deaths of more than one family member, and (c) both the deceased and bereaved were young. At the same time, these factors do not negate stresses associated with property loss: (a) having no place to live, (b) losing irreplaceable belongings, and (c) financial loss. However, a review of the literature showed that few of these assumptions had been tested empirically and that evidence of post-

Shirley A. Murphy, PhD, RN, is an associate professor at the Psychosocial Nursing Department, University of Washington, Seattle, WA.

From *Nursing Research,* September/October 1989, *38,* 294–297.

disaster psychological distress was conflicting, mainly because past studies had focused on the early recovery period (1–6 weeks) (Melick, 1985). When the project was begun in 1980, no longitudinal studies had been published, nor had conditions of loss, i.e., bereavement and property, been examined separately. Moreover, control groups were rarely included.

The search for theoretical models on which to base the research was frustrating since neither disaster nor bereavement theories produced an adequate fit. Therefore, a stressful life events model was selected. Three dimensions of stressful life events that promote understanding of health and recovery outcomes are (a) characteristics of the event and the meaning to the individual, (b) personal attributes of the individual, and (c) mediating processes (Hyman & Woog, 1982; Lazarus & Folkman, 1984).

The major goals of the study were to assess the relationships between disaster-related stress and mental and physical health outcomes, to examine the extent to which self-efficacy and social support would mediate the stress-health relationship, and to explore the effects of mass media coverage on recovery, using the multiple triangulation methods that were outlined by Denzin.

Data Triangulation

Multiple Data Sources

A total of 219 persons were contacted by a letter from the investigator for participation in 1981. Of these, 155 (71%) participated in 1981. In 1983, 134 persons were contacted for follow-up and 101 (75%) participated, for an overall attrition rate of 28%. All losses were documented officially, and bereavement and property losses were mutually exclusive among study participants.

Bereaved Groups Both a close family member and a close friend of each adult deceased disaster victim were recruited for the bereaved groups because of the potentially small sample of those who died (57 were adults). Thus, using a pair of subjects for each deceased victim potentially increased the sample size. A study participation criterion was that all bereaved subjects score 7 or higher on a 1 to 9 scale regarding centrality of relationship (1 = not close, 9 = very close). Names of bereaved family members were obtained from death certificates and a list of persons who gave court testimony required for processing provisional death certificates of persons presumed dead. Names of friends for both bereaved groups were obtained primarily from relatives who also confirmed closeness (centrality of the relationship) between these friends and the deceased. Study participants resided in ten cities in the United States and two cities in Canada.

Property Loss Groups Persons for the permanent property loss group were randomly selected from local telephone listings in 1981. The nature and extent of property loss was verified by tax assessment records. Criteria for inclusion in the study were total destruction of one's permanent residence or damage that necessitated moving at least temporarily. Persons for the recreation (second home) property loss group were randomly selected from a vacation homeowner's list. Their homes were completely destroyed, but all were unoccupied on the morning of the disaster.

No Disaster Loss Group Criteria for comparison group selection were no disaster loss and overall group similarity to the loss groups on personal characteristics of age, gender, occupation, and geographic location. To obtain some nondisaster loss participants who lived in the same eastern U.S. cities as some of the bereaved participants, bereaved participants suggested persons in their neighborhoods who had similar personal characteristics. These persons were then contacted by the investigator for study participation. Similarly, study participants residing in the Northwest also were invited to name their own controls, but these efforts were less successful. The investigator contacted local organizations likely to employ persons similar to the loss victims. Demographic characteristics of the multiple source sample in 1983 were similar to those in 1981. About 70% of the participants were women. The mean age of the sample was 34.5 years, and they could be characterized as white and above-average in educational attainment. The majority of participants had formal post-high school education and 15% held graduate degrees.

Multiple Measurement Techniques

Written informed consent was obtained prior to participation. The study instruments were arranged in three random orders and mailed one and three years postdisaster. Follow-up interviews were conducted with 44 persons from each of the five study groups.

Data were collected on 36 event, mediating, person attributes, and health and recovery variables shown in Table 1. Between-group comparisons were made on these variables using data collected in 1981 and 1983. Both cross-sectional and longitudinal analyses were conducted. The criteria for selection of measurement tools were based on constructs to be measured, availability of standardized instruments, and ease in administration to a high risk sample.

TABLE 1 Variables for Between-Group Comparisons in 1981 and 1983

	Time 1 (1981)	Time 2 (1983)
Event Variables		
Nature of loss	x	x
Rating of disaster loss compared with other losses	x	x
[a]Satisfaction with rescue operations	x	x
[a]Closeness of the deceased person at the time of death	x	–
[a]Relationship problems with deceased at the time of death	x	–
[a]Who can be blamed for the deaths	x	x
Effects of mass media coverage on recovery		
Geographic proximity to Mt. St. Helens	x	–
Concurrent stressful life events (43 items)		
Number of events in the past year	x	x
Impact of the event	x	x
Daily hassles (117 items)		
Persistence of hassles	x	x
Irritability experienced by hassles	x	x
Mediating Variables		
Number of confidants and contact per week	x	x
Number of close friends and contact per week	x	x
Number of family members and contact per week	x	x
Number of social groups and contact per week	x	x
Professional help sought	x	x
Perceived social support (15 items)	x	x
Person Attribute Variables		
Perceived self-efficacy (22 items)	x	x
Gender	x	x
Age	x	x
Education	x	x
Occupation	x	x
[a]Beliefs of preventability of death	x	–
Health/Recovery Variables		
Mental distress (90 items)	x	x
Physical symptoms (50 items)	x	x
Current health, change in health status and contact with health care systems (6 items)	x	–
Number and nature of illnesses since 1980	–	x
Perceived recovery (3 items)	x	x
Rating of current life situation	x	x
Comparison of pre and postdisaster change in income	x	x
Adequacy of income	x	x
Satisfaction with financial settlement	x	x

NOTE x = Data collected on variable during this time period.
[a] Data collected from bereaved participants only.

Investigator Triangulation

Because of considerable overlap between theoretical and methodological triangulations, the involvement of other investigators will be described generally, then one project will be described specifically.

Analysis of data collected at Time 1—one year postdisaster—showed that the bereaved group perceived their health, quality of life, and recovery to be poorer than did other study groups. Thus, the bereavement transition following catastrophic loss was of major interest. Secondary analyses of these data were undertaken by three additional investigators. Cowan examined predictors of bereavement outcome one year postdisaster (Cowan & Murphy, 1985). Kiger conducted a longitudinal reliability study of the Symptom Checklist 90-R (SCL-90-R) using a contrasted groups approach to evaluate internal consistency and test stability of the instrument (Kiger & Murphy, 1987). Chenell conducted a partial test of Bugen's (1977) theory of grief, based on central relationships between deceased and bereaved and beliefs of death preventability (Chenell & Murphy, 1985).

Chenell was unable to find any empirical tests of Bugen's (1977) theory in the literature. Bugen asserts that if the deceased/bereaved relationship is close, i.e., important, and if the bereaved believe that the death was preventable, then grief would be expected to be both *intense and prolonged*. If the relationship was not close and beliefs were that the deaths were unpreventable, grief would be *mild and brief*. Chenell compared grief symptom scores of those who held preventable beliefs with those who held unpreventable beliefs and also compared grief scores between the central relationship factor and the preventability factor. She found that grief responses were *intense and prolonged* for all circumstances tested. The peripheral relationship factor could not be tested because all bereaved reported a central relationship with the deceased (Chenell & Murphy, in review).

Theoretical Triangulation

Past disaster studies have tested communication theory (i.e., the role of rumors, information-processing, and decision-making), role dilemmas of emergency workers, and community resource models, but no individual adaptation models of recovery have been published. This section describes the formulation and testing of a magnitude of loss hypothesis and the test of two rival hypotheses to mediate disaster effects on health.

Magnitude of Loss Theory

A major hypothesis tested was that effects of loss are proportional to their magnitude. The magnitudes of loss expected to be greatest (ranked 1) to least (ranked 5) were: (1) bereavement resulting from deaths of persons presumed to be dead, i.e., the bodies were not found within five days following the disaster, (2) bereavement resulting from deaths of persons confirmed dead, (3) loss or severe destruction of one's permanent home, (4) loss of one's recreational (second) home, (5) no disaster-related loss. It was hypothesized that the greater the magnitude of loss, the greater the stress experienced and therefore the greater the negative effects on health. This hypothesis was tested with one-year postdisaster data and three-year postdisaster data. The hypothesis was supported in general, that is, statistically significant differences emerged from all tests on two stress and three health outcome variables between bereavement, property loss, and the nonloss disaster comparison group. However, not all differences were significant between presumed and confirmed death bereavement. Three major factors probably account for the latter finding. First, data were not collected until nearly one-year post disaster. Some additional bodies were found during the summer of 1980. Second, the state legislature passed a statute that allowed families of those presumed dead to claim financial benefits soon after the disaster rather than requiring them to wait the previously stipulated seven years. Again, this settlement, while positive for the families, undoubtedly affected what would have been a major difference between the two bereavement groups. Finally, group sizes were small, which may have accounted for a lack of statistical significance in some cases. In contrast, interview data revealed distinct differences between presumed and confirmed death bereavement.

Given the similarity between the two bereaved groups, they were combined for longitudinal analyses conducted after 1983. The results showed statistically significant differences over time by magnitude of loss on stress, health outcome, and recovery variables (See Murphy, 1986b.) Even though the bereaved group reported less stress and distress in 1983 than in 1981, their scores were significantly higher than the property loss and no disaster loss groups.

Rival Hypotheses: Self-Efficacy and Social Support

Although social support has been found to mediate (buffer) the effects of stress on health, studies confirming the buffering hypotheses have not tested rival hypothesis. Self-efficacy can be considered a rival hypothesis to social support because it is based on one's belief system—that a given behavior will lead to a desired outcome and that one is convinced he/she can initiate and execute the behavior required to produce the desired outcome (Bandura, 1977). Therefore, a major goal of the study was to test the effects of both constructs on health outcomes. In both the 1981 and 1983 data, self-efficacy had a statistically significant effect on mental distress whereas social support did not.

Methodological Triangulation

Multiple Statistical Techniques

The first critical issue in this study was to demonstrate the *independence* of the linked pairs of bereaved participants. This notion is in contrast to the usual expectation that scores from pairs of subjects will be correlated. While the bereavement for a pair of subjects was clearly linked to the same victim, the two bereaved subjects were assumed to be affected differently due to their relationships with the deceased (i.e., a wife-husband relationship differs from a mother-son relationship). Moreover, the relationship between two members of any given pair was not constant across pairs. Two statistical tests checked the assumption of independence of observation. First, a Pearson correlation tested the linear relationship between corresponding scores of each pair of subjects. Second, a random effects, one-way ANOVA was used. (The ANOVA had 28 levels of the linked-pairs variable with $n = 2$ subjects per level.) Results for the 10 major study variables showed that none of the Pearson r values and none of the F values were significant. Data from both members of pairs were then treated as independent observations in subsequent analyses (Murphy & Stewart, 1985–86).

The magnitude of loss hypothesis was also confirmed by the use of several statistical procedures. In 1981 the five study groups were compared on two stress and three health outcomes measures by one-way ANOVA and planned posthoc comparisons. The tests were followed by discriminant function analysis. In 1983, data collected from the same participants in 1981 were subjected to 3 X 2 ANOVA. The results of all three statistical procedures supported the magnitude of loss hypothesis. Bereavement was associated with greater mental distress and lower rates of perceived recovery than the property loss group; the property loss group had higher scores on mental distress than the no disaster loss comparison group. However, the two types of bereavement were not distinguishable in either one-way analysis of variance or discriminant function analysis.

Finally, a causal model was developed and tested using path analysis. The findings were consistent with other statistical tests. In 1981, magnitude of loss, satisfaction with financial settlement, self-efficacy, and mass media coverage accounted for 19% of the variance associated with negative rating of change regarding the disaster. Negative rating of change explained 29% of the variance in mental distress. In 1983, 36% of the variance at Time 2 was accounted for by mental distress reported at Time 1 (Murphy, 1989).

Interview Techniques

Interviews conducted with the same 44 persons one and three years postdisaster added many useful insights to the findings. The rationale for the interviews was to obtain in-depth information regarding perceived disaster stress, coping strategies used, and perceived recovery. A structured interview guide was used by one interviewer in 1981 and two interviewers in 1983. Following the 1983 interviews, responses obtained by both interviewers were compared for consistency.

Both unique and common bereavement stressors were reported (Murphy, 1986a). One unique stressor was the public nature of the disaster deaths. Bereaved persons did not feel prepared for the extensive publicity associated with the disaster which they perceived as invasion of privacy. Some initial, inaccurate media reports aroused anger and hostility. Other unique stressors were presumptive death—some persons' remains were found—and a "forced maturity" of young adults who lost both parents. A stressor common to the bereavement experience was the overwhelming sense of loss: "It was a senseless death, a continuation of grief," "I miss them—that's the bottom line."

Several factors were perceived as mediators of both unique and common stressors experienced by the disaster victims. For example, support provided by family members and friends—a factor not significant in the statistical analyses—was consistently believed to mediate stress. The passage of time, and the gradual acceptance of the inability to change the outcome were also reported to promote recovery. The interview data suggested that participants were "active copers." They searched libraries and bookstores for reading materials on grief and loss; more sought counseling after the first anniversary date than before; some joined together in lawsuits; several moved or rebuilt their homes; and some established scholarships or projects in memory of the deceased.

Perceived recovery was gradual. In 1983, bereaved persons reported some positive changes. For example, their dreams now seemed to be about earlier, happy times whereas in 1981, they reported distressing dreams and nightmares. By 1983, some were finally able to give away personal belongings of the deceased. However, the major theme was that the term *recovery* did not accurately convey their progress. Rather, most said they were "adapting" and could give examples of progress and adjustment, but that their lives were "forever changed." Persons in the property loss group reported multiple economic and legal problems and therefore delays in rebuilding their homes.

Thus, these representative examples provide evidence of the usefulness of Denzin's recommendation regarding multiple triangulation and are adaptable for the study of many traumatic life events.

References

Bandura A. (1977). Self-efficacy: Toward a unifying theory of behavioral change. *Psychological Review, 84,* 191–215.

Bugen, L. (1977). Human grief: A model for prediction and intervention. *American Journal of Orthopsychiatry, 47,* 166–174.

Campbell, D. T., & Fiske, D. W. (1959). Convergent and discriminant validation by the multitrait-multimethod matrix. *Psychological Bulletin, 56,* 81–105.

Chenell, S. L., & Murphy, S. A. (1985). *Belief of preventability of death among disaster bereaved.* Manuscript submitted for publication.

Cowan, M. E., & Murphy, S. A. (1985). Identification of postdisaster high risk bereavement predictors. *Nursing Research, 34,* 71–75.

Denzin, N. (1970). Strategies of multiple triangulation. In Denzin, N. (Ed.), *The research act* (pp. 229–313). New York: McGraw-Hill Book Co.

Hyman, R., & Woog, P. (1982). Stressful life events and illness onset: A review of critical variables. *Research in Nursing and Health, 5,* 155–163.

Kiger, J., & Murphy, S. A. (1987). Reliability assessment of the SCL-90-R using a longitudinal bereaved disaster population. *Western Journal of Nursing Research, 9,* 572–588.

Lazarus, R., & Folkman, S. (1984). *Stress, appraisal and coping* (pp. 22–224). New York: Springer Publishing Co.

Melick, M. E. (1985). The health of postdisaster populations: A review of the literature. In J. Laube & S. A. Murphy (Eds.), *Perspectives on disaster recovery* (pp. 179–209). Norwalk: Appleton-Century-Crofts.

Murphy, S. A. (1986b). Health and recovery status of natural disaster victims one and three years later. *Research in Nursing and Health, 9,* 331–340.

Murphy, S. A. (1989). An explanatory model of recovery from disaster loss. *Research in Nursing and Health, 12,* 67–76.

Murphy, S. A., & Stewart, B. J. (1985–86). Linked pairs of subjects: A method for increasing the sample size in a study of bereavement. *Omega, 16,* 141–153.

Methodological Triangulation in a Study of Nurse Retention

Lynne M. Connelly ■ Marge Bott ■ Nancy Hoffart ■ Roma Lee Taunton

Methodological triangulation, the application of diverse methods to generate and collect data about one phenomenon (Kimchi, Polivka, & Stevenson, 1991), is being used with increasing frequency by nurse researchers (e.g., Breitmayer, Ayres, & Knafl, 1993; Dreher & Hayes, 1993). This article reports an example of quantitative-qualitative triangulation, illustrating the procedures used and the benefits achieved.

Perspectives and Issues

Rossman and Wilson (1985) characterized three researcher stances relative to triangulation: purist, situationalist, and pragmatist. Purists focus on the paradigm level and hold that qualitative and quantitative approaches are derived from different, mutually exclusive epistemological and ontological assumptions about the nature of research and society. They assert that triangulation violates the philosophy, goals, and purposes of methods from different paradigms. Purists view triangulation as defensive research because it is performed to "see what happens," avoid conflicts, satisfy potential critics, and compensate for anticipated shortcomings (Leininger, 1992).

Situationalists focus on research methods and maintain that both approaches have value, but that each method is most appropriate for specific situations. Thus, situationalists will use both methods, but usually in a parallel manner or in different phases of a research project, with little integration of the procedures or findings. The situation dictates what method will be used and when (Rossman & Wilson, 1985).

Lynne M. Connelly, PhD, RN, is a colonel, Army Nurse Corps, and is chief, Department of Nursing Science, Army Medical Department Center & School, San Antonio, TX.

Marge Bott, RN, MA, is a senior research associate, School of Nursing, University of Kansas, Kansas City, KS.

Nancy Hoffart, PhD, RN, is an associate professor, School of Nursing, University of Kansas, Kansas City, KS.

Roma Lee Taunton, PhD, RN, FAAN, is a professor, School of Nursing, University of Kansas, Kansas City, KS.

From *Nursing Research,* September/October 1997, *46,* 299–302.

Finally, pragmatists argue for the integration of methods in a single study. They advocate use of all available techniques to answer questions of substantive importance and view triangulation not as an end in itself but as a vehicle that can lead to richer and more insightful analysis of complex phenomena (Rossman & Wilson, 1985).

An increase in the number of reports of triangulated studies suggests the purist stance is lessening and more scholars see triangulation as pragmatic. Breitmayer et al. (1993) used triangulation to confirm information and achieve a more complete understanding of phenomena under study. Other cited benefits include increased credibility and validity of study results owing to convergence and corroboration of data (Duffy, 1987; Rossman & Wilson, 1985). Many (e.g., Duffy, 1987; Morse, 1991) have asserted that triangulation enriches and elaborates a database in ways that show new dimensions and details about the phenomenon of interest. Triangulation also has been described as a strategy that can make sense of social phenomena, which in turn helps the researcher initiate new interpretations, suggest areas for further exploration, or recast the entire research question (Mathison, 1988).

As with any methodological approach, triangulation presents unique challenges and problems. First, using both quantitative and qualitative methods can be resource intensive, requiring substantial time, money, and investigator knowledge and skill (Duffy, 1987). Second, each method often is reduced to its elementary form and the bias-checking procedures are more likely to be applied inadequately (Steckler, McLeroy, Goodman, Bird, & McCormick, 1992). Third, several data analysis issues arise, including questions about how to combine numeric and textual data, how to interpret inconsistent and contradictory findings, what to do with overlapping concepts that are not clearly differentiated, whether or how to weight data sources, and whether to weight each method as equally sensitive (Mathison, 1988). A fourth problem relates to maintaining consistency of the unit of analysis across study components (Duffy, 1987). Finally, replication is difficult (Jick, 1979).

Application

This study was conducted as part of a larger project (Taunton, Boyle, Woods, Hansen, & Bott, 1997) designed to confirm and ensure completeness of an investigator-developed model of nurse retention. The model indicates that retention of staff registered nurses in an organization is related to four sets of predictor variables: manager characteristics (power, influence, and leadership style); organizational characteristics (distributive justice, promotional opportunity, and control over nursing practice); work characteristics (autonomy, instrumental communication, group cohesion, and routinization); and nurse characteristics (education and marital status). Opportunity elsewhere, also an exogenous variable, reflects staff nurses' perceptions of their marketability in the hospitals' external environment. These predictor variables influence retention indirectly through job stress, job satisfaction, commitment, and intent to stay. The variables in the model have been well established in the literature on nurse retention and turnover. However, previously studied models of turnover have explained on average less than 20% of the variance (Hinshaw & Atwood, 1982; Michaels & Spector, 1982: Price & Mueller, 1981).

In the final year of the project, a qualitative study was designed to examine whether a different research approach might produce additional variables that should be included in the model. Whether the qualitative findings would confirm the variables already in the model also was an important issue. A descriptive study was conducted to explore reasons for staying among nurses who had perceived themselves as "likely to leave" their hospital (Connelly, Hoffart, & Taunton, 1997). Potential subjects had scored in the lower third of the Intent to Stay scale in the first year of the project yet had remained working at the same hospital. We reasoned that these nurses would be most likely to offer significant information about retention.

At least two nurses from the four major specialty areas in each hospital were asked to participate. A total of 36 nurses were contacted, and 21 agreed to participate. Three major categories emerged from the qualitative analysis. These were (a) reasons for staying, (b) possible reasons for leaving, and (c) positive/negative aspects of employment. In the second category, informants shared possible reasons for leaving the hospital, such as caring for a child or parent. The last category included aspects of employment that informants did not see as reasons for staying or leaving but that they shared in the interviews about working at their facility. Included were a wide range of topics such as inadequate parking and implementing shared governance.

After the qualitative study was completed, the findings were compared with the model of nurse retention. Each of the three major qualitative categories contained codes that were compared with variables in the empirical model. The codes from each of the categories, along with representative quotes, were presented at a peer-debriefing session. The peer-debriefing group included three data collectors from the qualitative study and three nurses knowledgeable about nursing administration and the model. The qualitative codes and the quantitative variables in the model were compared at a general level. Many of the qualitative codes and the model variables were similar. However, in some cases the qualitative codes were conceptually broader than model variables. In other cases, there was no obvious match between codes and variables. A more systematic approach was needed to compare and integrate the findings from the two components of the study. Two researchers, the team leader of the qualitative study and a researcher who was familiar with the empirical model, developed an approach for triangulation that proved useful.

Matched Qualitative Codes and Quantitative Variables

To begin, each quantitative variable was written on a separate card with the definition and the specific items from the data collection instruments used to operationalize the variable. Each qualitative code was written on a card with three or more representative quotations from the interviews, with as much context as needed to clarify the meaning. The meaning of each code was compared with each variable definition. An example of the cards used for comparison is presented in Table 1. Through this analysis we identified qualitative codes with analogous quantitative variables as well as qualitative codes that were broader conceptually than the quantitative variables. (See Table 2 for examples.) In addition, the analysis showed quantitative variables with no corresponding qualitative codes and qualitative codes with no corresponding quantitative variables.

Search for Qualitative Data to Support Quantitative Variables

To further explore the broadly matched codes and variables as well as the unmatched codes and variables, the raw interview data were reviewed again. A more detailed analysis was conducted with the definition and instrument items operationalizing each variable in mind, with care not to read too much into informants' state-

TABLE 1 Example of Cards Used for Comparison of Qualitative Codes and Model Variables

Qualitative Code Cohesive Coworkers	Model Variable: Group Cohesion
Quotes that represented a feeling of closeness or sense of family among coworkers. "I guess [my reason for staying] would be the people I work with." "It's a very friendly bunch, helpful, we all help each other." "Oh, it's a great [work group]. I think there is a strong cohesiveness."	Definition: Degree to which members of the organization have close relationships with others in the work group Six items that address: Productivity Efficiency Morale Feelings of belonging Personal feelings about the group Feelings about working together

ments. When a quotation that provided support for a model variable was found, it was annotated and reviewed by members of the research team. This review helped ensure that qualitative data were not distorted or "made to fit" with the model. Thus, we were able to identify additional qualitative support for the following model variables: personal job stress, situational job stress, routinization, instrumental communication, distributive justice, and specific manager characteristics. (See Table 3 for example.)

However, two model variables still were not supported by the qualitative data: opportunity elsewhere and control over nursing practice. Although these two variables were implied in certain interview statements made by nurses, they were not stated clearly. Perhaps more probing questions could have elicited support for the variables, but the theoretical model was not used as a basis for interview questions to ensure data collectors did not lead the informants' responses inadvertently.

Qualitative Data without Matches

Finally, qualitative codes and quotes that had not previously been matched with a model variable were compared again with the model. Four qualitative codes still had no comparable model variables: location close to home, benefits, ability to give quality care, and ability to transfer among units within the hospital. Satisfaction with the quality of care had been in earlier versions of the theoretical model but was removed because it had not been a statistically significant predictor of retention. It is interesting to note that the ability to give quality care was mentioned, but not frequently, in the qualitative study. Exploration of whether there is a distinction between the quantitative variable, satisfaction with the quality of care, and the qualitative code, ability to give quality care, may be useful.

Because retention in this project was operationalized as remaining in the same job on the same unit, the ability to transfer among units within the hospital might be con-

TABLE 2 Examples of Comparison of Qualitative Codes with Model Variables

Result	Qualitative Codes	Model Variables
Qualitative codes analogous to model variables	Cohesive coworkers, loyalty and longevity, liked job	Group cohesion, commitment, enjoyment
Qualitative codes broader than model variables	Upper and middle management	Nurse manager influence, nurse manager leadership style, nurse manager power
Qualitative codes with no comparable model variables	Location close to home, benefits	None
Model variables with no comparable qualitative codes	None	Personal job stress, situational job stress

TABLE 3 Examples of Comparison of Model Variables to Raw Interview Data

Model Variable and Definition	Representative Quotations from the Raw Interview Data
Personal power: ability to control others through use of expert and referent power.	"I think once we got a manager in here who knew what she was doing, it helped a lot." "I mean, I feel like she is the boss, there's no grayness in my mind about who is in charge."

sidered as part of the variable "opportunity elsewhere." But in the quantitative project this variable was operationalized as an external variable: opportunities elsewhere in the community. For informants in the qualitative study, it was knowing that their managers were open to staff transfer that was perceived as a reason for staying where they were. Therefore, openness to internal transfer may be better developed as an organizational characteristic or an aspect of the manager's leadership style. The qualitative data suggested that the manager's openness to internal transfer deserves further examination.

Benefits of Triangulation

Triangulation helped us attain three benefits. First, the careful comparison of quantitative and qualitative data added support for the variables in the retention model. Second, the comparison also showed new dimensions about nurse retention, thereby contributing to a more complete understanding of nurse retention. The new dimensions warrant further exploration; for instance, the importance of employment at a location close to home, the need to consider pay and benefits as separate dimensions of satisfaction, and manager openness to transfer among units. Third, the researchers were able to make suggestions for revision of the quantitative instruments. For example, one item on the quantitative instruments addressed both pay and benefits. The participants in the qualitative study voiced concern about a wide range of benefits including insurance, day care, pensions, family leave, and others. These concerns were separate from comments made about pay.

After each component (qualitative and quantitative) of the study was independently completed, an approach to triangulation involving researchers knowledgeable about the respective components and methods was critical. It was helpful to focus on the "qualitative aspects" of the model variables, that is, the definition and the specific items from the instruments instead of just the name assigned to the variable. In addition, using several quotes rather than just the name assigned to the qualitative code was helpful. Staying open to what the informants were saying through the data also was essential. When raw data were reviewed for a second time, the researchers had to be careful not to read too much into the data in an unconscious attempt to locate support for the model variables.

The primary resource required to complete a triangulation analysis was researcher time and knowledge. Collection and analysis of the qualitative data involved many hours with considerable secretarial support for transcription of interview tapes. The team involved in the triangulation had experience in both quantitative and qualitative research methods, therefore additional resources were not required to acquire this expertise. Responsibility for the quantitative and the qualitative components of the investigation was assigned to a team member with expertise in the respective method. This enabled each to focus on one component, creating a sound design and attending to appropriate validity issues. It also ensured that inconsistent findings were explored in depth, rather than ignored, and that both the quantitative and qualitative approaches were weighted equally.

Application of our approach to triangulation confirmed key variables in a model of nurse retention and helped identify new variables for inclusion. In addition, areas of possible future exploration were identified. When researchers knowledgeable about the two methods being triangulated used a systematic approach, the challenges frequently associated with triangulation were overcome.

References

Breitmayer, B. J., Ayres, L., & Knafl, K. A. (1993). Triangulation in qualitative research: Evaluation of completeness and confirmation purposes. *Image: The Journal of Nursing Scholarship. 25,* 237–243.

Connelly, L. M., Hoffart, N., & Taunton, R. L. (1997). Why nurses stay: A qualitative study. *Surgical Services Management, 3*(5), 44–48.

Dremer, M. C., & Hayes, J. S. (1993). Triangulation in cross-cultural research of child development in Jamaica. *Western Journal of Nursing Research, 15,* 216–229.

Duffy, M. E. (1987). Methodological triangulation: A vehicle for merging quantitative and qualitative research methods. *Image: The Journal of Nursing Scholarship, 19,* 130–133.

Hinshaw, A. S., & Atwood. J. R. (1982). Anticipated turnover: A preventive approach. *Western Journal of Nursing Research, 4,* 54–55.

Jick, T. D. (1979). Mixing qualitative and quantitative methods: Triangulation in action. *Administration Science Quarterly, 24,* 602–611.

Kimchi, J., Polivka, B., & Stevenson, J. S. (1991). Triangulation: Operational definitions. *Nursing Research, 40,* 364–366.

Leininger, M. (1992). Current issues, problems, and trends to advance qualitative paradigmatic research methods for the future. *Qualitative Health Research, 2,* 392–415.

Mathison, S. (1988). Why triangulate? *Educational Researcher, 17*(2), 13–17.

Michaels C. E., & Spector, P. E. (1982). Causes of employee turnover: A test of the Mobley, Griffeth, Hand, & Meglino model. *Journal of Applied Psychology, 67,* 53–59.

Morse, J. M. (1991). Approaches to qualitative-quantitative methodological triangulation. *Nursing Research, 40,* 120–123.

Price, J. L., & Mueller, C. W. (1981). *Professional turnover: The case of nurses.* New York: Medical & Scientific Books.

Rossman, G. B., & Wilson, B. L. (1985). Numbers and words: Combining quantitative and qualitative methods in a single large-scale evaluation study. *Evaluation Review, 9,* 627–643.

Steckler, A., McLeroy, K. R., Goodman, R. M., Bird, S. T., & McCormick, L. (1992). Toward integrating qualitative and quantitative methods. An introduction. *Health Education Quarterly, 19,* 1–8.

Taunton, R. L., Boyle, D. K., Woods, C. Q., Hansen, H. E., & Bott, M. J. (1997). Manager leadership and retention of hospital staff nurses. *Western Journal of Nursing Research, 19*(2), 205–226.

Methodologic Mistakes in Grounded Theory

Holly Skodol Wilson ■ Sally Ambler Hutchinson

In 1992, one of the authors received a letter from the editor of a major, refereed nursing journal, lamenting the growing number of manuscripts submitted for publication that basically all reach the same conclusions about the various processes under study. The editor suggested the need for an article that would help researchers get beyond the trivial stage process, characteristically described by investigators as "getting in, getting on, doing it, finishing it, getting out, being transformed, or making meaning of the whole thing."

When we discussed this problem in view of our experience as manuscript reviewers, scientific investigators, and teachers of qualitative research, we realized that the journal editor had identified only one of the contemporary research variations subsumed under the banner of *grounded theory methodology* that is not a grounded theory. Becker (1993) stated that many studies purporting to produce grounded theory are really descriptive studies. She identified the following common pitfalls of portraying descriptive studies as grounded theory studies: not using theoretical sampling; not discovering the problematic situation; not doing concurrent data collection and analysis; using the wrong theoretical lens; and relying on computer programs to identify core variables based on frequency alone rather than integrative power.

This article goes beyond the journal editor's lament and the specific pitfalls identified by Becker to analyze additional methodologic mistakes in grounded theory research that detract from the credibility and value of authentic grounded theory approaches. We summarize the major "not a grounded theory" variations and offer illustrative examples. The examples serve as a heuristic and have been adapted and altered to protect the identities of investigators in any published or unpublished studies.

This inquiry is particularly timely given the current debate about any agreed upon "correct" rendition of grounded theory. Researchers are now obliged to specify whether the grounded theory approach they employ is the original 1967 Glaser and Strauss version, the 1990 Strauss and Corbin rendition, or the 1992 Glaser interpretation. Our intent is not to enter the current Glaser/Strauss debate nor to endorse either perspective. Instead, we address common problems that deviate considerably from the conceptual particulars of method and goal inherent in the Glaser/Strauss dispute.

Types of Methodologic Mistakes

Muddling Qualitative Methods

Grounded theory is only one of numerous accepted qualitative, naturalistic, interpretive methods. Ethnography, phenomenology, hermeneutics, ethnoscience, discourse analysis, ethnomethodology, thematic analysis, conceptual description, ethical and philosophical inquiry, and historical research all have their own philosophical underpinnings, methodological and analytic strategies, and outcomes.

As Stern (1993) pointed out, similarities across all interpretive methods and a certain amount of overlap are expected. Most of them, for example, rely primarily on interviews and observation as data collection strategies. The problem appears when the canons of a method are compromised through intentional or unintentional "muddling" (Baker, Wuest, & Stern, 1992). Muddling of methods refers to a situation in which the researcher compromises, for example, the integrity of the grounded theory approach and instead generates a typology, long verbatim biographical narratives, or an outcome associated with any number of alternative qualitative approaches. For example, in a study of head nurse management styles in a hospice service, one nurse investigator claimed to use participant observation and interviews to generate a grounded theory that described the management styles of "directing," "allowing," and "ne-

Holly Skodol Wilson, RN, PhD, FAAN, is a professor, Department of Mental Health, Community and Administrative Nursing, University of California, San Francisco, CA.

Sally Ambler Hutchinson, RN, PhD, FAAN, is a professor, University of Florida College of Nursing, Jacksonville, FL.

From *Nursing Research,* March/April 1996, *45,* 122–124.

gotiating." She noted that experienced hospice head nurses switch from one management style to another when managing various patient care situations. While this was a typology generated from qualitative data, it was not a grounded theory per se.

In another study, researchers claimed to generate a grounded theory of role response of drug-abusing mothers. The study results identified three such groups: Group 1, Group 2, and Group 3. Despite claiming to employ grounded theory methods, the investigators generated no theory but merely sorted data into three unnamed groups. Yet a third study purported to use grounded theory methodology to extract the context of past and current experiences from interviews of 245 adult survivors of sexual abuse. Findings were presented as long verbatim accounts of life histories and grouped under headings such as "Past and Current Abuse," "Childhood Traumas," and "Current Relationship Problems." While packed with rich, unanalyzed data, this product was not a grounded theory according to established criteria.

Generational Erosion

The term *generational erosion* (Stern, 1993) refers to an undermining of the original canons for grounded theory research. In 1967, Glaser, an innovative methodologist from Columbia University, and Strauss, a central figure from the School of Pragmatism at the University of Chicago, published their classic book, *The Discovery of Grounded Theory,* presenting their new method for theory generation. Over the next 20 years, they wrote books and articles that further explicated the method (Glaser, 1978; Strauss, 1987). Several nurses who studied with them or their students translated the method for students and other nurse scholars (Bowers, 1989; Chenitz & Swanson, 1986; Hutchinson, 1986; Quint, 1966; Stern, 1980; Wilson, 1993). In 1990, Strauss and Corbin (a Strauss graduate student and subsequent colleague) deviated from the original method. They suggested a new coding process using "a coding paradigm involving conditions, context, action/interactional strategies and consequences" (p. 96). Glaser's response to the Strauss–Corbin iteration was to label it "full conceptual description—a forced, preconceived product . . . which is fine, but is not grounded theory" (Glaser, 1992, p. 3). Glaser then presented his "corrected" version of generating grounded theory emphasizing "emergence."

Over the 20-year period from 1967 to 1987, nurse scientists with no firsthand contact with grounded theory's originators or their students began inventing rigid rules for judging the value of a grounded theory. Their "cooked up" translations, however, frequently break with the spirit of creativity inherent in the original grounded theory method and the philosophy of pragmatism undergirding the method. In critiquing manuscripts, these "translators" demanded that a visual diagram accompany all grounded theories and proclaimed that a sample size less than 12 is unacceptable, even when data collection methods have been triangulated. While we agree with John Dewey's view (1935), as cited by Strauss and Corbin (1990), that "If the artist does not perfect a new vision in his process of doing, he acts mechanically and repeats some old model fixed like a blueprint in his mind" (p. 6), the importation of rigid rules is counterproductive to the spirit of creativity and the generation of grounded theory. Although certain flexible methodologic guidelines, such as simultaneous data collection and analysis and purposive and theoretical sampling principles, are undisputed, credible grounded theory ultimately stands on its own as diverse, parsimonious, conceptual, and relevant to the data.

Premature Closure

This refers to the "underanalysis" of textual or narrative data. By definition, the grounded theory methodology requires that the researcher move from Level I in vivo or substantive codes (e.g., participants' own words for their experiences) through more abstract Level II categorical codes to Level III conceptual and theoretical codes (e.g., the building blocks of theory). At each level the theory becomes more refined, yielding a parsimonious integration of abstract concepts that cover behavioral variation. However, in the instance of premature closure, the researcher fails to move beyond the face value of the content in the narrative data. Consequently, the results of such a study never transcend the initial in vivo level of analysis; findings (grounded theory) are based solely on participants' descriptive phrases instead of concepts.

For example, in a study of spousal caregiving for an elderly disabled relative purporting to generate a grounded theory, one researcher organized her study findings according to the following major subheadings: Taking Care of Spouse, Taking Care of Self, Taking Care of Family, and Taking Care of the Home. In each of these sections representative of Level I coding only, she simply described the problems that participants related to her, thus prematurely closing off the additional analyses requisite for a grounded theory.

In another study, findings about parents whose school-age children are enuretic yielded an analysis organized by headings limited to parents' perceptions of and responses to their enuretic child. Although possibly producing useful descriptive information, these two examples are clearly not grounded theories.

Overly Generic

Overly generic refers to an analysis that relies on names for so-called "discovered" conceptual processes that are not situation-specific but, rather, are so general that they could apply to any experience or phenomenon. This particular mistake was most likely the one prompting the aforementioned journal editor's frustration over grounded theory reports. Creating this mistake in substantive theory development must be differentiated from an expressed intention to generate formal theory. A formal theory (see Glaser & Strauss, 1971) exists at the conceptual level of inquiry and explicates a process that transcends and derives from many substantive theories. While the concepts themselves may be general and generalizable, the theory is rich, complex, and replete with illustrations from multiple substantive areas of empirical inquiry.

The following examples, by contrast, are based on thin data, with minimal and poorly integrated properties, resulting in an overly general staged process applicable to anything and everything. For example, in a study of men recovering from heart attacks, the grounded theory reported was organized according to the following key processes: disintegration of identity, dealing with broken identity, and reconstructing identity. While somewhat conceptual, these processes could apply equally to a person disabled by a chronic illness or having experienced a traumatic event such as rape, divorce, or death of a loved one. The grounded theory produced is neither a formal one nor does it contribute to theoretic knowledge of a specific substantive area.

Importing Concepts

This occurs when an aspiring grounded theorist does not suspend preconceptions, disciplinary perspectives, and previous readings when examining the data and fails to provide an original and grounded interpretation. To illustrate, a nurse investigator studying dying AIDS patients did not see any way to think conceptually about his data except through the lens of Kubler-Ross's stages of dying. Another researcher, examining nurses' perceptions of critically ill children, collected 400 hours of observation data and conducted 30 interviews with staff nurses, but then resorted to the stages of nursing process (assessment, planning, intervention, and evaluation) for her explanatory schema. Generating grounded theory requires what Glaser has called "theoretical sensitivity," a quality that combines interpersonal perceptiveness with conceptual thinking.

Methodological Transgression

This refers to frank violations of the grounded theory philosophy and methodology. Rather than operate according to any version of grounded theory (even one that's been tinkered with), canons of quantitative, positivist method are slightly modified and applied to interview or textual data. This mistake is common when investigators have tacked on an open-ended question or two to a large survey questionnaire and find they need an analytic method. The outcome is a study report replete with conventional positivistic terminology, including random sampling, reliability and validity statistics, independent and dependent variables, and the like. Such studies customarily start with a conceptual framework and then try to match what appears in the data with the preexisting conceptual framework.

In one study of patients with lupus, the investigators began with a conceptual framework. They used cluster sampling procedures and a mailed questionnaire, identified an independent and dependent variable, and used the conceptual model for coding data. Then the themes they identified were transformed into categories for each of their three research questions and reported as percentages in each category. The data were analyzed using a one-way ANOVA.

The pitfall of methodological transgression must be differentiated from triangulation or the combining of qualitative and quantitative methods, a legitimate practice given certain complex research questions. The critical guideline is that each approach must be employed in accordance with its own philosophy and operational practices and must serve a particular purpose in the research. Findings from each approach must be reported in the language and style that are appropriate for the chosen method. Thus, a grounded theory that is part of a larger quantitative study will still read like a grounded theory, not as a frequency of occurrence.

Conclusion

The grounded theory methodology has a 30-year history of generating important insights and conceptual explanations across a highly divergent range of substantive areas and across numerous disciplines. Corruptions of the method in recent years place its credibility at risk, and the findings generated are earning a reputation as trivial or obvious. In this article, an attempt was made to offer some warning signs so that the six most common methodologic mistakes can be identified and avoided. A number of nurse scientists have published studies that in our view are excellent models of grounded theory. Examples of recent titles include: "Personal Risking" (Hitchcock & Wilson, 1992); "Mothering on Crack Cocaine" (Kearney, Murphy, & Rosenbaum, 1994); and "Filial Reconstruction" (Sohier, 1993). We hope that clarifying grounded theory's purpose and spirit will revitalize it as a highly useful approach to generate much needed knowledge of complex phenomena that are directly linked to the human world we seek to understand.

References

Baker, C., Wuest, J., & Stern, P. (1992). Method slurring: The phenomenology/grounded theory example. *Journal of Advanced Nursing, 17,* 1355–1360.

Becker, P. (1993). Common pitfalls of published grounded theory research. *Qualitative Health Research, 3*(2), 254–260.

Bowers, B. (1989). Grounded theory. In B. Sarter (Ed.), *Paths to knowledge* (pp. 33–58). New York: National League for Nursing.

Chenitz, W. C., & Swanson, J. (1986). *From practice to grounded theory.* Menlo Park, CA: Addison-Wesley.

Dewey, J. (1935). *Art as experience.* New York: Minton, Balch.

Glaser, B. (1978). *Theoretical sensitivity.* Mill Valley, CA: Sociology Press.

Glaser, B. (1992). *Basics of grounded theory analysis.* Mill Valley, CA: Sociology Press.

Glaser, B., & Strauss, A. (1967). *The discovery of grounded theory: Strategies for qualitative research.* New York: Aldine DeGruyter.

Glaser, B., & Strauss, A. (1971). *Status passage: A formal theory.* Chicago, IL: Adline Publishing.

Hitchcock, J., & Wilson, H. S. (1992). Personal risking: Lesbian self-disclosure to health professionals. *Nursing Research, 41,* 178–183.

Hutchinson, S. (1986). Grounded theory. In P. Munhall & C. Oiler (Eds.), *Nursing research, a qualitative perspective* (pp. 111–130). New York: National League for Nursing.

Kearney, M., Murphy, S., & Rosenbaum, M. (1994). Mothering on crack cocaine: A grounded theory analysis. *Social Science in Medicine, 38*(2), 351–161.

Quint, J. (1966). Awareness of death and the nurse's composure. *Nursing Research, 15,* 49–55.

Sohier, R. (1993). Filial reconstruction: A theory on development through adversity. *Qualitative Health Research, 13*(4), 465–492.

Stern, P. (1980). Grounded theory methodology: Its uses and processes. *Image, Journal of Nursing Scholorship 12,* 20–24.

Stern, P. (1993). Eroding ground theory. In J. Morse (Ed.), *Critical issues in quantitative research methods* (pp. 212–223). Thousand Oaks, CA: Sage.

Strauss, A. (1987). *Qualitative analysis for social scientists.* New York: Cambridge University Press.

Strauss, A., & Corbin, J. (1990). *Basics of qualitative research.* Newbury Park, CA: Sage.

Wilson, H. S. (1993). *Introducing research in nursing.* Redwood City, CA: Addison Wesley.

Self-as-Instrument in Qualitative Research

Lynn Rew ■ **Deborah Bechtel** ■ **Aida Sapp**

Qualitative nursing research is a systematic method of inquiry that enables the researcher to answer important questions about phenomena of concern to nursing. Such research is appropriate for generating nursing theory for further testing and application in practice (Fawcett & Downs, 1992). A qualitative design is based on philosophical assumptions and is conducted by applying corresponding rules. The relationship of the knower to the known is crucial to the study of human living experiences and provides an epistemologic position for qualitative inquiry.

Meticulous attention to how data are collected is a prerequisite to accurate, meaningful interpretation of those data. In qualitative methods of inquiry, the researcher not only collects data but also serves as the "instrument" through which data are collected. When reporting the results of qualitative inquiry, the researcher should provide a judicious description of the aspects of "self-as-instrument." Although nurse researchers have recently published details of steps they have taken to ensure scientific rigor (Sandelowski, 1986) and professional ethical behavior (Raudonis, 1992), few investigators have included details about the self as the primary, if not only, instrument for collecting data (Demi & Howell, 1991; Eyres, Loustau, & Ersek, 1992; Fleury, 1991). The purpose of this article is to describe in some detail the salient aspects of the investigator in using the self-as-instrument for data collection.

According to Harris, "The qualitative researcher seeks to enter the world of the participant, and to some degree regards himself or herself as a vessel or vehicle through which the participant makes known an intricate story of a 'slice' of the participant's life" (1990, p. 65). Understanding the following attributes can help the qualitative researcher describe the use of self as the primary instrument for data collection and underscores the need for rigor in collecting qualitative data.

Appropriateness

When the researcher is clear about the purpose of using self as the instrument for data collection and consistently poses questions in ways that are not ambiguous or open to multiple interpretations, confusion between the role of clinician and that of researcher is avoided. Boundaries appropriate for nursing intervention are then clearly differentiated from those of the researcher. In a grounded theory study of first birth in an intergenerational family, Bright (1992) emphasizes the importance of separating research and clinical roles. She clearly delineates her role as researcher by stating that she was not available to research participants for clinical consultation and referred participants to appropriate health care providers when needed.

Roberson (1992) studied 23 chronically ill rural African Americans to explore the meaning of compliance from the informants' perspective. During data collection she considered her responsibility to intervene when informants' descriptions conflicted with the medical advice they had received, but ultimately decided that "any intervention would have been inappropriate unless a clearly dangerous or harmful situation was revealed" (p. 14). Raudonis (1992) also discusses the inherent conflicts between her role as researcher and as clinician in conducting qualitative research with hospice patients. However, she states that ethical conflicts were resolved appropriately, in favor of the nursing imperative of advocacy taking precedence over the research imperative.

Authenticity

Authenticity is the researcher's ability to use one's personal history and awareness to perceive and to respond to another person (Paterson & Zderad, 1988) so that the researcher's behavior is congruent with personal attitudes, values, and beliefs. Genuinely caring about the informant's experience reflects the researcher's authenticity

Lynn Rew, EdD, RNC, FAAN, is an associate professor and assistant dean for Student Affairs, School of Nursing, The University of Texas at Austin, TX.

Deborah Bechtel, PhD, RNC, is an assistant professor, School of Nursing, Clemson University, Clemson, SC.

Aida Sapp, MSN, RN, CS, is a doctoral candidate, School of Nursing, The University of Texas at Austin, TX.

From *Nursing Research*, September/October 1993, *42,* 300–301.

and influences data analysis and interpretation. For example, in reporting results of a study of persons with terminal illness, Hall (1990) shares with readers her concern about how people face the end of life. She acknowledges her own experience with a diagnosis of metastatic cancer and the loss of both parents to this disease, thus illustrating the use of her personal history as the motivation to study and understand this experience in others.

Credibility

When the researcher's presentation of self is believed by the research participants, the trust and rapport essential to credibility of the team of researchers are established. Patton (1990) emphasizes that the qualitative approach to research depends greatly on the researcher's credibility as the "instrument of data collection and the center of the analytic process" (p. 461). In a grounded theory study of the experiences of survivors of suicide, Van Dongen (1990) reports that peer review and member checks are used to enhance the credibility of the researcher as instrument for data collection. Sowell, Bramlett, Gueldner, Gritzmacher, and Martin (1991) conducted a phenomenological study of survival and bereavement following the death of a lover from AIDS. They made phone contact with each potential participant prior to the interviews to establish credibility.

Intuitiveness

Intuitiveness is the ability of the researcher to synthesize the experience of the informant through immediate contact and empathy. This characteristic is described in phenomenological studies as the engagement of the self-as-instrument with the life experiences of those investigated (Swanson, 1991). Intuitiveness involves reflection and permits the researcher to discern meanings in terms of the whole (Lethbridge, 1991).

Receptivity

The researcher who is open and receptive to the lived experiences of those providing the data is willing to be taught by the participants and is open to their feedback (Swanson, 1991). Hinds, Chaves, and Cypess (1992) note the importance for the investigator to communicate willingness to interact with participants in a particular context. The authors add that the researcher can describe a specific context by noting all obvious and relevant aspects and incorporating the analysis of the interaction into the interpretation of findings.

Reciprocity

Reciprocity means that the researcher is on an equal footing with the research participants, who act as co-researchers. The researcher's primary goal is to understand the meaning of a phenomenon or experience, not to exert power over those from whom data are collected. Phenomenologists believe that it is essential to see the lived experiences of research participants as they are, not interpreted through the filter of the researcher's preconceptions (Cohen, 1987). By acknowledging previous knowledge, values, and beliefs, the researcher asserts that he or she is on a par with the participants (Campbell & Bunting, 1991).

Sensitivity

Sensitivity, the researcher's perception of phenomena as experienced by research participants, includes the ability to see and hear accurately what is reported as data. Self-as-instrument relies on a dynamic rather than static means of measuring a concept or phenomenon. Machines and paper-pencil tests are man-made inventions to enhance the natural sensory inputs of the researcher. All such measurements are vulnerable to individual interpretations. Just as the scientist sets the calibrations for machines (Grossman, 1991) and checks the internal consistency of paper-pencil tools, the qualitative researcher engaged in descriptive inquiry should record biases, feelings, thoughts, and historical circumstances in a journal or diary.

Qualitative research is becoming a more common approach to understanding the various phenomena of concern to nursing. Just as the musical instrument conveys harmony between artist and chord, so the qualitative researcher expresses the delicate blending of human experience and scientific understanding. The inherent value of human beings and their intersubjective experiences underscore the significance of the use of self-as-instrument in qualitative inquiry. No other entity could fully capture the multidimensionality and intricacy of the human experience.

References

Bright, M. A. (1992). Making place: The first birth in an intergenerational family context. *Qualitative Health Research, 2*(1), 75–98.

Campbell, J. C., & Bunting, S. (1991). Voices and paradigms: Perspectives on critical and feminist theory in nursing. *Advances in Nursing Science, 13*(3), 1–15.

Cohen, M. Z. (1987). A historical overview of the phenomenological movement. *Image: Journal of Nursing Scholarship, 19*(1), 31–34.

Demi, A. S., & Howell, C. (1991). Hiding and healing: Resolving the suicide of a parent or sibling. *Archives of Psychiatric Nursing, 5*, 350–356.

Eyres, S. J., Loustau. A., & Ersek, M. (1992). Ways of knowing among beginning students in nursing. *Journal of Nursing Education, 31*, 175–180.

Fawcett, J., & Downs, F. S. (1992). *The relationship of theory and research* (2nd ed.). Philadelphia: Davis.

Fleury, J. D. (1991). Empowering potential: A theory of wellness motivation. *Nursing Research, 40,* 286–291.

Grossman, D. G. S. (1991). Circadian rhythms in blood pressure in school-age children of normotensive and hypertensive parents. *Nursing Research, 40,* 28–34.

Hall, B. A. (1990). The struggle of the diagnosed terminally ill person to maintain hope. *Nursing Science Quarterly, 2,* 177–184.

Harris, B. L. (1990). Becoming deprofessionalized: One aspect of the staff nurse's perspective on computer-mediated nursing care plans. *Advances in Nursing Science, 13*(2), 63–74.

Hinds, P. S., Chaves, D. E., & Cypess, S. M. (1992). Context as a source of meaning and understanding. *Qualitative Health Research, 2*(1), 61–74.

Lethbridge, D. J. (1991). Choosing and using contraception: Toward a theory of women's contraceptive self-care. *Nursing Research, 40,* 276–280.

Paterson, J. G., & Zderad, L. T. (1988). *Humanistic nursing.* New York: National League for Nursing.

Patton, M. Q. (1990). *Qualitative evaluation and research methods* (2nd ed.). Newbury Park, CA: Sage.

Raudonis, B. M. (1992). Ethical considerations in qualitative research with hospice patients. *Qualitative Health Research, 2,* 238–249.

Roberson, M. H. B. (1992). The meaning of compliance: Patient perspectives. *Qualitative Health Research, 2,* 7–26.

Sandelowski, M. (1986). The problem of rigor in qualitative research. *Advances in Nursing Science, 8*(3), 27–37.

Sowell, R. L., Bramlett, M. H., Gueldner, S. H., Gritzmacher, D., & Martin, G. (1991). The lived experience of survival and bereavement following the death of a lover from AIDS. *Image: Journal of Nursing Scholarship, 23*(2), 89–94.

Swanson, K. M. (1991). Empirical development of a middle range theory of caring. *Nursing Research, 40,* 161–166.

Van Dongen, C. J. (1990). Agonizing questioning: Experiences of survivors of suicide victims. *Nursing Research, 39,* 224–229.

Validity Threats in Scheduled Semistructured Research Interviews

Sally Hutchinson ■ **Holly Skodol Wilson**

In contrast to the unscheduled, nonstandardized interview, where questions vary from situation to situation, and the scheduled standardized interview, in which the wording and sequence of questions is the same for all respondents, the scheduled semistructured interview requires certain types of information from all respondents, but allows flexibility in phrasing and order of questions based on the respondents' characteristics (Sellitz, Jahoda, Deutsch, & Cook, 1966). The validity of data from scheduled semistructured interviews, also termed "objectivity" by Davis (1980), "credibility" by Lincoln and Guba (1985), and "response errors" by many quantitative researchers, is the focus of this analysis.

Valid interview data are those that accurately portray what the investigator is attempting to study. The categories of validity threats that follow do not exhaust all the possible factors affecting validity of interview data but do provide a lens through which investigators can scrutinize their interview techniques.

Interview Questions

Interview questions that are not relevant to the research purpose represent one category of validity threats. The following example from a nursing study of cardiac patients illustrates this problem. The purpose of the research was to explore and describe heart transplant patients' experiences with cardiac biopsy. The first interview question was: "What is it like to be a heart transplant patient?" The second was, "How have things changed in your life since having your heart transplant?" Both questions would elicit good information in an interview about life as a heart patient, but they are too general to gather data related to the specific research purpose. A question such as, "Tell me about what it's like to have a cardiac biopsy?", is more directly related to the purpose of this particular study.

Irrelevant or tangential questions often arise from the researcher's past experience, favorite concepts or theories, or the existing literature rather than cues from the respondent. For instance, a researcher who intended to study children's emotional responses to a lumbar puncture asked children to name and describe all the equipment used in the procedure and their physical responses to the steps of the procedure (i.e., "What is on the tray?" "What is the needle for?" "What does the needle feel like?") These abrupt, factual questions cut off expression in some children and virtually no useful data of the children's overall experiences were collected.

Once relevant interview questions are formulated, they need to be sequenced so that they flow from general to specific. For example, an initial question such as, "Tell me about having a cardiac biopsy," is far more likely to elicit what is important to the patient than a specific question such as, "What special arrangements did you make on the day you came to the hospital?" The latter question may be important, but to ask it before a general question indicates that the researcher assigns it more importance than it may deserve in research that aims to learn about respondents' experience. In most qualitative research, open-ended questions are necessary in order to acquire the detailed data that permit theory generation or an interpretive analysis. However, open-ended questions may present problems in some studies, especially if quantification is a goal. One researcher conducted a study using structured interviews (120 questions) with families of persons with AIDS. The questions were open-ended (e.g., "What is it like to be a family member of an AIDS patient?"). These questions encouraged the family members to talk at great length. The interviewer was overwhelmed with "stories" and was unable to fill in the Likert Scale (ranking of very easy to most difficult) summary form. The answers to open-ended questions may not be translated easily to scales or dichotomous categories often used in quantitative analysis of interview data. Closed-ended questions, however, may not provide the necessary data for most qualitative analysis. Investi-

Sally Hutchinson, PhD, RN, FAAN, is a professor, College of Nursing, University of Florida Health Science Center, Jacksonville, FL.

Holly Skodol Wilson, PhD, RN, FAAN, is a professor, Department of Mental Health & Community Nursing, School of Nursing, University of California, San Francisco, CA.

From *Nursing Research,* March/April 1992, *41,* 117–119.

gators must consider carefully the structure of questions in relation to the research purpose and the recording format. Yet, as Chenitz and Swanson (1986) note: "There can be no cookbook recipes for interviewing . . . It is essential that the researcher be able to think in terms of an array of contingencies that may affect the content and form of the interview" (p. 84).

Timing of Interviews

The timing of interviews is critical to obtaining valid data and may need to be assessed in the beginning of a study and as the research progresses. One investigator who was interviewing widows about their dreams of their husbands found that widows of less than six months had difficulty focusing on the interview questions and wanted to discuss personal details about their loved ones and their relationship. However, interviews of women who had been widows six months or longer were less distressing and resulted in more focused and useful research data. Similarly, interviewing a patient who is in labor or awaiting a highly stressful procedure may be unethical, insensitive, and inadequate for obtaining useful research data.

Sufficient time should be devoted to greetings, establishing rapport, addressing respondent reluctance or idiosyncratic meanings, allowing for emotional catharsis, clarifying ambiguities, and providing for closure. Interviews should not be scheduled between other appointments and should end naturally, not because the researcher or the respondent must depart abruptly.

Researchers often design a quantitative and qualitative data collection protocol that requires administration of a set of standardized quantitative instruments followed by a semistructured interview at a second visit. To avoid bias, the standardized instruments are traditionally given on the initial visit. However, when respondents meet the researchers they may volunteer a wealth of spontaneous information. Research assistants or inexperienced investigators may not record this detail or may record it retrospectively, thus missing major insights. Thus, validity suffers if researchers adhere to rigid protocols at the expense of gathering quality data.

Good interviewers are flexible and able to conduct quality interviews in a variety of places. However, certain places are usually less conducive to obtaining valid information than others. For example, the Intensive Care Unit (ICU) with its disruptive sounds, sights, and lack of privacy presents many problems for interviewers and respondents alike. In addition, certain patients in an ICU are physiologically compromised, making interviewing difficult, if not impossible.

Interviewer Behaviors

Strong feelings such as attraction or revulsion bias the interviewer in that more or less time may be spent with the respondent to meet the researcher's needs rather than the needs of the study. One interviewer found a health care administrator attractive. In retrospect, she recognized that she did not ask him enough of the more controversial interview questions. She accepted brief answers and agreed too readily, "to have him approve of me." In another situation, an investigator avoided certain respondents, spent less time interviewing them and believed they were less credible. Close scrutiny of the investigator's feelings is necessary to avoid these potential sources of bias.

Good interviewers listen actively, pursuing leads and cues from respondents that allow them to formulate additional relevant questions. The interviewer who insists upon strictly following a prepared list of questions instead of following the respondents' beliefs of what is important usually produces less genuine results. Thus, good qualitative research requires a flexible interviewer.

An interviewer needs to be sensitive in listening for patterns or themes. Although the words or described events may initially appear irrelevant, at a theoretical level they may be very important. For example, if an elder respondent is always complaining about dinner being late, his nurse bathing him late, and his visitors coming late, an investigator may view him as a chronic complainer and wish he could move on to what the investigator would view as more relevant topics. However, a theoretically sensitive interviewer may notice that "waiting" appears to be a central theme in all of the elder's complaints and pursues what it means to always have to wait. Stories about seemingly unrelated events often have meaning and are relevant in retrospect. Clarifying questions may help assess the meaning.

Some interviewers are unwittingly influenced by existing literature, theory, or the jargon derived from them as a source for interview questions. They may ask questions about "social support needs," "coping strategies," or "barriers to mental health services." They may also begin to categorize the respondent's experiences and feelings into these theories or scientific jargon. In essence, they prematurely place the narrative data into predefined categories rather than listening for new ways of interpretation. In further interviews, they pursue such topics as "coping strategies" or "denial" rather than attempting to get to the respondents' interpretation of their behavior.

Nurses are socialized to care and to educate and may assume these roles to the detriment of their role as researchers. Ideally, the respondent teaches the interviewer, not vice versa. When typescripts of interviews reveal that the investigator has engaged in more narrative than the respondent, and when the content of that narrative is educational, therapeutic, or attempts at reassurance, the quality of research data suffers due to the changed role of the interviewer. Sharing information or honest reassurance is not totally inappropriate, but the predominant role of the interviewer should not be that of educator, therapist, or caretaker.

Problematic Respondent Behaviors

Sexual overtures and innuendoes occasionally occur during research interviews. Researchers may be shocked and even repulsed by this behavior. Rather than take control of the situation and gain useful information, they may terminate the interview. One young woman interviewed an older man about his decision to undergo chemotherapy for a probably fatal tumor. He repeatedly flirted, complimented her, and made suggestive comments. A review of the typed transcript of the interview showed that a number of strategies could have changed the conversational focus. The researcher could have briefly joked with the respondent and quickly returned to the interview guide. She could have commented on the flirtatious behavior: "You are a real flirt." An intervention such as naming and commenting on the behavior can shift the direction of an interview back to the research purpose when sexual innuendoes characterize the respondent's style.

Certain respondents, because of their idiosyncratic personalities or due to stressful circumstances, may assume an air of intimidation and/or hostility. In such situations, interviewers should ask if respondents would prefer not to be interviewed or continue the interview. If the choice is to continue, the interviewer should assess the meaning of the hostility and not respond personally. In one situation, an army physician who had a fatal illness barked his clipped answers to the interviewer. As the interview progressed, it became clear that this was consistent with his personality and was the way he interacted with the army, his family, and in social relationships. To enter his world and avoid a negative personal response was necessary in order not to lose valuable data by prematurely terminating the interview.

Cowles (1988) in her article about qualitative research on sensitive topics did not focus on threats to validity but offered strategies for dealing with extreme emotional responses from respondents. Interviews with survivors of murder-victims (Cowles, 1985), incest, child abuse, domestic violence, or death of a child may evoke hysterical crying and even screaming as the participants relive their feelings about the experience. In order to obtain valid and complete data, such interviews may require more time due to the need for emotional catharsis and recovery from the catharsis. In addition, the mental stress of the interview can affect what the interviewer believes was heard or not heard. Time to regain control, review the data, and formulate new approaches and/or interview questions is necessary.

An interviewer must be prepared for respondents' outbursts; one's own emotional response (Benoliel, 1975), and acknowledge the acceptance of both to the respondent in order to help make a very difficult situation more comfortable (Cowles, 1988). In addition, such psychological preparation by the interviewer will encourage respondents to feel free to share all their feelings.

Silences also need to be assessed by the interviewer. Some silences are pauses that enable respondents to get their thoughts together before replying to a question. Others may be hostile or ways of withholding information, which are a respondent's right. After careful assessment of the meaning of a silence, interviewers must decide whether to repeat the question, change the subject, or ask respondents if they are thinking, if the question is unclear, or if they would prefer not to answer. Sometimes asking the same question a different way or asking the question later in the interview will overcome a silence that occurred due to lack of clarity.

Jokes by the respondent may be used to avoid a subject, decrease tension, or relate on a personal level to the interviewer. If jokes are used as a substitution for a reply, the interviewer may say, "I know this can be a joking matter, but I am concerned about trying to understand." Brief joking by the interviewer can be appropriate, too, as shared joking often does imply equality, provides levity in tense situations, and may serve to increase respondent spontaneity.

On some occasions (e.g. a very young interviewer, or an interviewer who reminds the respondent of someone else) respondents may shift the focus of the interview to the interviewer. Young and/or inexperienced interviewers are likely to have difficulty returning to the topic at hand. A researcher may answer questions briefly and even share feelings or thoughts. A problem may occur, however, if interviewers allow the interview to become shifted from the research focus. Give and take conversations may be highly appropriate in unscheduled, unstructured interviews but are usually less efficient and effective in scheduled semistructured interviews as discussed here.

Recording Problems

Reluctance to transcribe interviews after they are completed is not uncommon. Transcription is tedious and time consuming. To delay, however, can directly affect the quality of research data. While typing or dictating, memories of a recently completed interview flood the investigator's mind and contribute new ideas, nuances, and perhaps relevant nonverbal behaviors, in addition to the investigator's personal feelings and responses used to monitor bias. Recording in a timely fashion to obtain accurate, in-depth information is essential to quality data.

Prop failure (Lyman & Scott, 1970), failure of technical equipment such as a tape recorder, is feared by all investigators. This problem can be avoided by using two tape recorders (Douglas' [1985] suggestion), by checking all equipment prior to each interview, and by having extra batteries and tapes. To jog their memories, interviewers should write down key points and issues that need to be clarified during taping. Interviewers' laments such as "I only wish I had asked about prior encounters with mental health professionals" or "I only wish I had followed up on what happened after she joined the support group" are less likely to occur if investigators write these notes to themselves.

In qualitative research each phase of an interview directly affects the validity of the final product. Proper interviewing is the "soul" of qualitative research (Downs, 1991). Only with good interviewing skills do we obtain good interview data; only with good interview data are we able to do a credible interpretation.

References

Benoliel, J. (1975). Research related to death and the dying patient. In P. J. Verhonick (Ed.), *Nursing Research* (vol. 1, pp. 189–227). Boston: Little, Brown.

Chenitz, C., & Swanson, J. (1986). *From practice to grounded theory.* Menlo Park, CA: Addison-Wesley.

Cowles, K. (1985). *Personal world expansion: Experiences of survivors of murder victims.* Unpublished doctoral dissertation, University of Illinois Health Science Center, Chicago.

Cowles, K. (1988). Issues in qualitative research on sensitive topics. *Western Journal of Nursing Research, 10,* 163–179.

Davis, A. (1980). Research as an interactional situation: Objectivity in the interview. *International Journal of Nursing Studies, 17,* 215–220.

Douglas, J. (1985). *Creative interviewing.* Beverly Hills, CA: Sage.

Downs, F. (1991). Personal Communication.

Lincoln, Y., & Guba, E. (1985). *Naturalistic inquiry.* Beverly Hills, CA: Sage.

Lyman, S., & Scott, M. (1970). *A sociology of the absurd.* New York: Appleton-Century-Crofts.

Sellitz, C., Jahoda, M., Deutsch, M., & Cook, S. (1966). *Research methods in social relations.* New York: Holt, Rinehart, & Winston.

Interviewer Training and Supervision

Clare Collins ■ **Barbara Given** ■ **C.W. Given** ■ **Sharon King**

Methodologists frequently cite three sources of error in survey research: (a) sampling error, or the error which occurs when a sample differs from the population from which it is drawn; (b) nonresponse error, or error attributable to the fact that information is not collected from all members of the population; and (c) response error, or error occurring when the respondents' answers to questions do not accurately measure what the researcher intends to measure (Fowler & Mangione, 1986). Response error includes error attributable to (a) questionnaire wording and design (Woodward & Chambers, 1983), (b) reluctance of the respondent to answer questions (Bradburn & Sudman, 1979; Woodward, Chambers, & Smith, 1982), and (c) variation among interviewers in how the interview is conducted (Fowler & Mangione). Adequate training and supervision of interviewers can reduce both subject reluctance to answer questions (Bradburn & Sudman) and variance attributable to differences among the interviewers (Fowler & Mangione).

Interviewer Variance

Interviewers differ in ability to establish rapport with the respondent, adherence to the interview schedule, correct use of appropriate question clarifications and probes, and care taken in editing and coding questionnaires (Woodward et al., 1982). In clinical nursing research studies, particularly those using longitudinal designs with clinicians conducting the research interviews, an additional source of variance may be introduced by a clinician's tendency to assume the role of intervenor during the research interview (Clinton et al., 1986). Observer bias, the tendency of interviewers to distort or inaccurately record data based on preconceived notions about how respondents will behave, has also been identified as a source of interviewer variance (Spool, 1978).

Research on Interviewer Training

Considerable evidence exists that respondents are influenced by variations in interviewer behaviors (Bradburn & Sudman, 1979; Cannell, Oskenberg, & Converse, 1977; Kish, 1962). However, little research has been conducted on the effectiveness of differing methods of interviewer training. Spool reviewed 25 years of research on training programs for observers of behavior and concluded that most training programs were based more on common sense than on theory or research.

In reviewing methods of interviewer training, Spool (1978) found the following components: (a) observation by trainees of model persons behaving in ways appropriate for the observational task; (b) practice with the interview task; (c) social reinforcement by the trainer in the form of constructive feedback; and (d) transfer of training, including application of the first three activities in increasingly complex and realistic situations. Two-thirds of the studies Spool reviewed examined only one training approach. Training interviewers as observers of behavior was found to be generally effective in reducing rating errors, but which components of training programs were effective could not be determined (Spool).

Fowler and Mangione (1986), in their large-scale field experiment with health survey interviewers, provided the first evidence on which specific training approaches were most effective in reducing interviewer bias by comparing training programs differing in length from one-half day to 10 days. In addition, three levels of field supervision were tested: minimal supervision, a review of completed interviews in conjunction with tape recording, and systematic feedback on interviews. Based on this experiment, they concluded: (a) giving interviewers less than 1 day of training resulted in inadequate interviewing skills; (b) increasing the length of the training program tended not to result in significant increments in basic interviewing skills; (c) intensive field supervision did not

Clare Collins, PhD, RN, is an assistant professor, College of Nursing, Michigan State University, East Lansing.

Barbara Given, PhD, FAAN, is a professor in the College of Nursing, Michigan State University, East Lansing.

C. W. Given, PhD, is a professor in the Department of Family Practice, Michigan State University, East Lansing.

Sharon King, PhD, RN, is an assistant professor in the College of Nursing, Michigan State University, East Lansing.

From *Nursing Research,* March/April 1988, *37,* 122–124.

alleviate the effects of poor interviewer training; (d) use of tape recording of interviewers was an effective form of field supervision.

The Interviewer's Task

The interviewer's task in the research interview includes instructing respondents about their role in the question-and-answer process, adhering carefully to the interview schedule and study protocol, and managing problems as they arise in the interview situation. Cannell et al. (1977) reported that most respondents in their study did not know what was expected of them in terms of the depth of the information sought by the interviewer. Respondents tolerated the research interview without a clear understanding of their task. Both the design of the questionnaire and the techniques used by the interviewer should clarify for respondents what is expected of them to perform the task properly and motivate the respondent to work diligently to recall and verbalize information (Cannell et al.). The task of the research interviewer is to reinforce acceptable respondent performance through use of feedback and to use neutral technique to remind respondents of their role if performance is unacceptable (Guenzel, Berckmans, & Cannell, 1983).

Respondents' requests for clarification of questions should be handled in the same way by all interviewers to assure that all respondents are asked questions in a similar way (Guenzel et al., 1983). Interviewers must be both rigid in their adherence (Cannell et al., 1977) to study protocols and flexible in handling situations when a departure from the interview schedule is inevitable (Clinton et al., 1986). More enthusiastic interviewers inspire subjects to greater response accuracy, but overly friendly interviewers may also serve to increase social desirability bias (Cannell et al.). The inability of interviewers to establish rapport with the respondent jeopardizes study results (Woodward et al., 1982) and is a particular problem in longitudinal study designs where attrition is a major concern.

Components of Interviewer Training

Building on the findings of Fowler and Mangione (1986) and the insights of Guenzel et al. (1983) and Woodward et al. (1982), we included the following components of interviewer training in our longitudinal study of family care giving: information specific to the research project and practice sessions where specific feedback is provided to the interviewer. Prior to training, all interviewers were asked to read the research proposal. In addition, we provided interviewers with a personal copy of an interviewer's manual for the study. The interviewer's manual contained general information about the study, a summary of the didactic material for the training sessions, and study procedures for questionnaire flow, confidentiality, eligibility determination of subjects, and coding of completed questionnaires. The interviewers' manuals were used as a source of information throughout the study when interviewers had technical or procedural questions. Interviewer training sessions were held on 3 days for a total of 10 hours, with practice sessions scheduled between training sessions.

The initial training session was opened with a discussion of the project aims, purpose, and phases. Although Diers (1979) reported that the techniques for obtaining data in research and nursing practice are essentially the same, our impression, and that of Clinton et al. (1986), is that there are distinct differences between interviewing techniques used in research and practice. Because our research interviewers were clinicians by background, we discussed the differences between research and clinical interviews in the initial training session (Table 1). This discussion was followed by instruction on general interviewing techniques and a question-by-question review of the study instrument.

In survey research, there is a commonly accepted set of guidelines for general interviewing techniques. Our instruction was based on the method of interviewer training outlined by Guenzel et al. (1983), which includes specific instruction about the interviewer's task, interview rules, and techniques for probing, clarification, and feedback. A particular benefit of this training approach is that it includes a method for systematic review of interviewer performance. Our modification of this method of performance evaluation is shown in Figure 1.

Between training sessions, interviewers conducted an interview with each other, conducted practice interviews with colleagues, listened to a taped interview, and taped an interview with a member of the project staff. Taped interviews were exchanged among interviewers and a peer evaluation was completed, using the interviewer performance rating tool. The second training session included a review and critique of the taped interviews, discussion of study procedures, and instruction about coding of questionnaires. Between the second and third training sessions, interviewers completed a taped interview with an actual subject, which was reviewed and critiqued at the third training session.

Field Supervision of Interviewers

Careful field supervision following intensive interviewer training is vital for improving and maintaining the quality of data collected by research interviewers (Fowler &

TABLE 1 Differences between Clinical and Research Interviews

Dimensions	Clinical Interviews	Research Interviews
Goal	Assessment/intervention	Collection of information
Questions	Individualized Nonuniform	Uniform
Rapport building	Established by empathic listening, reflection	Established by reenforcement of acceptable subject performance, role modeling
Elaboration	Encouraged by open-ended questions	Discouraged by controlled choices and use of specific probes
Interpretation	Data interpreted and summarized by clinician	Subject's specific response is recorded; few inferences are drawn

Mangione, 1986). Regular project staff meetings (Clinton et al., 1986) and the development of study protocols for handling problematic questions and situations (Guenzel et al., 1983) are vital if consistency among interviewers is to be maintained. Woodward et al. (1982) suggested the following general guidelines for field supervision of interviewers: make interviewers frequently reportable to supervisors, provide an opportunity for interviewers to express satisfaction and complaints with the task, and reward good performance through recognition.

In the early phases of data collection we conducted weekly debriefing meetings with interviewers during which issues and problems were discussed and resolved. The work records of interviewers, including number of

Total number of questions ________

1. QUESTION ASKING
   - A. Minor errors (small wording changes) ________
   - B. Major errors (wrong skip pattern, wrong choice from parenthesis, missed questions) ________
     Question numbers ____________ ________
   - C. $\frac{\text{Total number of questions} - (A + B)}{\text{Total number of questions}}$ ________ Percentage of questions asked correctly

2. INTERVIEWER FEEDBACK
   - A. Number of feedback phrases used ________
   - B. Number of incorrect feedback phrases used ________
   - C. $\frac{A - B}{\text{Total number of questions}}$ ________ Percentage of questions followed by correct feedback

3. PROBING FOR ANSWERS
   - A. Number of probes needed ________
   - B. Number of probes used ________
   - C. Number of incorrect probes ________
   - D. $\frac{B - C}{A}$ ________ Percentage of correct use of probes

4. EVALUATION COMMENTS:

FIGURE 1 Interview Evaluation Tool

subjects contacted, number of interviews completed, and average interview time, were reviewed weekly by the field supervisor. Review of the work records allowed the compilation of profiles of interviewer productivity and performance. These weekly meetings have been vital in maintaining interviewer consistency and enthusiasm.

Early in the data collection process and at scheduled intervals, interviewers conducted a self-evaluation using the interview evaluation tool of an actual taped interview. Tapes were also submitted to the field supervisor for review. The field supervisor provided written feedback to each interviewer and completed a questionnaire while listening to the taped interview. To date, our *interrater* agreement between each interviewer and the field supervisor has exceeded 97%.

As an additional safeguard on the accuracy of the data collected, an editor reviewed all completed questionnaires for coding accuracy prior to data entry and provided written feedback to the interviewer about coding performance.

Conclusions

Consistency among interviewers results in data that better reflect true variance among respondents. Conclusions drawn from these data serve to more accurately address the research questions and enhance the results of the researchers' efforts. The time and resources spent in the process of interviewer training and supervision should be adequately compensated by the increased confidence the investigator gains in the quality of the data collected and the accuracy of study findings.

References

Bradburn N., & Sudman, S. (1979). *Improving interview methods and questionnaire design.* San Francisco: Jossey-Bass Inc.

Cannell, C., Oskenberg, L., & Converse, J. (1977). Experiments in interviewing techniques: Field experiments in health reporting 1971–77. Hyattsville, MD: US Department of Health and Human Services, National Center for Health Services Research and Health Care Technology Assessment.

Clinton, J., Beck, R., Radjenovic, D., TayLor, L., Westlake, S., & Wilson, S. (1986). Time—series designs in clinical nursing research: Human issues. *Nursing Research, 35,* 188–191.

Diers, D. (1979). *Research in nursing practice.* Philadelphia: J. B. Lippincott Co.

Fowler, F., & Mangione, T. (1986). *Reducing interviewer effects on health survey data.* Hyattsville, MD: US Department of Health and Human Services, National Center for Health Services Research and Health Care Technology Assessment.

Guenzel, P., Berckmans, T., & Cannell, L. (1983). *General interviewing techniques.* Ann Arbor, MI: The University of Michigan, Survey Research Center, Institute for Social Research.

Kish, L. (1962). Studies on interviewer variance for attitudinal variables. *Journal of the American Statistical Association, 44,* 380–387.

Spool, M. (1978). Training programs for observers of behavior: A review. *Personnel Psychology, 31,* 853–888.

Woodward, C., & Chambers, L. (1983). *Guide to questionnaire construction and question writing.* Ottawa, Ont: Canadian Public Health Association.

Woodward, C., Chambers, L., & Smith, K. (1982). *Guide to improved data collection in health and health care surveys.* Ottawa, Ont: Canadian Public Health Association.

PART THREE

Measuring Differences and Change

Know Thy Data

Barbara S. Jacobsen

The teaching of statistical methods frequently focuses on inference and confirmatory analysis, in contrast to description and exploratory analysis. As Tukey (1980) points out, confirmatory data analysis is easier to teach and easier to computerize. The consequence of this emphasis on confirming rather than exploring is that researchers know their F-ratios and *p*-values, but do not know their data. Many researchers are eager to discuss their ANOVA tables, but when asked about graphs or plots of their data, they look blank or sometimes even irritated. They tend to see descriptive analysis as part of the process of cleaning data for a computer or as a step in checking statistical assumptions prior to hypothesis testing.

But simple description is good in itself. Rosemary Ellis (1977) pointed out the need for sound, factual knowledge relevant to certain variables that are commonly used in nursing research. For example, she noted the lack of published descriptive data about preoperative anxiety relative to its prevalence, intensity, the range of intensity, and even the shape of the distribution.

Confirmatory design and analysis may be easier to teach and computerize, but all too often it is learned in a mechanistic way and performed as a ritual. Resio and Verhonick (1973) warn that multivariate analytical techniques should not be viewed as the sole method of analysis. They urge researchers to take time to examine the data with graphs and their own eyes. But the terms "*p*-value" and "F-ratio" continue to induce a halo effect toward entire datasets. The actual data are still frequently ignored or conveniently put aside while statistical tests are conducted.

Barbara S. Jacobsen, MS, Ed, was an associate professor at the University of Pennsylvania School of Nursing, Philadelphia. She was involved in the use of computers to assist classroom teaching and in the analysis of data by researchers.

From *Nursing Research,* July/August 1981, *30,* 254–255.

False Interpretations

Failing to know one's data can lead to false interpretations of both confirmatory and summary statistics. Recently an excited researcher informed me that a computer had isolated a key variable on her questionnaire: number in household living with the patient. This variable correlated with everything, unfortunately sometimes in unexplained ways. For example, "number in the household" correlated positively with a measure of depression ($r = +.56$, $p < .001$). As the size of the household increased, so did the patient's depression. This finding struck the researcher as odd, but after all that was what the printout said. A scatter diagram then produced the following sort of plot:

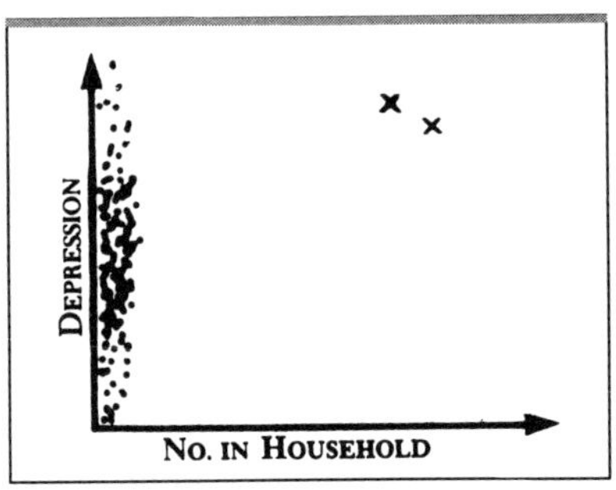

An examination of the questionnaires revealed that when two of the patients were asked how many people lived in their household, they reported huge numbers because they lived in institutions. The keypuncher simply entered the data as given, and it just so happened that both of these patients were very depressed. When outliers occur in such a fashion, increasing the range of one of the variables, the correlation coefficient increases, sometimes drastically. When the two outliers were removed, r changed to $+.07$, $p > .10$.

Extreme scores can have an opposite effect on r, reducing the coefficient to make it appear as though no relationship exists between two variables. In the following type of scatter diagram with 30 cases, $r = .2$. When the outlier in the extreme lower right corner was removed, r increased to .4.

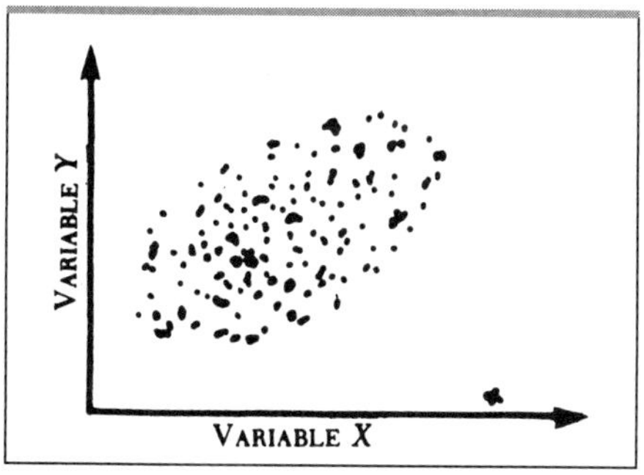

The correlation coefficient is not the only statistic that is sensitive to outliers—so are the mean, the standard deviation, the regression coefficient, and the *t*-ratio. A single outlier can invalidate a *t*-test. It is not difficult to find examples in the research literature where investigators have ignored extreme scores for their parametric tests.

What should researchers do to become better acquainted with their data? First, they can carry out descriptive analyses as they proceed instead of waiting until data collection is completed. If you are updating your histograms every week, then acquaintance with your data is unavoidable. Second, researchers can use a variety of descriptive approaches, such as frequency tables, stem and leaf displays, histograms, box and whisker plots, spider webs, scatter diagrams, contingency tables, residual plots, and others. Choose the methods that are appropriate for your data and, if you wish, carry out confirmatory analyses at the same time. Third, use a computer to help with your descriptive analyses.

The use of a computer to help explore your data as you collect them implies that a codebook must be prepared before data collection begins. It is true that a computer must often be helped along a bit more with descriptive methods by the researcher's prior judgments (for example, the appropriate size of class intervals or categories). These judgments in turn require basic knowledge of your data as an ordered array. Descriptive analyses can be time-consuming if you use pencil and graph paper, but a computer can produce quick and inexpensive graphs and plots. . . .

What should researchers look for in tables and graphs? They should examine the data for outliers. Both Chatterjee and Price (1977) and Tukey (1977) offer guidelines for classifying an observation as an outlier. The computer package BMDP from the Health Sciences Computing Facility, UCLA, offers suggestions for detection of outliers in a stepwise multiple regression (Dixon and Brown, 1979). If outliers exist, researchers may elect several routes:

- Eliminate them. In many other fields, such as engineering, outliers are often assumed to be measurement or recording errors and are routinely eliminated. In research on human beings, however, far-out observations may exist. Each case should be examined before it is eliminated—it may be simply a recording or keypunch error. The researcher has to decide whether to eliminate the case entirely from the sample or just delete that variable. Perhaps the researcher may decide to report the data both ways—with and without the outlier. In any event, the researcher should report how many outliers were eliminated.
- Collect more data points. The effect of extreme scores is reduced with a larger sample. More "outliers" may keep turning up, and what appeared to be a stray observation after 20 cases may seem more typical after 100 cases.
- Retain the outliers. As noted earlier, their effect diminishes as sample size increases. If you collect more data, there may be no need to eliminate them. Simply mentioning their existence may suffice. If sample size is small and you wish to retain these far out observations, use nonparametric methods. Statistics such as the rank correlation coefficient or the Mann-Whitney U are relatively insensitive to outliers.
- Use the outliers for case studies or as clues to further analysis. As Chatterjee and Price (1977) note, troublesome observations can sometimes be more informative than well-behaved observations. You may want to focus attention on these cases immediately or in a future study.

Besides outliers, unexpected irregularities in a distribution can also suggest further exploration. Thus, researchers should examine the shapes of their distributions for gaps, differences in variabilities, and asymmetries. And when they are correlating variables, the nature of the relationships need to be checked. For example, in a study currently being conducted, a certain interview item asked patients for an opinion about the importance of emotions relative to their disease. The bulk of the responses on a seven-point scale tended to be either one or seven. This apparently U-shaped distribution suggested an analysis contrasting the two extreme groups. Contingency tables can be helpful in such a situation. Simply using the mean here (4.4) would have ignored this pattern.

Differences in variabilities between distributions may lead a researcher to question the adequacy of the assumption of equal variances necessary for some parametric tests, but even more important, these differences in variabilities may be noteworthy in themselves. Many statistical packages such as SPSS (Nie et al., 1975) routinely test for homogeneity of variances before performing *t*-tests, but researchers tend to look upon these statistics only in terms of whether to use a pooled or separate variance t-ratio. A researcher may want to ask why groups are unequal in variation, once chance has been ruled out as unlikely. Perhaps an intervention should be examined further, if it produces a much greater variation of response in an experimental group.

An informal analysis of residual plots may prove to be the most important part of a regression analysis (Chatterjee and Price, 1977). These plots can help enormously in uncovering patterns in the data that lead the researcher to question the adequacy of assumptions such as linearity or homoscedasticity; however, they can also offer suggestions about the data and the structure of the relationships that may lead to a better model. Residual plots can also provide clues as to appropriate transformations for data. Chatterjee and Price emphasize that a large value of P^2 or a significant F statistic does not ensure that the data are fitted well (1977). They offer many instructive graphs illustrating how computing only summary statistics and performing a confirmatory analysis can obscure data. Residual plots are easily obtained from many computer packages, for example, SPSS and BMDP.

Exploratory Attitude

Tukey (1980) says that exploratory data analysis is in part an attitude. Many researchers view descriptive techniques as oil-lamp methods, a step backward; while computer-calculated p-values are the "real" statistics. The problem for instructors of statistics and research design courses is how to foster a willingness to explore data while not neglecting their obligation to teach confidence intervals and significance tests. One solution may be to provide more opportunities for students to "play" with data, besides solving specific problems given in textbooks. The source of the data is irrelevant; it could be produced by computer simulation, a class project, or an actual dataset contributed by a researcher. By increasing student involvement in becoming acquainted with data, they will begin to think of descriptive analysis as important in itself. Perhaps they will even equate it with having fun.

References

Chatterjee, S., and Price, B. *Regression analysis by example.* New York, John Wiley & Sons, 1977.

Dixon, W. J., and Brown, M. B., eds. *BMDP-79: Biomedical computer programs, P-Series.* rev. ed. Berkeley, University of California Press, 1979.

Ellis, R. Fallibilities, fragments, and frames: Contemplation on 25 years of research in medical-surgical nursing. *Nurs Res, 26*,177–182, May–June, 1977.

Nie, N. H., and others. SPSS: *Statistical package for the social sciences.* 2d ed. New York, McGraw-Hill Book Co., 1975.

Resio, D. T., and Verhonick, P. J. On the measurement and analysis of clinical data in nursing. *Nurs Res, 22*, 388–393, Sept.–Oct. 1973.

Tukey, J. W. *Exploratory data analysis.* Reading, Mass., Addison-Wesley Publishing Co., 1977.

Tukey, J. W. We need both exploratory and confirmatory. *Am Statist, 34*, 23–25, 1980.

*, **, and ***; Statistical Nonsense at the .00000 Level

Malcolm J. Slakter ■ **Yow-Wu B. Wu** ■ **Nancy S. Suzuki-Slakter**

We have all read and/or written journal articles where the tests of significance have been decorated in Christmas tree fashion with *, **, or ***. The .05 level is usually assigned * to indicate significant; the .01 level receives ** for very significant; and the .001, *** for extremely significant. A more popular alternative these days is to simply assign the p value spewed out by the computer when the statistical test is performed. For example, one might see $p = .0023$, or $p = .037$. Both *, **, ***, and p values are examples of setting the alpha level *after* the test of significance instead of before. This is statistical nonsense!

Why is this statistical nonsense? Because it represents several misinterpretations of the test of significance (Bakan, 1966; Sawyer & Peter, 1983; Smith, 1983). In this paper, we would like to emphasize two misinterpretations that have important practical implications for readers and writers of nursing research articles.

The first misinterpretation of the test of significance is the confusion of statistical significance with practical or clinical significance. The second misinterpretation is even more serious, as it concerns the assumption that power is irrelevant in the design and analysis of research. The historical reasons for this confusion are reviewed briefly by Sedlmeier and Gigerenzer (1989, pp. 314–315).

Confusion of Statistical Significance with Clinical Significance

Bakan (1966, p. 428) lists "taking the p value as a 'measure' of significance" as the first common misinterpretation of the test of significance, e.g., thinking of a p value of .05 as less significant than a p value of .01. Smith (1983) is even more explicit in pointing out the confusion of statistical significance with "practical meaningfulness" (p. 320), and the false assumption that small p values imply large effects or a strong relation (pp. 318–320).

In order to better appreciate the confusion of statistical significance with clinical or practical significance, we need to review the equivalence of a $(1 - \alpha)$ confidence interval with a corresponding test of the null hypothesis at the α level; e.g., in testing $H_0: \mu_1 - \mu_2 = 0$ versus $H_1: \mu_1 - \mu_2 \neq 0$, *if the $(1 - \alpha)$ confidence interval does not include 0, we reject H_0 at the α level; otherwise we fail to reject.* For example, in calculating the .95 confidence interval for the difference between two means if we find $6 < \mu_1 - \mu_2 < 13$, we would reject $H_0: \mu_1 - \mu_2 = 0$ at the .05 level because the interval does not include 0. On the other hand, if the .95 interval were $-2 < \mu_1 - \mu_2 < 7$, we would fail to reject H_0 at the .05 level because the interval does not include 0. One final note, the width of a confidence interval provides insight into the precision of the study. All things being equal, the shorter the width of the interval, the more precise (powerful) the study. (For a more in-depth look at confidence intervals, see Slakter, 1972.)

Now let us consider the results of a hypothetical study in which knowledge about AIDS was compared between RNs and non-RNs. First, assume the .999 confidence interval was: $.0003 < \mu_{RN} - \mu_{NRN} < .0007$. Since this .999 confidence interval does not include 0, we can reject the null hypothesis of no mean difference at the .001 level, and declare that we have statistical significance. But do we have clinical significance? Hardly. Even though the p level is quite small, there are not too many applications where differences of the magnitude of .0007 are apt to have clinical significance. However, suppose the results instead had produced the following .95 confidence interval: $15 < \mu_{RN} - \mu_{NRN} < 30$. Clearly, there is apt to be more clinical significance here *even though the alpha level is higher at. 05!* What is going on here? Obviously the first result is much more precise (width = .0007 − .0003 = .0004) than the second result (width = 30 − 15 = 15), undoubtedly because of a much larger sample size, which invariably determines the degree of precision. As another example, assume in a hypothetical correlational study that we are testing $H_0: \rho = 0$ versus $H_1: \rho \neq 0$. Consider a

Malcolm J. Slakter, PhD, is a professor, Department of Counseling and Educational Psychology, State University of New York at Buffalo.

Yow-Wu B. Wu, PhD, is an assistant professor, School of Nursing, State University of New York at Buffalo.

Nancy S. Suzuki-Slakter, PhD, is an educational psychologist in Honolulu, HI.

From *Nursing Research,* July/August 1991, *40,* 248–249.

.999 confidence interval of $.0006 < \rho < .0009$, where we would reject H_0 at the .001 level against a .95 confidence interval of $.6 < \rho < .7$, where we would also reject H_0 but "only" at the .05 level. Which is apt to have more clinical significance? The very precise (width = .0009 – .0006 = .0003) large sample study with H_0 rejected at the .001 level, or the less precise (width = .7 – .6 = .1) smaller sample study with H_0 rejected at the .05 level? So now we must come to grips with one important fact: *p* values are as much a function of sample size as they are of effect size or strength of relation. More precisely, *if the sample size is large enough, the null hypothesis of no treatment effect or no relation will always be rejected at any alpha level—as small as you want to make it* (Bakan, 1966, pp. 425–426). Therefore, it is exceedingly important to recognize that statistical significance does not guarantee clinical significance, and more to the point, *the magnitude of the p value (.05, .01, .001, .00029, or whatever) is no guide to clinical significance.*

Assuming Power Is Irrelevant in the Design and Analysis of a Research Study

The second misinterpretation involved with setting the alpha level after the test of significance rather than before is more serious. Unless alpha is preset, we are unable to decide on a sample size that will provide adequate power for detecting clinical significance. Hence, without power calculations we invariably end up with a sample size based on convenience, which in turn leads to studies that are (a) either too precise (powerful), resulting in everything being statistically significant whether or not it has clinical significance (e. g., $.0003 < \mu_{RN} - \mu_{NRN} < .0007$), or (b) studies that are apt to be too imprecise where it is almost impossible to detect statistical significance even when there is great clinical significance.

Unfortunately, in practice the evidence is quite clear that studies tend to be too imprecise. In a summary of articles from various research journals in which the power of studies was examined, Sedlmeier and Gigerenzer concluded that most had low average power (1989, pp. 310–314). They stated:

"In general, these studies reveal an apparently paradoxical state in research. Given the high premium placed by both researchers and journal editors on significant results . . . it seems strange that research was planned and conducted to give only a low chance of a significant result if there was a true effect. *Researchers paradoxically seem to prefer probable waste of time, money, and energy to the explicit calculation of power*" (p. 311). (Italics added.)

How Does One Avoid Wasting Time, Money, and Energy?

In designing a study, the sample size must be calculated for a given alpha to provide adequate power for a given clinically significant effect size or relation. This, of course, requires: (a) a preset alpha (and no indulgence in *, **, ***, or *p* value nonsense), (b) a preset β or the power $(1 - \beta)$, and (c) a decision on what constitutes clinical significance. Rather than delve further into the mechanics of this approach, the reader is referred to the following excellent sources: Cohen (1988), Goodwin (1984a, 1984b), Jacobsen & Meininger (1986), and Slakter (1972).

Summary

Researchers who report statistical significance with *, **, ***, or *p* values are confusing statistical significance with clinical significance and are wasting time, money, and energy with studies that are either too precise, or more likely too imprecise. Therefore, researchers who value their time, money, and energy should avoid this outmoded statistical procedure, and preset alpha to engage in the power calculation.

References

Bakan, D. (1966). The test of significance in psychological research. *Psychological Bulletin, 66,* 423–437.

Cohen, J. (1988). *Statistical power analysis for the behavioral sciences* (2nd ed.). Hillsdale, NJ: Lawrence-Erlbaum.

Goodwin, L. D. (1984a). The use of power estimation in nursing research. *Nursing Research, 33,* 118–120.

Goodwin, L. D. (1984b). Increasing efficiency and precision of data analysis. Multivariate vs. univariate statistical techniques. *Nursing Research, 33,* 247–249.

Jacobsen, B. S., & Meininger, J. C. (1986). Randomized experiments in nursing: The quality of reporting. *Nursing Research, 35,* 379–382.

Sawyer, A. G., & Peter, J. P. (1983). The significance of statistical significance tests in marketing research. *Journal of Marketing Research, 20,* 122–133.

Sedlmeier, P., & Gigerenzer, G. (1989). Do studies of statistical power have an effect on the power of studies? *Psychological Bulletin, 105,* 309–316.

Slakter, M. J. (1972). *Statistical inference for educational researchers.* Menlo Park, CA: Addison-Wesley.

Smith, K. (1983). Tests of significance: Some frequent misunderstandings. *American Journal of Orthopsychiatry, 53,* 315–321.

Testing for Experimental Effects in the Pretest-Posttest Design

Marlene J. Egger ■ Jean R. Miller

Researchers using pretest-posttest control group experimental designs are faced with the decision of choosing one of at least eight possible applications of *t* tests, including matched pairs, and two-sample *t* tests applied to raw gains, percentage changes, uncorrected posttest value, and variance-stabilized transformations of these variables. Some researchers avoid *t* tests in favor of analysis of covariance (ANCOVA) or blocked analysis of variance (Burckhardt, Goodwin, & Prescott, 1982). Nonparametric analogues of all these tests further complicate the decision.

A plethora of literature discusses the pitfalls inherent in common methods and lists caveats, but little attention has been given to algorithms for determining the appropriate analysis for the data at hand. Furthermore, ignorance of the relationships between gain scores, paired *t* tests, ANCOVA, and the assumptions of these tests lead to incorrect statements in the literature, such as "paired *t* tests should be preferred to tests of gain scores." In fact, the two procedures can be identical (Polit & Hungler, 1983). The real problem is that different analyses may produce different conclusions. It is crucial to choose an analysis logically, based on the statistical characteristics of the data, and *not* because the test procedure makes the results look more significant than some other test procedure does.

The purpose of the present paper is to provide a unified, logical exposition of analytic techniques that tests for treatment effects on groups in the pretest-posttest problem, to clarify potential pitfalls, and to provide a decision-making tree for easy determination of the appropriate test.

Marlene J. Egger, PhD, is assistant professor, Division of Biostatistics, Dept. of Family and Community Medicine at the University of Utah, Salt Lake City.

Jean R. Miller, PhD, RN, is Associate Dean for Research and Development at the College of Nursing, the University of Utah, Salt Lake City.

From *Nursing Research,* September/October 1984, *33,* 306–312.

T Tests

Some commonly conceived analytical strategies, diagrammed in Figure 1, use the notation of Campbell and Stanley (1963). Parametric tests (*t* tests, ANOVA, ANCOVA) will be considered, but their nonparametric analogues could be substituted if the data look nonnormal. The simplest parametric analysis conceivable would use a two-sample *t* test to compare the posttest scores of the experimental and control groups. Strategies 1a, 1b, and 1c are weak since they fail to check for baseline noncomparability between groups and correct for small individual differences at baseline. In particular, Strategy 1c provides no control for the Hawthorne effect, in which improvement occurs seemingly due to the sole fact that the individual participated in a study. Thus, if improvement is statistically significant in both the experimental and control groups, this strategy provides no measure of the degree of improvement attributable to the experimental condition.

Strategy 1d measures the degree of improvement for each individual by gain scores (i.e., posttest minus pretest differences), and these gains are compared across groups. A baseline comparison should also be performed. If significant baseline differences exist, Strategy 1d may or may not be sufficient to control for them, since it is a special case of the more general control for baseline values provided by ANCOVA Strategies 1h and 1j. For the moment, a competing strategy, 1e, might be to perform the same tests on the ratio of posttest/pretest scores. This strategy is the same as the percentage improvement[1] for the purpose of hypothesis testing. For example, measuring management success in terms of salary raises would in general require the study of percentage increases as well as dollar gains.

[1] Strictly speaking, percentage improvement = $\frac{\text{Post} - \text{Pre}}{\text{Pre}} \times 100$,
but this equals

$$100 \times \frac{\text{Post}}{\text{Pre}} - 100,$$

so the statistical tests will produce identical *p* values.

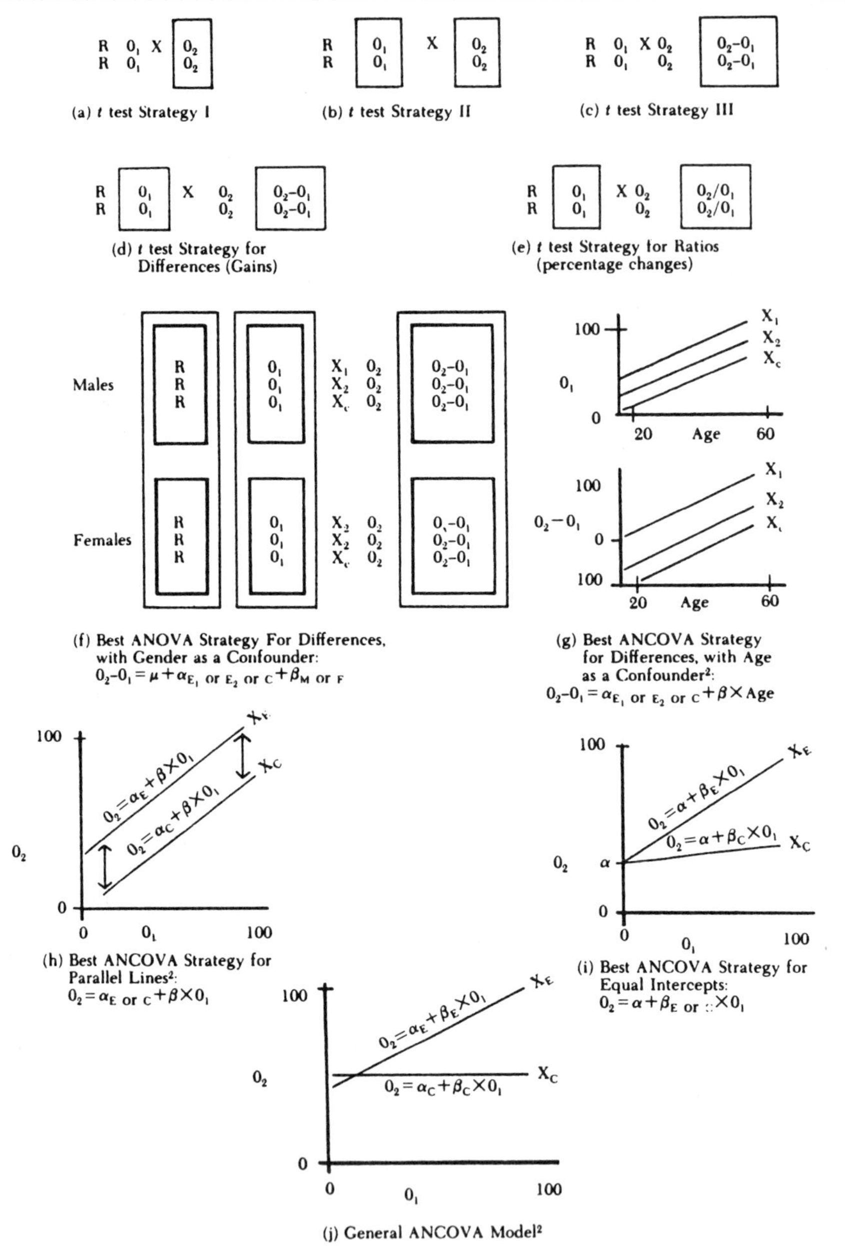

[1] Using Campbell and Stanley's (1963) notation, 0_1 and 0_2 are pretest and posttest values. *R* indicates randomization of subjects to experimental groups and X, X_1, X_2 are treatments. A blank, C, or X_c represents the concurrent controls or subjects given the reference treatment.

[2] Pretest analysis to check for noncomparability of groups should still be performed in strategies 1(g) through 1(j). Randomization to treatment and control groups is still assumed here.

FIGURE 1 Conceivable Analyses for the Pretest-Posttest Control Group Design[1]

Once a t-test strategy has been selected (usually d or e), the second part of the decision tree, Figure 2 (see pages 104–105), can be used to check distributional assumptions and to determine the correct computational form of the test.

When more than two groups must be compared or confounding variables must be controlled, similar strategies use analysis of variance (ANOVA) as in Figure 1f. In fact, the square of the pooled-variance t statistic is exactly an F statistic. For example, the two-way ANOVA in Figure 1f allows the effects of gender to be removed before experimental conditions are compared. The computation is different from, and inferentially superior to, t tests or one-way ANOVA done for males and females separately. More complicated aspects of ANOVA are discussed by statistical texts on experimental design (e.g., Cochran & Cox, 1957).

Analysis of Covariance

T tests are not always sufficient to control for pretest differences since they force the pretest-posttest relationship to be summarized by a simple gain or percentage change score. ANCOVA generalizes the t test by permitting more detailed description of the pretest-posttest relationship and changes resulting from the experimental condition. This analysis is different from the ANCOVA familiar to most researchers, in which gain scores are adjusted for continuous confounding factors such as age. Description of t tests as special cases of ANCOVA can provide the basis for a logical decision-tree approach to help choose an analysis for a pretest-posttest experimental design.

Ignoring confounder variables, the general ANCOVA Model 1j is:

$$\text{expected posttest value} = \text{adjusted mean (group height)} + \text{slope} \times \text{pretest value, or,}$$

$$E(0_2) = \alpha_E + \beta_E \times 0_1,$$

in the treatment group, and

$$E(0_2) = \alpha_C + \beta_C \times 0_1$$

for controls.

Pretest values are assumed to have been chosen by the researcher, and individuals' deviations from these equations are assumed to be independent and normally distributed with equal variances. Mathematically, ANCOVA is simply a generalization of ANOVA and regression. Elashoff (1969) discussed the implications of these assumptions, the first of which is usually broken in practice. Any number of treatment groups can be compared by ANCOVA. For simplicity, the subsequent discussion will assume that one treatment group is being compared to one control group.

An experimental condition may have an incremental effect on the pretest-posttest equations above, moving each point on the line a constant distance up or down. The overall height of a pretest-posttest line in ANCOVA is characterized by intercept α_E or α_C, the actual height of the line at the posttest axis. Alternatively, the experimental condition may have a stronger effect for some pretest values than others, consequently changing the tilt of the pretest-posttest line. Tilt is characterized by the slopes β_E and β_C. The slopes are related to the reliability of the test and are exactly equal to the correlation coefficients[2] between pre- and posttests if the pre- and posttest standard deviations σ_1 and σ_2 are equal within each group.

The parallel line ANCOVA model of Figure 1h models experimental conditions with only incremental effects and is the model commonly called ANCOVA. Thus, the improvement attributable to the treatment group is the vertical distance $\alpha_E - \alpha_C$. This difference is more precise than the difference in mean gains.

Equal intercepts Model 1i applies to experimental conditions that change the tilt but not the height at the posttest axis. The crossed-line Model 1j is used for experimental conditions that produce both effects on the pretest-posttest line. In both of these models, the experimental condition changes either the correlation between pretest and posttest values or the variability of the posttest.

An obvious example of the crossed-line model is a treatment or experimental condition consisting of an announcement to the class that anyone with a pretest score above 50 is expected to do much better on the posttest. Higher pretesters would be expected to do better on the posttest, simply by suggestion. The experimental condition is thus directly confounded with the pretest values. One situation where crossed ANCOVA lines occur is a biological assay, comparing the dose-response curve of a new drug to a standard, when the new drug's mechanism of action is dissimilar to the mechanism of action of the standard. In that case, the new drug cannot be considered to have an effect equivalent to the effect of some dilution of the standard drug. The most extreme example of crossed pretest-posttest lines would be the case where the experimental condition yields the best posttest scores for low pretesters, and the control or reference condition yields the best posttest scores for high pretesters. In this case, mean gain scores are likely to be equal, even though ANCOVA will find significant differences in slopes and intercepts.

---

[2] This is exactly true only for the general ANCOVA Model 1j.

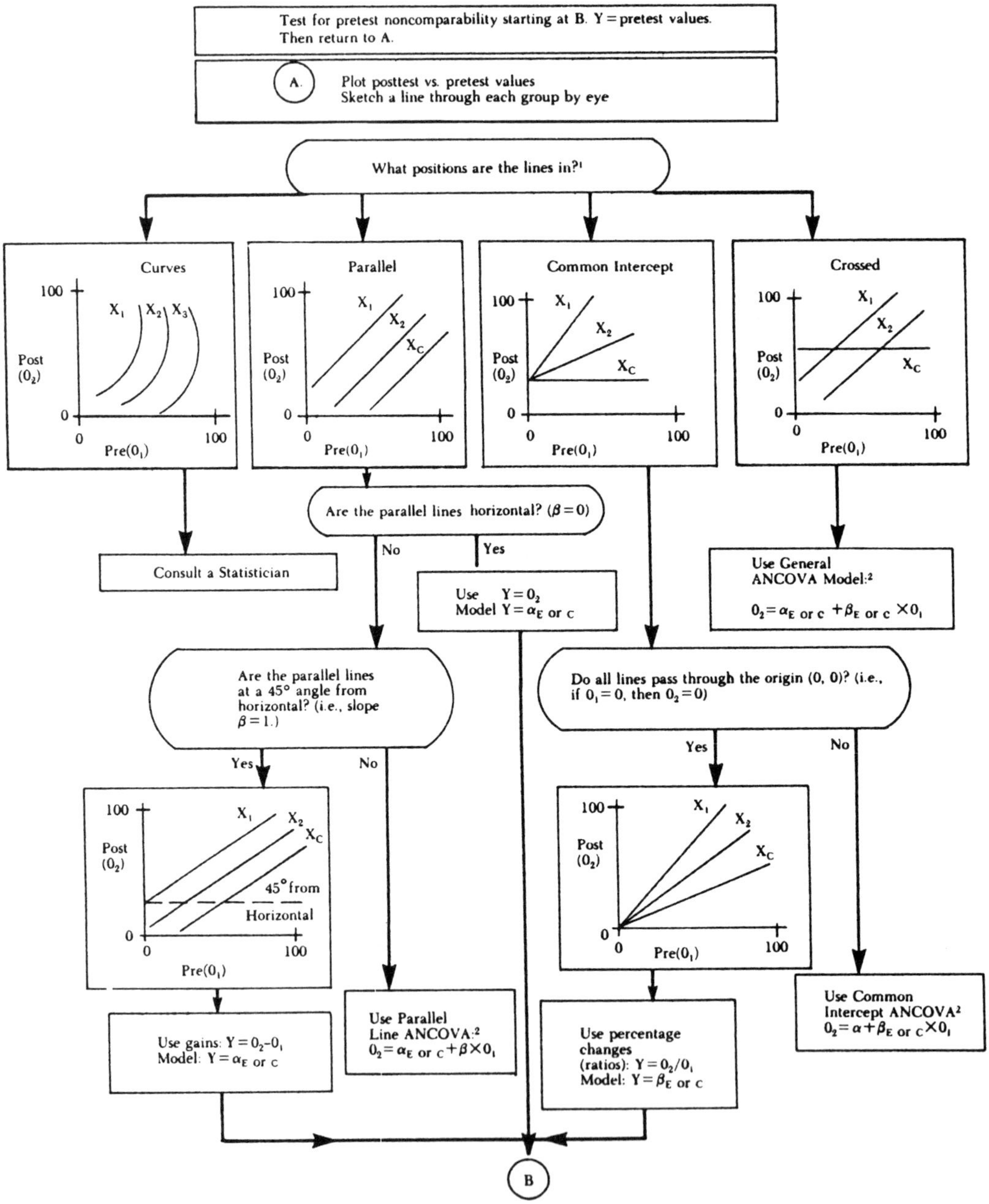

FIGURE 2 Decision Tree

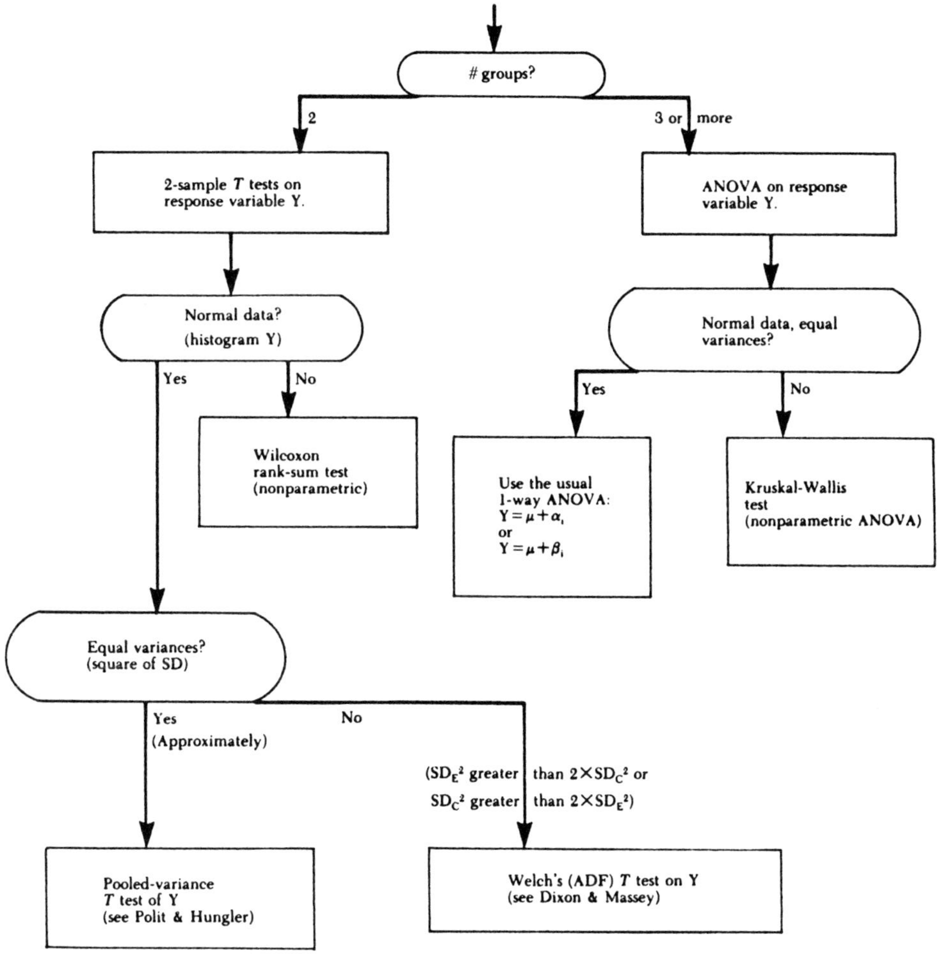

[1] If positions of lines are not obvious, there are statistical tests to identify them. Consult a statistician.

[2] Residuals $O_2 - \hat{\alpha} - \hat{\beta} O_2$ from ANCOVA should always be histogrammed to check the normality assumption. If the histogram is not approximately symmetric and bell-shaped, consult a statistician.

FIGURE 2 ***(CONTINUED)***

ANCOVA Analyses Equivalent to T Tests

In the special case where slopes $\beta_E = \beta_C = 1$, the lines tilt at 45° from the horizontal, and the parallel line ANCOVA model reduces to:

$$E(0_2) = \alpha_i + 0_1, \text{ or}$$

expected posttest value = height + pretest value.

This could equivalently be expressed:

$$E(0_2 - 0_1) = \alpha_E,$$

for the treatment group, and

$$E(0_2 - 0_1) = \alpha_C,$$

for the controls.

Thus, when a plot of the data reveals parallel pretest-posttest lines with slopes equal to 1, all the information about the experimental effect is contained in the gain scores. The appropriate analysis is either the pooled variance *t* test on gains or Welch's test (Dixon & Massey, 1969), depending on whether the standard deviations of the gains in the treatment and control groups are equal or unequal (Fig. 2). In this case, the correct ANCOVA analysis is identical to the correct analysis on gains (1d) and therefore ANCOVA cannot improve on the poor reliability of gain scores. This is contrary to the claim of Burckhardt et al. (1982).

Similarly, ANCOVA Strategy 1i reduces to *t* tests on percentage changes (i.e., Strategy 1e) in the special case where $\alpha_E = \alpha_C = 0$. The ANCOVA model is then: expected posttest value = group slope × pretest value; or

$$E(0_2) = \beta_E \times 0_1,$$

for the experimental group, which can be rewritten as:

$$E(0_2/0_1) = \beta_E,$$

and similarly for the control group. Thus, when a plot of the data reveals pretest-posttest lines, both originating at the point (0,0) on the graph, *t* tests on percentage changes should be used as in Figure 3, page 107.

If terms for confounder variables such as age and sex are added to the general ANCOVA model, Figures 1f and 1g are also found to be special cases of ANCOVA. Thus, all of the useful hypothesis-testing strategies, 1d through 1j, may be identified by plotting the posttest versus pretest values and inspecting the slopes and intercepts of the regression lines. A systematic approach can be done from the general ANCOVA model to a special case by a series of statistical tests on the slopes and intercepts, although eyeball inspection is often adequate as specified by the logical decision tree of Figure 2.

A Comment on Nonparametric Tests

Although parametric tests have been discussed almost exclusively, similar considerations apply to nonparametric tests (Siegel, 1956). The sign test has very poor power, and is not generally used. Wilcoxon tests are about 95% efficient relative to *t* tests if the data were actually from a normal distribution. Nonparametric tests can have considerably better power than *t* tests for some non-normal distributions, such as the exponential distribution (Lehmann, 1975). Nonparametric methods also exist for ANCOVA (Conover & Iman, 1982).

Examples

Results of a pretest-posttest control group experimental design are obtained and plotted as in Figure 3a. Following the decision-tree logic (Fig. 2), a line is drawn through each group's data by eye: $0_2 = 35 + 0_1$ for the treatment group (*x*) and $0_2 = 10 + 1.1 \times 0_1$ for the controls (*o*). (See Appendix, page 108.) These lines are not horizontal but parallel, each with slopes approximately equal to 1, so the use of gain scores $0_2 - 0_1$ is appropriate. The decision tree now requires the gains for each group to be histogrammed, and group means and standard deviations (SD) calculated. Suppose that in the example, the histogram is roughly bell-shaped in each group, and the variances, or squares of the standard deviations, are $SD_E^2 = 20.1$, $SD_C^2 = 41.3$. The decision tree indicates that nonparametric tests will not be used and the variances are not approximately equal, so Welch's *t* test is the appropriate statistical test of the gain scores. If the slopes had been equal but more different from 1, the correct approach would have been the parallel line ANCOVA.

Figure 3b shows a similar example, this time with (roughly) $0_2 = 75 + .01 \times 0_1$ for the treatment group and $0_2 = 35 - .02 \times 0_1$ for the controls. These lines are roughly parallel and nearly horizontal (i.e., the posttest values fall into one clump for controls and a higher clump for the treatment group, regardless of the pretest values). For example, guests at a cocktail party have their blood alcohol measured. Half are randomly assigned to a no-alcohol group, and half to a one-drink-per-hour group; everyone's blood alcohol is retested 24 hours later. Posttest values in each group should be fairly uniform, regardless of pretest values. Since pretest values are irrelevant here, *t* tests (or their nonparametric analogues) on posttest values 0_2 are appropriate.

Lines drawn through the data for Figure 3c are neither parallel nor have a common intercept. They fall into the category of crossed lines since they would have crossed if the maximum possible score had not been 100. Hence, the control group doesn't change appreciably from pretest to posttest (roughly $0_2 = 0_1$), but the treated group shows substantial improvement for low pretesters ($0_2 = 50 + 0.5 \times 0_1$). Equality of slopes and intercepts is statistically tested, and the general ANCOVA model is used. Use of gain scores in this example would be less powerful (less likely to detect a difference between treat-

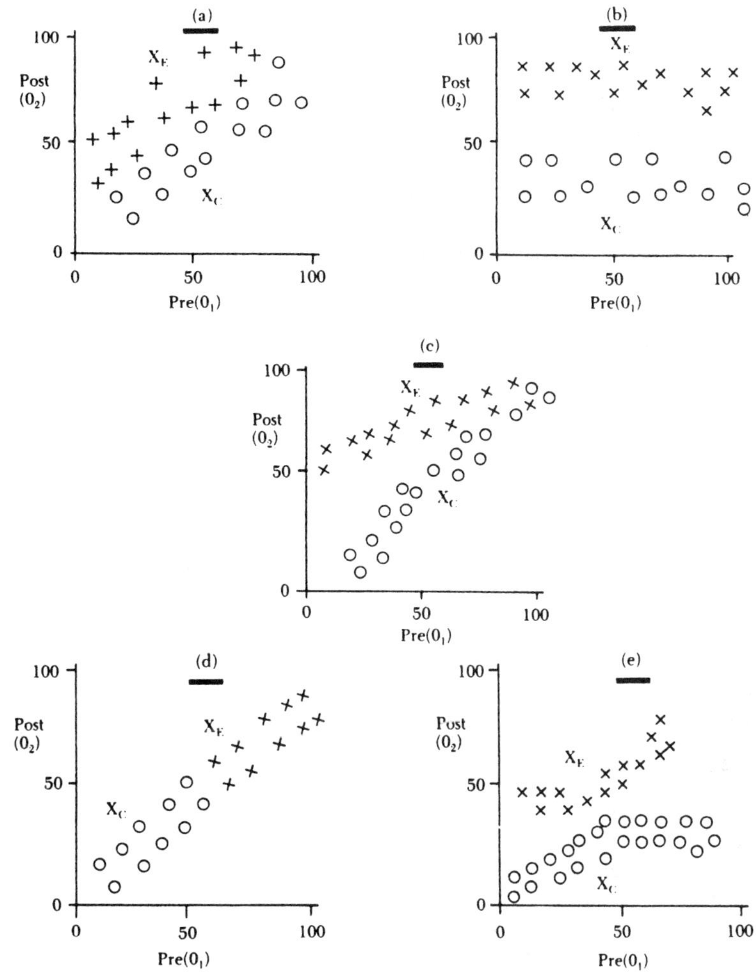

FIGURE 3 Examples

ment group and controls) because of the proximity of the two groups for high pretest scores.

Figure 3d has been widely discussed in the literature (Cox & McCullagh, 1982; Lord, 1967, 1969). Theoretically, since both treatment and control groups lie on the same line through the origin, $0_2 = 0.7 \times 0_1$, any logical path through the decision tree should lead to the same conclusion: no differences between groups. For example, the lines could be described as parallel lines (equal slopes), not horizontal, with slopes $\neq 1$. The parallel line ANCOVA tests the group means adjusted for the common slope, and should detect no statistically significant differences between intercepts (heights) (i.e., no differences between treatment and control groups). Alternatively, starting from the fact that the lines have common intercepts, and that they pass through the (0,0) point, the percentage change or ratio model is appropriate and should conclude that the average posttest-pretest ratios are not significantly different (in fact, they are both 0.7) in the two groups.

The worst possible strategy would be to use the gains model. It is likely to find statistically significant differences between the two groups because it is making the wrong correction for noncomparability of the groups at pretest time. However, Lord (1969) pointed out that any statistical analysis of such data is imperiled by the baseline noncomparability, since each strategy requires extrapolation from the data in each group to the higher or lower pretest values where data have not been collected.

If the true trend changed unexpectedly, as in Figure 3e, all the previous analyses would be invalidated by an incorrect extrapolation. No statistical technique can completely patch up the results of bad randomization. The most important insight here came not from any statistical strategy, but simply from plotting the data and observing that both groups fell without overlap along the same line.

A Priori Considerations

An adequate number of subjects is crucial to the outcome of any experimental design. Too few subjects cause clinically meaningful differences between groups to be statistically undetectable, even if the decision-tree logic is carefully followed. Too many subjects cause clinically negligible differences to be statistically significant. Further, sample size calculations done before the start of the study usually refer to gain scores or percentage changes. For samples of more than 20 subjects per group, these calculations will be conservative even if ANCOVA is the ultimate analytical strategy. However, since these calculations do not apply to the test of baseline (0_1) differences between groups, the researcher will want to scrutinize the test of noncomparability carefully to verify that statistically nonsignificant differences between groups at the pretest were also clinically nonsignificant.

Some researchers prefer to block subjects by pretest values and randomize to treatment and control groups within blocks, rather than using post hoc ANCOVA. Feldt (1958) showed that compared to parallel line ANCOVA with pretest and posttest variances equal in each group, such a blocked factorial ANOVA design is marginally more powerful when the correlation between pretest and posttest scores is less than 0.4. However, this margin totals about four patients per hundred. Feldt did not consider the cases of unequal variances or nonparallel ANCOVA models. If his assumptions can be verified by a pilot study or previous reports in the literature, or if the posttest versus pretest relationship may be curvilinear, the blocked factorial experimental design should be considered at the study design stage.

Conclusions

Analysis of data from the pretest-posttest design might be capsulized by the injunction "Plot the data!" A slightly more descriptive summary would be:

1. Plot the posttest versus pretest scores to determine their empirical relationship.

2. Following the decision-tree logic, increase statistical power by making all the asumptions that appear reasonable (e.g., slopes = 1 or equal intercepts).

3. Apply the simplest appropriate test to the data.

4. If a clinically meaningful treatment effect is obvious on the plot, but the appropriate test finds the effect nonsignificant, or vice versa, consult a statistician.

Careful adherence to the logic of the pretest-posttest design in the analysis phase protects the researcher from analytical blunders that change the conclusions of the study, or worse, leave one vulnerable to the accusation of fixing the numbers to prove a theory.

References

Burckhardt, C. S., Goodwin, L. D., & Prescott, P. A. (1982). The measurement of change in nursing research: Statistical considerations. *Nursing Research, 31,* 53–55.

Campbell, D. T., & Stanley, J. C. (1963). *Experimental and quasi-experimental designs for research.* Boston: Houghton Mifflin.

Cochran, W. G., & Cox, G. M. (1957). *Experimental designs* (2nd ed.). New York: John Wiley & Sons.

Conover, W. J., & Iman, R. L. (1982). Analysis of covariance using the rank transformation. *Biometrics, 38,* 715–724.

Cox, D. R., & McCullagh, P. (1982). Some aspects of analysis of covariance. *Biometrics, 38,* 541–554.

Dixon, W. J., & Massey, F. J., Jr. (1969). *Introduction to statistical analysis* (3rd ed.). New York: McGraw-Hill.

Elashoff, J. D. (1969). Analysis of covariance: A delicate instrument. *American Educational Research Journal, 6,* 383–401.

Feldt, L. S. (1958). A comparison of the precision of three experimental designs employing a concomitant variable. *Psychometrika, 23,* 335–353.

Lehmann, E. L. (1975). *Nonparametrics: Statistical methods based on ranks.* San Francisco: Holden-Day.

Lord, F. M. (1967). A paradox in the interpretation of group comparisons. *Psychological Bulletin, 68,* 304–305.

Lord, F. M. (1969). Statistical adjustments when comparing pre-existing groups. *Psychological Bulletin, 72,* 336–337.

Polit, D. F., & Hungler, B. P. (1983). *Nursing research: Principles and methods* (2nd ed.). Philadelphia: J. B. Lippincott.

Siegel, S. (1956). *Nonparametric statistics for the behavioral sciences.* New York: McGraw-Hill.

APPENDIX

Determining the Equation of a Line

1. Draw a line through one group's data by eye.
2. Pick two points on that line, as far apart as is practical, and list their pretest and posttest (x and y) coordinates.

Point	Pretest (x)	Posttest (y)
1	20	32
2	80	98

3. Calculate the slope (m) of the line from the two points:

$$m = \frac{rise}{run} = \frac{y_2 - y_1}{x_2 - x_1}, \quad \text{e.g.,} \quad = \frac{98 - 32}{80 - 20} = 1.1$$

4. Using the two-point formula, the equation of the line is:

$$y - y_1 = m(x - x_1),$$

or

$$y = mx - mx_1 + y_1;$$

e.g.,

$$y = 1.1x - 1.1(20) + 32,$$

$$y = 10 + 1.1x.$$

Increasing Efficiency and Precision of Data Analysis: Multivariate vs. Univariate Statistical Techniques

Laura D. Goodwin

A review of research articles published in *Nursing Research* and other research-oriented journals in nursing and related health professions during the past several years indicates a frequent use of data analysis techniques that are less efficient and precise than other alternatives. More specifically, several of these articles reported the use of multiple univariate strategies when multivariate strategies would have been a better choice. The purpose of this paper is to discuss the advantages of multivariate over univariate techniques for several representative situations. This discussion is not an exhaustive treatment of multivariate statistics. Rather, it is intended to review some commonly used multivariate approaches to data analysis, and to point out their general advantages in typical situations—the use of multifactor or factorial analysis of variance (ANOVA), or separate one-way or single-factor ANOVAs; the use of multivariate analysis of variance (MANOVA), or separate univariate ANOVAs; and the use of multiple regression analysis, or separate simple correlational analyses. Other somewhat less typical multivariate vs. univariate choices will also be discussed.

General Advantages of Multivariate Techniques

There are three general advantages in using a single multivariate analysis to test the hypotheses in a research study: (1) ability to keep alpha at a known and accurate level; (2) an increase in power; and (3) ease in computation and interpretation.

Alpha Considerations

One very important reason for using multivariate techniques rather than separate univariate techniques is to keep control over alpha (α), the probability of a Type I error. For example, consider the related but simpler choice of conducting a one-way ANOVA or multiple *t* tests when there are more than two group means to be compared to test a null hypothesis of the type H_o: $\mu_1 = \mu_2 = \ldots = \mu_J$. If multiple *t* tests are conducted (and there would be

$$\frac{J(J-1)}{2}$$

of them, where *J* equals the number of groups), the alpha level for the entire set of *t* tests would be much greater than the nominal, or tabled, alpha level desired to use for a single comparison. As Keppel (1982) and Kirk (1968) pointed out, the actual probability of obtaining at least one significant comparison by chance (i.e., alpha level) for a set of independent *t* tests is: $\alpha = 1 - (1 - \text{“}\alpha\text{”})^c$, where α is the Type I error probability for a set of *t* tests; "α" is the nominal Type I error probability or Type I error level per comparison; and *C* is the number of comparisons to be made (i.e., the number of separate *t* tests). This formula refers to the alpha level for a set of multiple independent *t* tests. The corresponding probability for nonindependent multiple comparisons is difficult to estimate (but certainly is greater than the alpha level for any single comparison), thereby compounding the problem even further (Kirk, 1968). And, in most uses of multiple *t* tests for a given set of data, the *t* tests are not independent of each other because the various means enter into more than one test.

As an example of this problem, consider a situation where one is comparing average cognitive achievement scores for four groups of nursing students, each group having been taught the same lesson plan by a different type of instructional method. The levels of the independent variable (type of instructional method) might be (1) lecture only; (2) films only; (3) lecture and films; or (4) self-instructional module. The basic null hypothesis is H_o: $\mu_L = \mu_F = \mu_{L+F} = \mu_M$. If the desired alpha level for the hypothesis test were .05, and six separate *t* tests were conducted on the data, the actual alpha for the set of six tests would be at least:

$$\begin{aligned} \alpha &= 1 - (1 - .05)^c \\ &= 1 - (.95)^6 \\ &= 1 - .74 \\ &= .26 \end{aligned}$$

Laura D. Goodwin, PhD, is an associate professor at the University of Colorado at Denver, School of Education, Denver, CO.

From *Nursing Research,* July/August 1984, *33,* 247–249.

Alpha thus is spuriously inflated. A much better strategy would be to conduct a single one-way ANOVA, followed by appropriate multiple comparison tests if the overall *F* is statistically significant at the preset alpha level. (For a discussion of multiple comparison techniques, see Hopkins & Anderson, 1973; Keppel, 1982; or Kirk, 1968.)

This same principle applies to the use of multivariate strategies as opposed to separate univariate strategies in more complex designs. If a study with multiple independent variables is conducted, a multifactor or factorial ANOVA is preferable to separate ANOVAs for each independent variable. Consider an extension of the above example, in which two other independent variables might be added to the design: sex (male vs. female) and age (20–25; 26–30; 30–35). There are now three main effect null hypotheses to be tested:

$$H_o: \mu_L = \mu_F = \mu_{L+F} = \mu_M$$
$$H_o: \mu_M = \mu_F$$
$$H_o: \mu_{20-25} = \mu_{26-30} = \mu_{30-35}$$

If three separate one-way ANOVAs instead of a single three-way ANOVA were conducted, the alpha level for the entire set of tests would be spuriously inflated, for the same reason as was shown in the simpler example. Further, the separate univariate ANOVAs approach precludes the direct testing of the first- and second-order interaction hypotheses, resulting in a loss of power and information.

A final example of the benefits of multivariate over separate univariate techniques in relation to keeping control over the alpha level is illustrated by the choice of using a multivariate analysis of variance (MANOVA) or separate ANOVAs when there are multiple dependent variables in the study. Consider another extension of the hypothetical study, this time incorporating three dependent variables—cognitive learning achievement, attitudes toward the content area, and skill levels. Three separate three-way ANOVAs could be conducted, one for each of the dependent variables, or MANOVA could be used. The MANOVA approach would keep the alpha level at a known and constant rate for the entire set of univariate tests subsumed under it. Thus, it provides an overall protection for alpha by accurately estimating the probability of a Type I error across the package of dependent variables considered simultaneously (Gabriel & Hopkins, 1974). If the *F* ratio for MANOVA is statistically significant at the preset alpha level, the results of the three univariate ANOVAs would be examined to determine the effects of the independent variables on each dependent variable separately. (This is similar to using multiple comparison techniques to study pairwise comparisons among means, following the detection of a significant *F* ratio from a one-way ANOVA.) Thus, the significant MANOVA *F* ratio allows more confident interpretation of the results of the univariate analyses. A nonsignificant MANOVA *F* ratio indicates that it would be inappropriate to examine further the univariate *F* ratios for statistical significance, since the actual alpha level for any one of those tests would be greater than the initial preset, nominal alpha level. Gabriel and Hopkins summed up the undesirable effect on alpha of using multiple univariate ANOVAs in a study with multiple dependent variables:

> In repeated applications of univariate ANOVA, the probability of one or more Type I errors in the set of analyses is unknown in all but the limiting and unrepresentative cases—where all outcome measures intercorrelate zero or where all intercorrelate perfectly. If the *K* measures exhibit perfect correlation, the overall probability of one or more Type I errors is simply α. If all criteria intercorrelate zero, the probability of one or more Type I errors is $1 - (1 - \alpha)^K$. These extremes are never in evidence except in contrived situations. [1974, pp. 378–79]

Power Considerations

The second reason for preferring multivariate techniques over separate univariate techniques is related to power (the probability of rejecting the null hypothesis if it is false). Consider, again, the use of three separate one-way ANOVAs versus a single factorial ANOVA in the example given above with three independent variables and one dependent variable. The General Linear Model that underlies each separate one-way ANOVA is:

$$X_{ij} = \mu + \alpha_j + e_i$$

Where X_{ij} = a person's (the ith person in group j) score on the dependent variable

μ = the grand mean (a constant for each person), estimated by $\bar{X}..$

α_j = the group effect for group J (i.e., the elevation or depression of a person's score due to the fact that she is in a particular treatment group), estimated by $(\bar{X}_j - \bar{X}..)$

e_{ij} = the error component (difference between the person's score and the average score for the group she is in), estimated by $(X_{ij} - \bar{X}_j)$.

The estimation of MS_B (Mean Squares Between) is based on the variance in the data due to α_j, the group or treatment effect, while MS_W (Mean Squares Within) reflects the within-group variance due to error (e_{ij}). One major way to increase power is to reduce MS_W, and thereby increase the F ratio (MS_B/MS_W). By using the factorial ANOVA approach, the General Linear Model for the single three-way ANOVA becomes:

$$X_{ijkm} = \mu + \alpha_j + B_k + Y_m + \alpha B_{jk} + \alpha Y_{jm} + BY_{km} + \alpha BY_{jkm} + e_{ijkm}$$

where B_k represents the group effect for the second independent variable; Y_m represents the group effect for the third independent variable; and αB_{jk}, αY_{jm}, BY_{km}, and αBY_{jkm} represent the interaction effects between each pair of independent variables as well as among all three together.

Here, the error component (MS_W) will be reduced by "pulling" what was part of error in the one-way model into the components associated with the additional main effects and interaction effects. That is, the additional independent variables can account for some of the original within-groups or error variance (assuming the presence of main effects and/or interactions involving these variables), thus reducing the MS_W for the F test of the major null hypothesis of interest. This, then, increases the power for that test.

Closely related is the advantage of adding a covariate to an ANOVA, that is, using analysis of covariance (ANCOVA, another multivariate strategy) if one has available a covariate that correlates well with the dependent variable, and if the additional assumptions involved in ANCOVA can be met. ANCOVA increases the power over ANOVA by reducing MS_W (Cook & Campbell, 1979; Kirk, 1968; Winer, 1971). The reduction is approximately:

$$MS_{W'} = MS_W(1 - r^2)$$

where $MS_{W'}$ is the adjusted MS_W from ANCOVA; MS_W is the unadjusted MS_W from ANOVA; and r^2 is the squared correlation between the covariate and the dependent variable. Thus, if there was an available covariate (such as pretest scores in a pretest-posttest comparison group study) that correlated .60 with the dependent variable (posttest scores), the MS_W in ANCOVA would be reduced to approximately .64 [i.e., $(1-.6^2)$] of its original size.

In general, then, multivariate techniques can result in an increase in power as compared to the power in separate univariate techniques, provided the additional variables incorporated into the analysis have some relationship to the dependent variable. (The additional variables usually do have some relationship to the dependent variable, since that expected relationship dictated the decision to include them in the first place.) The relationship to the dependent variable results in variance accounted for that otherwise would be included as error variance in the analysis.

Computation and Interpretation Considerations

A final reason why multivariate strategies are preferable to separate univariate strategies is that they represent a more efficient way of conducting analyses and interpreting results. In the simple, non-multivariate comparison of a one-way ANOVA versus six separate t tests, the one-way ANOVA is certainly a simpler and more efficient computational approach. In the comparison of the factorial, three-way ANOVA versus three separate univariate ANOVAs, the multivariate ANOVA requires just one ANOVA; further, and more important in this example, the three-way ANOVA allows the detection of the presence of interactions among the independent variables and thereby increases the information yield. It would be extremely cumbersome, inefficient, and imprecise to attempt to test each main effect and interaction effect via separate one-, two-, and three-way ANOVAs, although the use of such an approach can be found in recently published research articles. In the comparison of MANOVA versus separate ANOVAs when there are multiple dependent variables, the economy of the more complex multivariate techniques is again illustrated. In a single analysis, all of the same information is obtained that would be obtained via the separate ANOVAs and the added important advantage of the overall protection of the alpha level is provided.

Another multivariate versus separate univariates comparison that illustrates computational and interpretation advantages is the use of multiple regression analysis instead of multiple simple correlational analyses when the association between a number of independent variables and a single dependent variable is studied. Likewise, canonical correlation is a multivariate strategy that allows simultaneous examination of the relationships among multiple independent and multiple dependent variables. In both cases, the multivariate approaches afford a simpler and more economical way of obtaining all of the information desired, and facilitate interpretation of the many interrelationships among the variables. (For a good discussion of multiple regression, see Chatterjee & Price, 1977; Kerlinger & Pedhazur, 1973; Weisburg, 1980; and, for a discussion of canonical correlation, see Cooley & Lohnes, 1971; and Harris, 1975.)

Summary

In deciding upon an appropriate analysis strategy during the planning phase of a research study, it is important to specify all of the independent and dependent variables to be included. From there, a technique should be chosen that will yield all of the information desired in the most efficient, precise, and powerful way. Frequently, the method of choice in nursing research will be a multivariate technique, since so many studies involve numerous variables whose effects on, or relationships with, other variables are of interest, as well as involving additional variables that should be taken into account for control or generalizability purposes.

Not discussed in this paper, but worth mention, is the fact that all of these techniques involve various underlying assumptions (e.g., normality, homogeneity of variance, and independence in ANOVA) that must be met in order to use the techniques appropriately. If the assumptions are not met, the researcher might want to consider the use of nonparametric techniques—and there are both univariate and multivariate techniques available to choose from (Hollander & Wolfe, 1973; Siegel, 1956). The general advantages of a multivariate technique rather than separate univariate techniques would apply in terms of nonparametric statistics as well as parametric statistics.

Increasing the accuracy, power, and efficiency of data analysis strategies should be a major concern to researchers. An otherwise very well-designed study can suffer from a poor choice of statistical techniques in terms of inaccurate estimations, lack of power to detect "true" significant difference, or cumbersome and inefficient reporting of results. Multivariate statistical techniques were developed to handle the analysis of data in studies with complex and multivariate data sets, and should be used whenever possible.

References

Chatterjee, S., & Price, B. (1977). *Regression analysis by example.* New York: John Wiley.

Cook, T. D., & Campbell, D. T. (1979). *Quasi-experimentation: Design and analysis issues for field settings.* Chicago: Rand McNally.

Cooley, W. W., & Lohnes, P. R. (1971). *Multivariate data analysis.* New York: John Wiley.

Gabriel, R. M., & Hopkins, K. D. (1974). Relative merits of MANOVA, repeated measures ANOVA, and univariate ANOVAs for research utilizing multiple criterion measures. *Journal of Special Education, 8,* 377–389.

Harris, R. J. (1975). *A primer of multivariate statistics.* New York: Academic Press.

Hollander, M., & Wolfe, D. A. (1973). *Nonparametric statistical methods.* New York: John Wiley.

Hopkins, K. D., & Anderson, B. L. (1973). A guide to multiple-comparison techniques: Criteria for selecting the method of choice. *Journal of Special Education, 7,* 319–327.

Keppel, G. (1982). *Decision and analysis: A researcher's handbook* (2nd ed.). Englewood Cliffs, NJ: Prentice-Hall.

Kerlinger, F. N., & Pedhazur, E. J. (1973). *Multiple regression in behavioral research.* New York: Holt, Rinehart & Winston.

Kirk, R. E. (1968). *Experimental design: Procedures for the behavioral sciences.* Belmont, CA: Wadsworth.

Siegel, S. (1956). *Nonparametric statistics for the behavioral sciences.* New York: McGraw-Hill.

Weisburg, S. (1980). *Applied linear regression.* New York: John Wiley.

Winer, B. J. (1971). *Statistical procedures in experimental design* (2nd ed.). New York: McGraw-Hill.

Increasing the Precision of Data Analysis: Planned Comparisons vs. Omnibus Tests

Yow-Wu B. Wu ■ Malcolm J. Slakter

The issue of increasing the power of statistical tests and the precision of estimation has been addressed recently in nursing research literature (e.g., Cobb, 1985; Goodwin, 1984a, 1984b). In discussing the increasing of power and precision, Goodwin (1984b), stated that multiple *t* tests will inflate the alpha rate; therefore, "A much better strategy would be a single one-way ANOVA, followed by appropriate multiple comparison tests if the overall *F* is statistically significant at the pre-set alpha level."

The underlying question is how to increase the power and at the same time control the Type I error. The purpose of this article is to compare the power (precision) for a given alpha level of two approaches: planned comparisons (i.e., multiple *t* tests) vs. an omnibus test (i.e., single one-way ANOVA), "... followed by appropriate multiple comparisons tests if the overall *F* is statistically significant at the pre-set alpha level." Guidelines for using thesc two techniques will also be provided.

An Example of the Two Approaches

Goodwin (1984b, p. 247) introduces the following relevant example:

> As an example of this problem, consider a situation where one is comparing average cognitive achievement scores for four groups of nursing students, each group having been taught the same lesson plan by a different type of instructional method. The levels of the independent variable (type of instructional method) might be (1) lecture only; (2) films only; (3) lecture and films; or (4) self-instructional module.

The omnibus test would examine the null hypothesis H_0: $\mu_1 = \mu_2 = \mu_3 = \mu_4$, and if H_0 were rejected an appropriate multiple comparison test would follow.

Yow-Wu B. Wu, PhD, is an assistant professor in the School of Nursing, State University of New York at Buffalo.

Malcolm J. Slakter, PhD, is a professor in the Department of Counseling and Educational Psychology, State University of New York at Buffalo.

From *Nursing Research,* July/August 1990, *39,* 251–253.

The planned comparison approach, however, would instead focus attention on comparing a few specified subsets of means. These comparisons or contrasts would enable the researcher to increase the power while at the same time controlling the Type I error. To illustrate, with planned comparisons the researcher might examine differences between all possible pairs as follows:

$$H_{01} : \mu_1 = \mu_2$$
$$H_{02} : \mu_1 = \mu_3$$
$$H_{03} : \mu_1 = \mu_4$$
$$H_{04} : \mu_2 = \mu_3$$
$$H_{05} : \mu_2 = \mu_4$$
$$H_{06} : \mu_3 = \mu_4$$

To continue the comparison of these two approaches, the concept of a contrast must be introduced.

Contrasts

Common to both approaches is the concept of a contrast or comparison between two sets of means. More specifically, a contrast (ψ) is a weighted sum of group means ($\psi = \Sigma C_j \mu_j$) in which the sum of these weights equals zero ($\Sigma C_j = 0$), and not all of the weights are zero. (See Table 1 for the coefficients of the contrasts described in the example above.) The estimated contrast is denoted as $\hat{\psi}$ where $\hat{\psi} = \Sigma C_j \hat{\mu}_j$ and in a one-way ANOVA the estimated variance of the contrast $\hat{\psi}$ is

$$\hat{\sigma}^2_{\hat{\psi}} = MS_w \Sigma \frac{C_j^2}{n_j}$$

See Kirk (1982, chap. 3) or Slakter (1972, chap. 18) for further discussions on contrasts.

Omnibus Test

An omnibus (overall) test is used to test the differences existing among *all* possible contrasts under a certain prespecified alpha level, usually .05 or .01. The hypothesis to be tested for a one-way ANOVA may be written as $H_0 : \mu_1 = \mu_2 = \ldots = \mu_j$. If the null hypothesis is rejected the researcher can use an appropriate multiple comparison technique to see if any contrasts of interest are significantly different from zero. For example, assume a researcher is interested in examining the comparative effectiveness of four different pain relief drugs. If the researcher

TABLE 1 Statistical Hypotheses, Associated Coefficients, and Type I Error Rate

Contrast	Null Hypothesis	Coefficients for Groups 1	2	3	4	Individual Alpha Rate (α_1)
1	$H_0: \mu_1 = \mu_2$	1	−1	0	0	.0083
2	$H_0: \mu_1 = \mu_3$	1	0	−1	0	.0083
3	$H_0: \mu_1 = \mu_4$	1	0	0	−1	.0083
4	$H_0: \mu_2 = \mu_3$	0	1	−1	0	.0083
5	$H_0: \mu_2 = \mu_4$	0	1	0	−1	.0083
6	$H_0: \mu_3 = \mu_4$	0	0	1	−1	.0083
						.0498*

NOTE: Each individual alpha is determined by the researcher; in this case it is assigned by .05/6.
* Total $\alpha \leq .05$

has no idea of which drug is most effective, an omnibus test would be used and an appropriate multiple comparison technique would follow if the omnibus test were significant. Although there are different types of multiple comparisons (e.g., Kirk, 1982, chap. 3), the Scheffé (1953) technique has many advantages. For example, Scheffé showed that the omnibus H_0 will be rejected if and only if there is at least one contrast that will be significantly different from zero with the Scheffé technique. In other words, the test on H_0: $\mu_1 = \mu_2 = \ldots = \mu_j$ is essentially an omnibus test that uses the Scheffé interval to test the equality of all imaginable contrasts to zero. The Scheffé confidence interval is stated as follows in Formula 1:

$$\hat{\psi} - R\hat{\sigma}_{\hat{\psi}} < \psi < \hat{\psi} + R\hat{\sigma}_{\hat{\psi}}$$

where $R^2 = (J - 1)\, F_{J-1,\, N-J;\alpha}$ for a one-way ANOVA.

The width of the confidence interval which determines the precision (power) of the test is a function of R and $\hat{\sigma}_{\hat{\psi}}$. The shorter the width, the more precise the estimate and the more powerful the test. Therefore, the approach which provides the shorter confidence interval for ψ will provide more precision (power) for the researcher.

Planned Comparisons

Frequently, the researcher has a small set of contrasts of interest in mind prior to the collection of data. These a priori hypotheses can be examined with t tests to decide whether the contrasts differ from zero, and at the same time the alpha level for the entire set of tests can be easily controlled (Miller, 1981, pp. 8, 11). This approach is referred to as the method of planned comparisons. In a planned comparisons study, researchers can set the total alpha at a certain level and assign each individual alpha as $\alpha \leq \alpha_1 + \alpha_2 + \ldots + \alpha_k$ where k is the number of comparisons and α_i = alpha level for comparison i. To illustrate, in our four-group study with contrasts on the six possible pairs, assume the researcher wants the total alpha level ≤.05. Each of the six individual tests can be set at .05/6 or .0083 (see Table 1).

The contrasts can be independent (orthogonal) or dependent, and the hypotheses can be directional or nondirectional. For a nondirectional null hypothesis; i.e.,

$$H_0 : \psi = 0,$$

H_0 will be rejected if the following confidence interval in Formula 2 does not include zero:

$$\hat{\psi} - t_{N-J;\alpha/2}\hat{\sigma}_{\hat{\psi}} < \psi < \hat{\psi} + t_{N-J;\alpha/2}\hat{\sigma}_{\hat{\psi}}$$

For a directional hypothesis, i.e.,

$$H_0 : \psi \leq 0 (\text{or } H_0 : \psi \geq 0),$$

H_0 will be rejected if

$$\frac{\hat{\psi}}{\hat{\sigma}_{\hat{\psi}}} \geq t_{N-J;\alpha} (\text{or } \frac{\hat{\psi}}{\hat{\sigma}_{\hat{\psi}}} \leq -t_{N-J;\alpha})$$

Planned Comparisons versus Omnibus/Scheffé Test

To examine the comparative power (precision) of planned comparisons and the omnibus test, the confidence intervals in Formulas 1 and 2 must be examined. Note the estimated contrast and the estimated standard error of the contrast are the same in both Formula 1 and Formula 2. Therefore, the comparative width of the confidence interval is determined by the size of either R or $t_{N-J;\alpha/2}$. Based on the example used by Goodwin (1984b, p. 247) to argue for the omnibus approach, we present a comparison between R and $t_{N-J;\alpha/2}$ to demonstrate that planned comparisons will actually provide shorter confidence intervals and thus greater power (precision). Recall that Goodwin's example had four groups, $\alpha = .05$, and examined all six possible pairwise comparisons (note that comparisons need not be confined to pairs; they can compare one mean against the other three, or two against two, etc.).

Table 2 indicates that in a four-group study, when cell frequencies are greater than or equal to four in each group, $t_{N-J;\alpha/2}$ will be less than R, i.e., planned comparisons will have shorter confidence intervals than the Scheffé test. (In a real study, it is unlikely there would be less than four cell frequencies.) In other words, in this case the planned comparisons are more powerful than the omnibus/Scheffé approach. In addition, note that all these null hypotheses are nondirectional. If, for example, one or more of these hypotheses had been directional, the power with planned comparisons would have been even greater.

Miller (1981, p. 69) indicated if k (the number of comparisons) and d (the degrees of freedom between groups or J – 1 in the one-way ANOVA) are at all similar in size, planned comparisons will be more precise than the omnibus/Scheffé test. Only if k is much larger than d will the omnibus/ Scheffé test be more precise. In our example, even though k was twice as large as d, the result was still in favor of using planned comparisons.

A clinical example of using planned comparisons follows. A researcher intends to compare the onset time of two newly developed anesthetic drugs (A, B) to the currently used drug (C). The researcher's interest is to find out: (a) will these two new drugs have shorter onset time than the currently used drug? (b) will Drug A or Drug B have shorter onset time than Drug C? (c) is there onset time difference between Drug A and Drug B?

Four planned comparisons are recommended for the above questions. The first two questions can be answered by directional tests. The first question will be tested by contrasting the mean onset time of Drugs A and B against Drug C ($\psi_1 = 0.5\mu_A + 0.5\mu_B - \mu_C$) and the second question can be tested by two contrasts ($\psi_2 = \mu_A - \mu_C$ and $\psi_3 = \mu_B - \mu_C$). The third question can be examined by using a nondirectional test to detect the difference of onset time between Drug A and Drug B ($\psi_4 = \mu_A - \mu_B$).

To better understand the difference in approaches, consider an analogy to the microscope. The omnibus approach is similar to looking at a slide under the low power (magnification) of the microscope. It allows us to examine a large field (*all* possible contrasts, almost all of which, such as $\psi = \mu_1 - .9907\mu_2 - .0093\mu_3$, are of no practical interest) under low power. On the other hand, the planned comparison approach is similar to looking at the slide under high power (magnification). It allows us to examine a small field (k contrasts) with high power.

Guidelines for Use

Comparisons of group means to examine the treatment effects are of major interest to researchers. We compared planned comparisons and omnibus/Scheffé tests at a given alpha in terms of their power (precision) and conclude:

- Whenever a researcher can specify the contrasts of interest before the collection of data, planned comparisons should be considered instead of the omnibus/Scheffé approach in order to increase precision.
- If the researcher has k planned comparisons, to maintain an overall alpha level, say α, individual alphas should be assigned to the individual tests so that they sum to α; e.g., α/k to each individual test.
- In general, unless k (the number of comparisons) is considerably larger than d (the number of degrees of freedom between groups), planned comparisons will be more powerful.
- To determine specifically which approach will have higher power (precision), compare R and $t_{N-J;\alpha/2}$. If R is larger, planned comparisons will be more powerful;

TABLE 2 Comparison of the Values of R and $t_{N-J;\alpha/2}$ in Calculating Confidence Intervals for All Possible Pairs with Four Groups

Number of Subjects in Each Group (n)	Total N	$v = N - J$	R	t_{v}; (X)417*
2	8	4	4.45	5.25
3	12	8	3.49	3.52
4	16	12	3.24	3.16
5	20	16	3.12	3.01
11	44	40	2.92	2.77
31	124	120	2.84	2.68
∞			2.79	2.64

*$t_{v;\alpha} \cong Z_\alpha + \frac{(Z_\alpha^3 + Z_\alpha)}{4(v-2)}$ (e.g., See Slakter 1972, p. 337).

if $t_{N-J;\alpha/2}$ is larger, the omnibus/Scheffé will be more powerful.

- These guidelines can be used for unequal *n* or in higher order designs.

References

Cobb, E.B. (1985). Planning research studies: An alternative to power analysis. *Nursing Research, 34,* 386–388.

Goodwin, L.D. (1984a). The use of power estimation in nursing research. *Nursing Research 33,* 118–120.

Goodwin, L.D. (1984b). Increasing efficiency and precision of data analysis: Multivariate vs univariate statistical techniques. *Nursing Research, 33,* 247–249.

Kirk, R.E. (1982). *Experimental design: Procedures for the behavioral sciences* (2nd ed.). Belmont. CA: Wadsworth Publishing Co.

Miller R.G. (1981). *Simultaneous statistical infererence* (2nd ed.). New York: Springer–Verlag.

Scheffé, H. (1953). A method for judging all contrasts in the analysis variance. *Biometrika, 40,* 87–104.

Slakter, M.J. (1972). *Statistical inference for educational researchers.* Menlo Park, CA: Addison–Wesley.

Examining Amount and Pattern of Change: Comparing Repeated Measures ANOVA and Individual Regression Analysis

Souraya Sidani ■ Mary R. Lynn

Analysis of longitudinal data has traditionally been directed toward identifying differences, if any, in the values of variable(s) between groups and over time, and toward determining the point at which change has occurred. The direction or pattern of change, however, has seldom been explored (Burchinal & Appelbaum, 1991). The purpose of this paper is to describe and compare two statistical approaches for the analysis of longitudinal data, repeated measures analysis of variance (ANOVA) and individual regression analysis (IRA). Data from a small experimental study are presented to illustrate the differences between these two approaches for analysis of longitudinal data.

Repeated Measures ANOVA

Repeated measures ANOVA is a statistical technique to analyze the separate and interactive effects of two or more independent variables on a dependent variable (Kerlinger, 1986). It is often used in split-plot factorial designs where repeated measurements are obtained on all subjects. Repeated measures ANOVA can be applied in three experimental conditions: (a) Subjects are randomly assigned to two or more treatment conditions, with observations taken on subjects within each treatment group over time. (b) All subjects are exposed to all treatment conditions, and repeated measurements are taken on all subjects within each treatment condition. (c) Subjects are divided into groups, with each group receiving only one level of one treatment and all levels of another treatment (Kirk, 1968). Since it is the assessment of change over time (conditions a and b) that is of particular interest to nursing, the discussion of repeated measures ANOVA in this paper will be confined to these conditions. It is important to note that the use of repeated measures ANOVA is not limited to experimental and quasi-experimental research designs; however, it can be validly applied in nonexperimental designs where observations over time are obtained on naturally occurring groups of subjects (such as single- vs. two-parent families). In these instances, time and group or treatment condition become variables of interest, and their independent and interactive effects on the criterion variable are analyzed.

The statistical model forming the basis for repeated measures ANOVA analysis is an extension of the linear model. Using time and group as the independent variables, the repeated measures ANOVA model states:

$$y = a0 + T + G + TxG + e,$$

where y is the score of an individual on the criterion variable, a0 is the general mean (of all groups across all points in time), T is the effect of the time variable, G is the effect of the group variable, TxG is the interactive effect of the time and group variables (working together), and e is an error term (Kerlinger, 1986). The effect of G is commonly called the *between-subjects* or *group* effect; the effect of T is commonly called the *within-subjects* or *time* effect. In repeated measures ANOVA, the effects of the variables are assessed at the group level. An *F*-statistic is computed for each of the three effects and tested for significance. For a detailed discussion of the computational formulas, refer to Kerlinger (1986), Downie and Heath (1974), and Kirk (1968).

With the appropriate degree of freedom, a significant *F*-statistic indicates that there is a difference in the mean values of the criterion variable. The difference could be among the groups (group effect); over time regardless of group membership, where the mean values change in a similar pattern for the groups (time effect); or over time within each group, where the mean values change across the different time periods, although the pattern of change is not the same in all the groups (interaction effect). The direction of these differences is not known. To find out which of the mean values contributes most to the overall significant difference, a series of post-hoc comparisons is done, wherein means of the groups are compared within each point in time (Bray & Maxwell, 1985).

Repeated measures ANOVA presents a major advantage for the analysis of longitudinal data over univariate analyses because it allows for the assessment of the independent

Souraya Sidani, MS, RN, is a doctoral candidate, University of Arizona, College of Nursing, Tucson, AZ.

Mary R. Lynn, PhD, is an associate professor, University of North Carolina at Chapel Hill, Chapel Hill, NC.

From *Nursing Research,* September/October 1993, *42,* 283–286.

and simultaneous effects of two or more variables, including time. This multivariate analysis is an accurate representation of real-life situations where variables are rarely, if ever, independent of one another. Despite its advantage, the use of repeated measures ANOVA has limitations that result from the strict assumptions underlying the statistical analysis. These assumptions are:

1. The within-group variance should be equal across the different data collection points (homogeneity of variance) to maintain independence of the observations (Kerlinger, 1986). Chi-square statistic is used to test for the equality of variance. If the computed chi-square value is not significant, the assumption of homogeneity of variance is met, and the *F*-statistic described above is referred to for interpretation of results. If the computed chi-square value is significant, the assumption of homogeneity is violated; in this case, other *F*-tests (such as Wilks's *F*-test) are evaluated. The Wilks's *F*-test is less stringent and does not require homogeneity of variance.

2. The spacing of the time points must be the same for all the subjects (Francis, Fletcher, Stwebing, Davidson, & Thompson, 1991).

3. There should be an equal number of observations per subject (Francis et al., 1991). When this assumption is not met, subjects with missing data at any point in time are excluded from the analysis, thus reducing statistical power.

Replacing missing data with either the subject's overall mean value on the variable, or the subject's mean value over the two values adjacent (i.e, before and after) to the missing one, is controversial. This solution reduces variance and consequently the *F*-statistic value, which weakens the validity of the results.

Individual Regression Analysis

Individual regression or growth curve analysis is a statistical technique that permits description of the individual pattern of change in a variable of interest over time. In individual regression, individual refers to a single person, group, or organization, based on the identified unit of analysis (Burchinal & Appelbaum, 1991; Rogosa, Brandt, & Zimowsky, 1982). Individual regression is more frequently used in descriptive correlational designs in which repeated measurements are obtained on each subject (such as in developmental studies) than in experimental or quasi-experimental designs, although its use in the latter case is acceptable. When used in experimental or quasi-experimental research, individual regression offers the researcher the opportunity to compare the pattern of change of individuals within each treatment group or treatment condition.

As in repeated measures ANOVA, the linear model forms the basis for individual regression analysis. In IRA, the linear model poses that the individual's score or value on a variable is a function of his score on another variable; this functional relation is represented by a regression line and is expressed by the following equation:

$$y = a + b\left(X\right) + e,$$

where y is the score of the individual on the criterion variable, a is the intercept of the regression line (i.e., the value of y when x = 0), b is the slope of the regression line (indicating the direction and strength of the functional relationship), and e is the error term (i.e., error of prediction/measurement). In IRA, the criterion variable is regressed on the time variable[1]; this functional relation is represented by a regression line (in which time is on the x axis and the criterion variables are on the y axis), and the regression equation for each subject is specified as:

$$Y_{it} = a_i + B\left(t\right),$$

where Y_{it} is the predicted subject's value on the criterion variable over time, a_i is the intercept, B is the slope, and t is the time variable. The intercept represents the value of the variable at baseline (i.e., when t = 0). The slope is of most importance in IRA; it represents the pattern and rate of change in the criterion variable. As in regression analysis, the values of B are evaluated for direction and magnitude. Negative slopes imply that values of the variable decrease with time, while positive slopes imply that values of the variable increase with time. High values of B (close to −1 or +1) indicate that the criterion variable changes rapidly and drastically over time; moderate values (± .2 to ± .4) indicate that the criterion variable changes slowly and undramatically over time; values equal to zero indicate no change in the criterion variable over time. Moreover, *t*-tests can be performed to determine if the slope for each subject is statistically different from zero, thus making it possible to model the pattern of change for each individual. Individual differences can then be described and evaluated.

---

[1]A time variable, representing all the points of data collection, is created for each subject. The values of this time variable should be consecutive, ranging from 1 to t, t being the total number of data collection points. For example, if variable X is measured at three points in time for each subject, the data are arranged in the following way:

Subject Number	Time	X
1	1	X1
	2	X2
	3	X3
2	1	X1
	2	X2
	3	X3

When the research purpose is to compare the pattern of change among groups (whether experimental or naturally occurring), the intercept and slope are estimated for each subject in the total sample, then tested for group differences using *t*-test or ANOVA, with group being the independent variable and the intercept or slope serving as the dependent variable. A significant group effect using the intercept as the dependent variable indicates a difference among the groups at baseline, which is similar to the group effect in the repeated measures ANOVA. A significant group effect using the slope as the dependent variable indicates a difference in the pattern of change among the groups, which is similar to the interaction effect in repeated measures ANOVA. Similar analyses can be conducted when the purpose is to determine differences in the pattern of change across various treatment conditions.

The advantages of using IRA can be summarized as: (a) The pattern of change can be modeled, and change as a process can therefore be examined; and (b) individuality in the pattern of change is maintained and described, although analysis of aggregate data is also possible. While there are no statistical assumptions that must be met when conducting IRA, two assumptions have been mentioned: All subjects must have equal numbers of data points, and a linear equation should be used to model the data. Rogosa et al. (1982) argued against the first assumption, explaining that IRA is concerned with identifying a pattern of change represented by a single line that best fits the data at hand. Two data points are enough to draw a line; therefore, a missing data point(s) should not be crucial to the identification of the pattern. Although the issue of missing data points is debatable, including subjects with missing data points is justified when qualitative change is of concern and maximal sample retention is needed (Suter, Wilson, & Naqvi, 1991). The second mentioned assumption regarding linearity can be maintained by using polynomial functions to best fit the data when the pattern of change is nonlinear (Lessne & Hanumara, 1988).

It should be noted that the use of IRA is limited under two conditions. First, IRA is limited when the variable or attribute being studied does not maintain the same dimension across measurement occasions. It is essential that the criterion variable retain the same meaning over time; otherwise, change in the variable cannot be validly inferred (Burchinal & Appelbaum, 1991; Rogosa et al., 1982). The second limiting condition for the use of IRA is when the values of the criterion variable demonstrate drastic changes occurring in opposite directions over consecutive points in time; for example, it increases at Time 1, decreases at Time 2, then increases at Time 3. In such cases, the best fitting slope (using least squares) will fail to show any significant change, unless the pattern of change is divided into segments (measurement times) that are then analyzed separately.

IRA offers valuable information to researchers when used in analyses of longitudinal data. The specific contributions of IRA are that the individual pattern of change can be modeled and examined, the specific direction and rate of change can be identified, and the interindividual differences in the pattern of change can be analyzed. Consequently, change can be viewed as a process when IRA is used.

Comparison between the Two Approaches

Repeated measures ANOVA and IRA have commonalities and differences when used as analytic strategies in the analysis of longitudinal data. They are both used in the analysis of longitudinal data in which measurements on the same criterion variable are taken on consecutive occasions, where it is assumed that the dependent variable is measured with minimal measurement error, and where there is concern about identifying change over time, with time being the key variable.

The differences between repeated measures ANOVA and IRA exist at both the theoretical and practical levels. The theoretical difference between them arises from the dimension of change to be examined, that is, whether it is the quantitative or the qualitative aspect of change that is of interest. Repeated measures ANOVA tests the differences among a variable's values at different points in time: The quantitative amount of change is of importance. IRA looks at the variable's values over continuous data points: The pattern or trajectory of change (qualitative aspect), and not the differences over time, is what is of interest and is, therefore, examined (Burchinal & Appelbaum, 1991; Francis et al., 1991). Additionally, repeated measures ANOVA focuses on differences between groups over time. In repeated measures ANOVA, means of individuals within groups over time, and means of groups within time points, are compared; the type of analysis is geared toward examining interindividual differences. Even though IRA can be used to compare pattern of change among individuals or groups, the main purpose of IRA is to identify change within individuals, that is, intraindividual change.

At the practical level, differences between the two measures are embedded within the statistical techniques used and the assumptions required. In repeated measures ANOVA, analysis is based on aggregate data; group means are compared and individual differences are not examined, but are considered a major source of error. IRA, as the name implies, is based on individual data; individual differences are examined. Repeated measures ANOVA requires equal spacing and equal number of observations for the subjects; this condition is not necessary in IRA. Finally, because these techniques are so different they produce different results and consequently lead to different conclusions. Therefore, selection of whether to use repeated measure ANOVA or IRA is determined by two factors: the aspect of change that is to be analyzed and the unit of analysis for the study.

Example

To illustrate the similarities and differences between the use of the two methods, analysis of data from an experimental study will be presented. The purpose of this pilot study was to determine the effect of sedative music on respiratory rate in 10 patients with chronic obstructive airway diseases. Each subject was randomly exposed to the treatment (listening to music for 20 minutes) and to the control condition (resting for 20 minutes). Measures included pretest and posttest assessment of respiratory rate, along with monitoring of respiratory rate five times during each of the two conditions. In this study there were two outcomes of interest: (a) the comparison between the control and treatment conditions to evaluate the effectiveness of sedative music in reducing respiratory rate and (b) the exploration of the rate and the pattern of change in respiratory rate to better understand the effect on the individuals. Therefore, it was necessary to employ both repeated measures ANOVA and IRA.

The data met the following assumptions required for doing a repeated measures ANOVA: Homogeneity of variance was maintained, spacing of data points was equal for all subjects, and an equal number of observations per subject were available. As can be seen from the results presented in Table 1, there are a significant independent treatment condition and time effects. From these findings it can be concluded that the mean respiratory rate in the treatment phase is different from the mean respiratory rate in the control phase, and respiratory rate changes over time. However, no conclusions can be drawn regarding direction, magnitude, and timing of the change.

In the IRA analysis, respiratory rate was regressed on time and the slope was estimated for each subject in each of the treatment and control phase. Table 2 presents the individual *b*-values for respiratory rate.

Results from the IRA analysis are interpreted at the individual level. For example, for Subject 1, respiratory rate decreased significantly and rapidly during the treatment phase, while it remained unchanged in the control phase. For Subject 2, respiratory rate decreased significantly and steeply in both the treatment and control phases. For Subject 3, no significant change was observed in either phase. For Subject 4, no significant change was observed, but the trend was toward a decrease in respiratory rate during both phases. The IRA results for the remaining individuals can be examined, and the pattern of change (or no change) can be described for each.

In the IRA, differences in the pattern of change between the treatment and control phase were also examined. Results of one-way analysis of variance, where the *b*-values (representing individual patterns of change) were treated as the dependent variable and the treatment-control phase as the independent variable, indicated no significant difference in the mean of the *b*-values (–.22) in both phases. It can be concluded that the pattern of change in respiratory rate is similar in the treatment and control phases and, as noted by considering the mean *b*-value of –.22, it decreases with time.

The results obtained by the two methods can be compared to illustrate what use each method offers in the analysis of this type of data. In both methods, respiratory rate was found to change with time; using IRA, respiratory rate was found to decrease during both the treat-

TABLE 1 Results of Repeated Measures ANOVA on Pilot Data from Effects of Sedative Music Study

Variable	Effect	*df*	*F*
Respiratory rate	Treatment condition	(1.9)	5.66*
	Time	(7.63)	2.15*
	Condition X time	(7.63)	1.69

*$p < .05$

TABLE 2 Results of IRA on Pilot Data from Effects of Sedative Music Study

Subject Number	Treatment Phase		Control Phase	
	b-VALUE	*t*-TEST	*b*-VALUE	*t*-TEST
1	–.82	–4.5*	.03	.1
2	–1.25	–7.7*	–0.90	–6.0*
3	–.39	–1.5	.07	.3
4	–.17	–.5	–.53	–1.7
5	.28	.9	.10	.2
6	.28	.8	.03	.1
7	.21	.6	–.32	–1.7
8	–.46	–2.5*	–.32	–1.3
9	.25	.7	.35	.9
10	–.14	–.3	–.71	–2.0*

*$p < .05$

ment and control phases. Results regarding effect of phase on respiratory rate were not consistent across the two methods: The effect of treatment condition was found to be statistically significant when repeated measures ANOVA was used, and not significant when IRA was used. Lack of convergence of these results should be expected theoretically because repeated measures ANOVA examines differences in the amount of change, while IRA examines the pattern of change. Consequently, rather than looking at these two methods as separate, independent methods for the analysis of change, they can be looked at as complementary methods.

References

Bray, J. H., & Maxwell, S. E. (1985). *Multivariate analysis of variance.* Newbury Park, CA: Sage.

Burchinal, M., & Appelbaum, M. I. (1991). Estimating individual developmental functions: Methods and their assumptions. *Child Development, 62,* 23–43.

Downie, N. M., & Heath, R. W. (1974). *Basic statistical methods* (4th ed). New York: Harper & Row.

Francis, D. J., Fletcher, J. M., Stwebing, K. K., Davidson, K. C., & Thompson, N. M. (1991). Analysis of change: Modeling individual growth. *Journal of Consulting and Clinical Psychology, 59* (1), 27–37.

Kerlinger, F. N. (1986). *Foundations of behavioral research* (3rd ed). Fort Worth: Holt, Rinehart & Winston.

Kirk, R. E. (1968). *Experimental design: Procedures for behavioral sciences.* Belmont, CA: Brooks/Cole.

Lessne, G. J., & Hanumara, R. C. (1988). Growth curve analysis in marketing: Method and application. *Journal of Marketing Research, 25,* 391–396.

Rogosa, D., Brandt, D., & Zimowsky, M. (1982). A growth curve approach to the measurement of change. *Psychological Bulletin, 92,* 726–748.

Suter, W. N., Wilson, D., & Naqvi, A. (1991). Using slopes to measure directional change. *Nursing Research, 40,* 250–252.

Using Slopes to Measure Directional Change

W. Newton Suter ■ Dwight Wilson ■ Alice Naqvi

One long-lived methodological puzzle faced by most nursing researchers is the measurement and analysis of change. Readers of *Nursing Research* know that suggestions for analyzing change have been made by Burckhardt, Goodwin, and Prescott (1982), Egger and Miller (1984), and Feldman and Ventura (1984). There appears to be no generally accepted method to statistically analyze change in the behavioral sciences. The title of the classic Cronbach and Furby (1970) statement on the subject ("How We Should Measure 'Change'—Or Should We?") raises the question of whether research designs that yield change scores should *ever* be used. Fortunately, during the past decade behavioral statisticians have developed new methods for the analysis of change and refined older methods. The purpose of this article is to describe one such method—a very simple one—and show how it was applied to the analysis of data collected over three years in a test of the self-care model of nursing in a geriatric nursing care facility. This method is described in greater detail by Kraemer and Thiemann (1989) and is hereafter referred to as the Kraemer-Thiemann strategy.

The Use of Slopes

Simply, the Kraemer-Thiemann strategy for analyzing change involves regressing each participant's dependent (criterion) variable on time (first test, second test, third test, etc.) and using the computed slope as the outcome variable. For example, consider a participant who had a baseline (pretest) pain rating of 8, a posttest rating of 7, a first follow-up rating of 5, and a second follow-up rating of 4. Regressing the y-values of 8, 7, 5, and 4 on the x-values (time) of 1, 2, 3, and 4 yields a slope of 1.4.

W. Newton Suter, PhD, is assistant professor, Department of Educational Leadership, University of Arkansas at Little Rock, Little Rock, AR.

Dwight Wilson is associate chief of nursing service, Extended Care, Veterans Administration Center, Palo Alto, CA.

Alice Naqvi is chief of nursing service, Veterans Administration Center, Palo Alto, CA.

From *Nursing Research,* July/August 1991, *40,* 250–252.

Computationally, the slope is the product of the (a) correlation coefficient between x-values and y-values and (b) the ratio of the standard deviation of x-values over the standard deviation of y-values. This slope, easily computed on many handheld calculators, functions as the primary outcome measure, and group differences can be tested by usual methods (e.g., the t-test or Mann-Whitney U test). The usual assumptions of population normality and population homogeneity of variance apply to the t when used to test for differences between slopes. Further, the t statistic can be used to test whether the slope is significantly different from 0, that is, whether there is any linear trend from baseline to endpoint.

The Kraemer-Thiemann strategy is most appropriately applied to randomized controlled clinical trials involving repeated measurements across time. The technique is especially useful when the multiple observations have low coefficients of test-retest reliability (stability) and when there are missing or censored data. The strategy assumes linear relationships as well as independent errors and equal variances across repeated measurements, an assumption reasonably assured by blinded assessments (Kraemer & Thiemann, 1989).

The concept of using a single statistic to summarize repeated observations over time is not new. Applications of the slope model to data with low test-retest correlations and missing observations, however, is receiving increasing attention. The Kraemer-Thiemann strategy is one option that begins to fill the gap created by a lack of sound procedures for analyzing repeated measures—particularly those relatively unreliable measures prone to error and which are often missing due to uncontrollable circumstances.

Advantages of Slopes

Whether data are "soft" (low retest reliabilities) or "hard" (high retest reliabilities), the use of slopes of response on time maximizes sample retention. Participants who have internally missing data or missing endpoint measures need not necessarily be discarded since only two data points are needed to compute a slope. Also, investigators may want to include in the dataset the number of internally missing data points, the number of valid observations, whether endpoint data were collected, whether testings were evenly spaced, etc. One can easily test whether such data characteristics are related to slopes and make better decisions about data exclusion and generalizability based on this information.

It is with the soft data that one advantage of the Kraemer-Thiemann strategy becomes pronounced, particularly when more than two observations per subject are collected. This advantage concerns the enhancement of power over and above that power achieved with maximal sample retention. The general principle, according to Kraemer and Thiemann, is that the greater the number and spacing of repeated observations, the greater the enhancement of effect size and power. Using actual data from a two-group (drug vs. placebo) experiment testing the effects of benzodiazepines on tardive dyskinesia with 17 subjects and 6 repeated measures (Csernansky, Tacke, Rusen & Hollister, 1988), Kraemer and Thiemann showed that the traditional *t*-test-on-endpoints approach yielded an effect size of .19 and a significance level of .344. The *t*-test-on-change-score approach, by contrast, increased the effect size to .65 and yielded a significance level of .106. The slope approach nearly doubled the effect size to 1.20 and, interestingly, produced a statistically significant *t* value with an associated probability level of .045. The Kraemer-Thiemann slope approach when used with soft data, in other words, decreases error variability, hence increases statistical power without tampering with sample size.

Slopes in Nursing Research

The usefulness and simplicity of the Kraemer-Thiemann strategy for comparing group differences by examining change over time can be illustrated by describing one dataset on which the technique was applied. The dataset used for this illustration was especially prone to mortality and problems associated with incomplete measurements over time, hence was well suited for the Kraemer-Thiemann strategy because it maximizes sample retention and, consequently, power.

The illustrative study tested the self-care model in a geriatric nursing care facility. (The description of this study is restricted to how the slope model might be applied to actual data; readers wanting detailed information about methodology and findings should request this from one of the authors.) Participants were randomly assigned to either an experimental group (self-care) or a control group (traditional care). The participants were given up to six repeated measurements (including a pretest) on 16 variables over a three-year period. Of the 146 initial participants, 62% were alive at the endpoint of the study. Many of these participants were, for one reason or another, unable to provide complete data over the six repeated testings. The average age of these participants was 78.10 years ($SD = 12.75$).

To simplify this presentation, the use of only one criterion variable—the Beck Depression Inventory (BDI)—will be described. In addition to a maximum of six BDI raw scores, values on the following five variables pertaining to the BDI for each participant were included in the restructured data set: (a) the number of internally missing data points, (b) the valid number of observations, (c) the time at which the subject entered the study, (d) the *Y*-intercept based on the regression of response on time, and (e) the slope based on the regression of response on time.

The slope was the primary outcome measure, and the *Y*-intercept provided information about starting points and initial group comparability. It also functioned as a covariate in the analysis of covariance to test for differences between slopes. The other variables were useful in the determination of relationships between the primary slope outcome and factors associated with the repeated measurement. The number of internally missing data points and the number of valid observations provided information about the generalizability of the slope outcome as a function of the number of available measurements. Coding the time of entry into the study enabled an analysis of slope and its relationship to temporal factors.

In addition, sociodemographic variables were included, not only for the purpose of describing the sample, but for the purpose of learning about treatment interactions. For example, the question "Do younger patients progress at different rates than older patients?" can be tested by correlating slopes with age.

The power of the Kraemer-Thiemann strategy is evidenced by comparing the results of a slope analysis with a traditional endpoint (single observation) analysis. Using only BDI scores and a subset ($N = 36$) of the larger data set (those with three or more valid observations), the mean endpoint BDI for the experimental group was 7.11 ($SD = 6.89$) compared to a mean endpoint of 11.06 ($SD = 7.67$) for the control group. The *t*-test revealed that this difference, although in the predicted direction, was not statistically significant, $t = 1.62$, $p > .05$. Slope analysis using the same subjects, by contrast, revealed a statistically significant difference in the predicted direction between groups. The mean slope for the experimental group was .06 ($SD = 1.64$) compared to a mean slope of 1.46 ($SD = 1.79$) for the control group, $t = 2.46$, $p < .05$.

(Many datasets include multiple dependent variables, hence it is recommended that a multivariate analysis of variance be done on all slope outcomes prior to computing separate *t*-tests.)

The above example shows that treatment effects using soft data may go undetected without the use of powerful methods associated with multiple observations per subject. The use of slopes as a measure of directional change, seemingly rarely used in nursing research, provides a simple yet powerful option to researchers who pose questions that can be answered by directional change.

Limitations and Alternatives

The reader at this point may be concerned about the use of slopes as a measure of nonlinear relationships. Kraemer and Thiemann (1989) described these concerns well: "What if one patient has a long latency before there is perceptible change, while another responds immediately and then stabilizes, and a third simply follows a linear trend?" (p. 153). They also addressed these concerns well by reference to the "horse-racing" analogy. They stated, "One horse hesitates . . . Another takes the race out . . . The third builds up speed . . . Should we take the running patterns of these horses into consideration when we judge who won the race? It is certainly not customary to do so" (p. 153).

It must be emphasized that the use of a slope model is not the ultimate technique for the measurement of change. It is merely one method in an array of strategies that deserves methodological attention. The array of alternative strategies and their limitations is described by Cook and Campbell (1979), the most traditional being the analysis of variance with gain scores (either simple or standardized) and the analysis of covariance using a pretest as the covariate.

The advantages of collecting three or more observations per subject is described by Rogosa, Brandt, and Zimowsky (1982), who advocated a time path, growth curve approach to measuring change. The reader must not assume, of course, that newer, more sophisticated techniques to analyze change are necessarily better. For example, Kraemer and Thiemann (1989) noted that the use of multiple observations and slopes with hard data such as weights, cell counts, and stable performance scores will not likely increase power over that provided by a traditional test on posttest-only scores.

The answer to the question initially posed by Cronbach and Furby (1970) in their seminal article is Yes! We *should* measure change, and do so in the most powerful way possible. The use of slopes as a measure of directional change with soft data provides one such powerful method.

References

Burckhardt, C. S., Goodwin, L. D., & Prescott, P. A. (1982). The measurement of change in nursing research: Statistical considerations. *Nursing Research, 31,* 53–55.

Cook, T. D., & Campbell, D. T. (1979). *Quasiexperimentation: Design and analysis issues for field settings.* Chicago: Rand-McNally.

Cronbach, L. J., & Furby, L. (1970). How we should measure "change"—or should we? *Psychological Bulletin, 74,* 68–80.

Csernansky, J. G., Tacke, U., Rusen, D., & Hollister, L. E. (1988). The effect of benzodiazepines on tardive dyskinesia symptoms. *Journal of Clinical Psychopharmacology, 8,* 154–155.

Egger, M. J., & Miller, J. R. (1984). Testing for experimental effects in the pretest-posttest design. *Nursing Research, 33,* 306–312.

Feldman, M. J., & Ventura, M. R. (1984). Evaluating change using noninterval data. *Nursing Research, 33,* 182–184.

Kraemer, H. C., & Thiemann, S. (1989). A strategy to use soft data effectively in randomized controlled clinical trials. *Journal of Consulting and Clinical Psychology, 57,* 148–154.

Rogosa, D., Brandt, D., & Zimowsky, M. (1982). A growth curve approach to the measurement of change. *Psychological Bulletin, 90,* 726–748.

Strengthening Experimental Design by Balancing Potentially Confounding Variables across Treatment Groups

Richard Zeller ■ Marion Good ■ Gene Cranston Anderson ■ Dean L. Zeller

Simple random assignment of subjects to treatment and control groups provides two major benefits to experimental research: (a) balance of known and unknown subject idiosyncracies across groups and (b) unbiased estimates of both treatment effects and random error variation. However, simple random assignment does not guarantee that groups will be comparable. For example, studies using simple random assignment (hereafter referred to as random assignment) are at risk for producing groups that are imbalanced in one or more levels of confounding covariates (Silverman, 1985). This is especially true of small studies, but it is also a concern in large ones (Cook & Campbell, 1979). Minimization is a method of assignment to groups that reduces the amount of bias by controlling for as many known extraneous sources of variation as possible. It produces groups that are comparable in size and distribution of potentially confounding covariates (Pocock, 1979; Pocock & Simon, 1975; White & Freedman, 1978).

This article is written for nurse researchers who are designing randomized clinical trials both as their research programs mature and as the demand for tested nursing interventions increases. Building on the work of Conlon and Anderson (1990), this report includes a rationale for using minimization in intervention studies and describes the development and testing of the minimization-8 (min-8) computer program for assigning subjects to as many as eight groups. Nurse researchers who use minimization will have a powerful, rigorous, and feasible research advantage.

Richard Zeller, PhD, is a professor of sociology, Bowling Green State University, Bowling Green, OH.

Marion Good, PhD, RN, is assistant professor of nursing, Frances Payne Bolton School of Nursing, Case Western Reserve University, Cleveland, OH.

Gene Cranston Anderson, PhD, RN, FAAN, is an Edward J. and Louise Mellen Professor of Nursing, Frances Payne Bolton School of Nursing, Case Western Reserve University, Cleveland, OH.

Dean L. Zeller, MS, is an instructor of computer science, Bowling Green State University, Bowling Green, OH.

From *Nursing Research,* November/December 1997, *46,* 345–349.

In 1974, Taves introduced and tested minimization, a method of randomly assigning subjects to comparable groups in which levels of selected potentially confounding covariates are evenly distributed (balanced). Taves provided support for the proposition that minimization improves the validity of clinical trials by preventing two sources of error that reduce comparability of (a) systematic selection/assignment bias and (b) chance skewing (imbalance) of potentially confounding covariates across groups. He concluded that in clinical trials little or no theoretical reason exists to continue using traditional methods of randomization such as a table of random numbers or a tossed coin.

Although the problem of incomparable groups has been addressed by several adaptive assignment models such as randomized block (Kirk, 1982), urn (Bagchi & Pal, 1985; Rudy, Vaska, Daly, Happ, & Shiao, 1993; Schouten, 1995; Wei, 1978), permuted block (Lachin, Matte, & Wei, 1988; Zelen, 1974), and big stick design (Soares & Wu, 1983), these methods are cumbersome and the number of covariates that can be controlled must be restricted. Minimization is more efficient and flexible for use in clinical studies that frequently have numerous confounding variables.

A variety of minimization methods has been proposed. Differences among methods are based on method of computation (Begg & Iglewicz, 1980; Conlon & Anderson, 1990; Taves, 1974), inclusion of a probability factor (Klotz, 1978; Pocock & Simon, 1975; Signorini et al., 1993; Soares & Wu, 1983), self-adjustment after subject mortality (Nordle & Brantmark, 1977), and minimization not only across covariates but also across clinical sites (Akazawa et al., 1991; Akazawa, Kamakura, Sakamoto, Odaka, & Nose, 1994; Odaka, Akazawa, Watanabe, Nose, & Ogura, 1994; Signorini et al., 1993; Therneau, 1993). These authors and others (Birkett, 1985; Green & Byar, 1978) found support for the effectiveness of minimization assignment designs, usually testing them with computer simulations. Other investigators discussed the statistical properties of minimization strategies (Lachin, Matte, & Wei, 1988: Ohashi, 1990; Therneau, 1993), whereas two others documented that minimization strategies increase the power of statistical tests (Green & Byar, 1978; Johnson, Tolley, Bryson, & Goldman, 1982).

Studies are unanimous in concluding that minimization reduces the potential for systematic selection bias and chance skewing.

Articles about minimization have been in the literature for over 20 years; however, articles describing minimization are written for statisticians and published in sources rarely read by nurse researchers. Additionally, those nurse researchers who know about the method may perceive it as too slow and inflexible for use in the clinical research arena. Perhaps easy access to software for a simple minimization computer program is needed to encourage nurses to efficiently assign subjects to several comparable groups.

The major advantage of minimization is research control of selected potential covariates in clinical studies. A potentially confounding covariate, or simply covariate, is an extraneous variable that is expected to be significantly correlated with the dependent variable and if unbalanced across groups may be a source of error that confuses interpretation of the trial results. Many possible covariates may affect outcomes in clinical trials. For example, patient conditions such as medical diagnosis, stage of disease, or type of medical or surgical treatment are important to control in clinical trials. Other potential covariates include lifestyle variables such as smoking and drinking or parental decisions such as whether to breastfeed or bottlefeed. All of these potential covariates can be controlled with min-8.

Minimization-8 (Min-8) Software Program

Min-8 is based on the *min* software program for two groups, which was created by Conlon in 1989 (Conlon, 1993; Conlon & Anderson, 1990). The min-8 program was developed by Dean Zeller (1995), who created a new computer algorithm that assigns each case so that groups are comparable and error variance of the covariates is minimized across multiple groups. Both programs were developed to meet the requirements of studies funded by the National Institute of Nursing Research.

Min-8 can quickly assign each clinical subject to one of several groups after the subject has been selected and assessed for the selected covariates. The researcher cannot predict group assignments because the computer calculates them internally based on the balance of a subject's characteristics in relation to data on numerous covariate levels in several groups. To further ensure that min-8 assignment of subjects is a "blind" procedure, the investigator can select the first few cases from a table of random numbers and delete subjects who must be excluded from the analysis. Min-8 can be used on a personal, laptop, notebook, or palmtop computer but is more portable and less expensive in a smaller palmtop computer.

In using min-8, the investigator selects the potential covariates and identifies levels of each. For example, levels of using a certain medication such as an antidepressant might be *yes* and *no*. Min-8 balances use of the antidepressant across the groups by assigning so that each group has a similar number of subjects who use an antidepressant and subjects who do not. Min-8 calculates a tentative frequency for each affected covariate level in each group, should the new subject be assigned to that group. The subject is assigned to the group that would result in the lowest sum of squares across groups. In the case of a tie between two or more groups, the random number generator in min-8 randomly assigns the new subject to one of the tied groups. The result is that groups are of the same size and covariate composition, differing by only one or two subjects at the maximum. The covariates are therefore held constant, which decreases the covariate error variance. Documentation is available to interested readers on the Web site.

The following hypothetical example is provided to illustrate the similarity of groups after assignment with min-8. Thirty subjects with chronic asthma were assigned to three groups (relaxation, music, and control) while minimizing on (controlling for) three covariates (smoking, gender, and use of a bronchodilator). The study was planned to test the effects of the two interventions, relaxation and music, on number of episodes of dyspnea. Because minimization was used, the three groups were similar in levels of these covariates. For example, each group had a similar number of heavy smokers, females, and subjects using a bronchodilator. Thus, the effect of these variables on the frequency of dyspnea episodes was held constant. In addition, the three groups were similar in size throughout the study, another important advantage of minimization.

Monte Carlo Computer Simulation

A Monte Carlo simulation was used to compare the effects of min-8 and random assignment on comparable groups in 300 "studies." A Monte Carlo simulation produces many iterations of a research procedure and produces a sampling distribution that can be used in evaluating the procedure. To determine differences in comparability of groups, this simulation compared min-8 assignment with random assignment of subjects to four treatment groups: A, B, C, and D. Three covariates labeled X, Y, and

Z were constructed. Each covariate had two levels: 1 and 2. Comparable groups was operationally defined as the mean error variance (variance) of covariate levels across groups.

Simulation data were created for the 300 studies, each with four groups. There were 50 studies in each of six different conditions. Conditions 1 and 2 were very small studies with 20 subjects or 5 subjects per group; conditions 3 and 4 were small studies with 40 subjects or 10 subjects per group, and conditions 5 and 6 were medium-sized studies with 100 subjects or 25 subjects per group. Examination of Table 1 shows that in Conditions 1, 3, and 5, subjects were assigned using random assignment, and in Conditions 2, 4, and 6, subjects were assigned using min-8. A total of 16,000 subjects were included in the simulation. To ensure that min-8 was effective with different distributions of covariate levels, the statistician varied the proportions of subjects assigned to the levels of each covariate. Subjects in each level were then randomly assigned to groups using either randomization or min-8.

To compare the effect of method of assignment on comparable groups as indicated by a lower mean covariate error variance, the mean and standard deviation of subjects in each covariate level were calculated. With 6 covariate levels in each of 300 studies, there were 1,800 means and standard deviations. Standard deviations for each size study were then categorized and plotted on the horizontal axes of the graphs in Figure 1 so that, for example, those of .25 or less were designated as 0, those of .26 to .75 were categorized as .5, and those of .75 to 1.25 as 1. The percent of standard deviations per category was calculated for each condition and plotted on the vertical axes. Figure 1 presents three graphs (A, B, C), one for each size study (N = 20, 40, 100).

The results of the simulation are presented as the percent distribution of standard deviation categories for the randomly assigned studies and for the studies assigned by min-8. An examination of Figure 1A shows that when N = 20, the mean standard deviation in the min-8 assigned studies (.45) was smaller than the mean standard deviation from the randomly assigned studies (1.35). To calculate mean error variances, the mean standard deviations were squared. The mean error variance was .20 for min 8 and 1.82 for random assignment. Therefore, when N = 20, min-8 assignment resulted in a mean error variance that was nine times smaller than that of random assignment.

Figure 1B presents the percent distribution of standard deviation categories when N = 40. Again, the mean standard deviation in the min-8 assigned studies was smaller than that following random assignment. The mean error variance for min-8 assignment was .21, whereas the mean error variance for random assignment was 3.72. Therefore, when N = 40, the min-8 error variance was 18 times smaller than the random assignment error variance.

Figure 1C presents the percent distribution of standard deviation categories when N = 100. Again, the min-8 average standard deviation (.24) was smaller than that for random assignment (10.89). In this case, when N = 100, the min-8 mean error variance was 45 times smaller than that of random assignment. These comparisons show that in small- to medium-sized studies there are dramatic reductions in error variance with min-8 and the magnitude of these reductions increase with sample size.

Discussion

An examination of the simulation data clearly indicates that groups were more comparable when using min-8 rather than random assignment because the mean covariate error variance was substantially less. This supports the proposition that minimization prevents chance skewing, that is, the imbalance of potential covariates across groups. The use of min-8 allows confident dis-

TABLE 1 Monte Carlo Simulation of Six Conditions: Studies, Method of Assignment, and Size

Condition	No. of Studies	Assignment Method	*N*/Study	*N*/Group	Total *N*/Condition
1	50	Random	20	5	1,000
2	50	Min-8	20	5	1,000
3	50	Random	40	10	2,000
4	50	Min-8	40	10	2,000
5	50	Random	100	25	5,000
6	50	Min-8	100	25	5,000
Totals:	300	—	—	—	16,000

NOTE: Min-8 = Minimization-8.

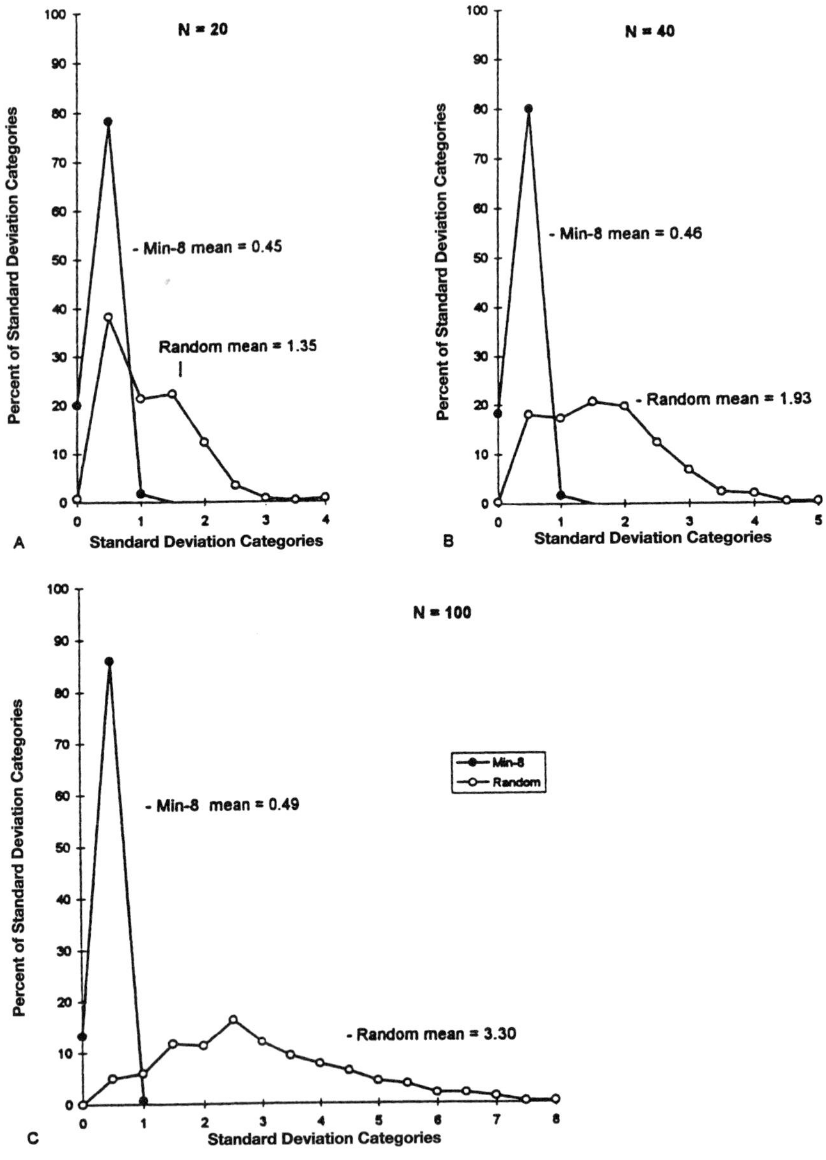

FIGURE 1 Percentage Distribution of Standard Deviations of Covariates Comparing Min-8 With Random Assignment in Studies of Different Size

missal of the effects of selected covariates on the outcome of experimental studies regardless of sample size. This clear advantage is added while preventing bias during selection, assignment, or both. In other words, researchers can neither predict nor choose the group to which the next subject will be assigned, and thus, a new subject cannot be selected, assigned, or both, based on characteristics that would support the study hypotheses. The particular importance of these controls for clinical trials was recognized by Pocock (1979). He noted that because patients usually become available for entry one at a time in clinical trials, patient assignment is an ongoing process rather than a procedure that is performed at one time point, and therefore careful monitoring is needed.

Random assignment gives each subject an equal chance of being assigned to any treatment group, which results in the probable balance of both known and unknown sources of error across groups. This has been a major benefit of the experimental model in creating credible causal inferences for the past century. Both minimization and random assignment are based on the reasonable assumption that no correlation is expected between the unknown characteristics of any one subject and the next. However, random assignment merely provides the *probable* balance of known and unknown sources of error across groups. In contrast, the min-8 (and min) programs virtually guarantee an adequate balance of covariates or known sources of error, which is of far greater value to the validity of causal inferences in a randomized clinical trial. Thus, the min and min-8 programs result in an experimental design of increased power, decreased error variance, and increased inferential accuracy.

The min-8 program has been placed in the public domain, and investigators may obtain it on the World Wide Web at the following addresses: http://www.cs.bgsu.edu/~dzeller/min8.html. Plans for future development include expanding the program to allow an increase in the number of groups and covariates, improving the generators and graphic interface, and adding a probability factor.

From a methodological perspective, using more than eight covariates rarely improves the power of the design owing to a diminishing return as the number of selected covariates increases. This is especially true in clinical trials with a modest sample size. Although the min-8 program will allow for 20 covariates if necessary, often 3 to 4 is enough. Decisions about the number of covariates selected and which ones to select rest with the researchers who must be able to justify their choices based on an in-depth review of the scientific literature, careful preliminary work in the clinical setting, and strong intuition.

Min-8 is superior to random assignment in ensuring that potentially confounding covariates are as equivalent as possible across treatment and control groups. Although the original min program is sufficient when subjects are assigned to only two groups, the min-8 program is needed when researchers plan an experimental design with more than two groups. These researchers can now conduct randomized controlled trials without the fear of distorting effects from imbalanced covariates because this effective, feasible, and inexpensive way to assign subjects to several groups has been developed.

References

Akazawa, K., Kamakura, T., Sakamoto, M., Odaka, T., & Nose, Y. (1994). Patient registration and treatment allocation in multicenter clinical trials using a FAX-OCR system. *Methods of Information in Medicine, 33,* 530–534.

Akazawa, K., Odaka, T., Sakamoto, M., Ohtsuki, S., Shimada, M., Kamakura, T., & Nose, Y. (1991). A random allocation system with the minimization method for multi-institutional clinical trials. *Journal of Medical Systems, 15,* 311–319.

Bagchi, A., & Pal, A. K. (1985). Asymptotic normality in the generalized Polya-Eggenberger urn model, with an application to computer data structures. *SIAM Journal on Algebraic and Discrete Methods, 6,* 394–405.

Begg, C. B., & Iglewicz, B. (1980). A treatment allocation procedure for sequential clinical trials. *Biometrics, 36,* 81–90.

Birkett, N. J. (1985). Adaptive allocation in randomized controlled trials. *Controlled Clinical Trials, 6,* 146–155.

Conlon, M. (1993). Minimization software [Computer software]. [On-line]. Available FTP://www.stat.ufl.edu/pub/min-1.0.tar.Z.

Conlon, M., & Anderson, G. C. (1990). Three methods of random assignment: Comparison of balance achieved on potentially confounding variables. *Nursing Research, 39,* 376–379.

Cook, T. D., & Campbell, D. T. (1979). *Quasiexperimentation: Design & analysis issues for field settings.* Boston: Houghton Mifflin.

Green, S. B., & Byar, D. P. (1978). The effect of stratified randomization on size and power of statistical tests in clinical trials. *Journal of Chronic Disease, 31,* 445–454.

Johnson, M. E., Tolley, H. D., Bryson, M. C., & Goldman, A. S. (1982). Covariate analysis of survival data: A small-sample study of Cox's model. *Biometrics, 38,* 685–698.

Kirk, R. E. (1982). *Experimental design: Procedures for the behavioral sciences* (2nd ed.). Belmont, CA: Brooks/Cole.

Klotz, J. H. (1978). Maximum entropy constrained balance randomization for clinical trials. *Biometrics 34,* 283–287.

Lachin, J. M., Matte, J. P., & Wei, L. J. (1988). Randomization in clinical trials: Conclusions and recommendations. *Controlled Clinical Trials, 9,* 365–374.

Nordle, O., & Brantmark, B. (1977). A self-adjusting randomization plan for allocation of patients into two treatment groups. *Clinical Pharmacology Therapeutics, 22,* 825–830.

Odaka, T., Akazawa, K., Watanabe, Y., Nose, Y., & Ogura, H. (1994). A flexible random allocation program for multi-institutional clinical trials. *Journal of Medical Systems, 18,* 39–53.

Ohashi, Y. (1990). Randomization in cancer clinical trials: Permutation test and development of a computer program. *Environmental Health Perspectives, 87,* 13–17.

Pocock, S. J. (1979). Allocation of patients to treatment in clinical trials. *Biometrics, 35,* 183–197

Pocock, S. J., & Simon, R. (1975). Sequential treatment assignment with balancing for prognostic factors in the controlled clinical trial. *Biometrics, 31,* 103–115.

Rudy, E. B., Vaska, P., Daly, B. J., Happ, M. B., & Shiao, P. (1993). Permuted block design for randomization in a nursing clinical trial. *Nursing Research, 42,* 287–289.

Scholten, H. J. A. (1995). Adaptive biased urn randomization in small strata when blinding is impossible. *Biometrics, 51,* 1529–1535.

Signorini, D. F., Leung, O., Simes, R. J., Beller, E., Gebski, V. J., & Callaghan, T. (1993). Dynamic balanced randomization for clinical trials. *Statistics in Medicine, 12,* 2343–2350.

Silverman, W. A. (1985). *Human experimentation: A guided step into the unknown.* New York: Oxford University Press, Inc.

Soares, J. F., & Wu, C. F. J. (1983). Some restricted randomization rules in sequential designs. *Communications in Statistics: Theory & Methods, 12,* 2017–2034.

Taves, D. R. (1974). Minimization: A new method of assigning patients to treatment and minimization control groups. *Clinical Pharmocology and Therapeutics, 15,* 443–453.

Therneau, T. M. (1993). How many stratification factors are "too many" to use in a randomization plan? *Controlled Clinical Trials, 14,* 98–108.

Wei, L. J. (1978). An applicant of an urn model to the design of sequential controlled clinical trials. *Journal of the American Statistical Association, 73,* 559–563.

White, S. J., & Freedman, L. S. (1978). Allocation of patients to treatment groups in a controlled clinical study. *British Journal of Cancer, 37,* 849–857.

Zelen, M. (1974). The randomization and stratification of patients to clinical trials. *Journal of Chronic Disease, 27,* 365–375.

Zeller, D. L. (1995). Minimization-8: A computer algorithm for minimizing the variance of covariates across experimental treatment groups [Computer software]. dzeller@cs.bgsu.edu; rzeller@bgnet.bgsu.edu.

Time-Series Analysis: An Alternative for Nursing

Bonnie Lou Metzger ■ **Samuel Schultz II**

Nursing is both science and professional service. Its scientific legitimacy becomes explicit when nursing knowledge is used to guide and enchance practice. The primary guiding force of nursing's scientific inquiry must be the nature of the phenomenon, not an idolization of a specific scientific technique. The crucial question is whether the specific technique of inquiry actually illuminates the phenomenon of interest. Indeed, there is some question whether or not we have become idolizers of experimental design and inferential statistics at the expense of *representative* (Petrinovich, 1979) design and analysis, true paramorphic models of our clinical realities. Perhaps in our zeal to use available paradigms from the behavioral sciences, we allow the methodological and analytical tail to wag the clinical dog. Why, though so many phenomena of interest to nursing research are time-dependent by nature, do time-series methods rarely appear in our journals? The purpose of this article is to explore the fundamental components of time-series methods and their use for nursing.

Most of the phenomena of interest to nursing are intimately related to time. Nursing assessments are heavily based on rate, pattern, and change. Selecting points in time and measuring changes in behavior occurring along the delineated interval is not unique to nursing or even modern man. However, the freedom to examine and not discard as random error the unique fluctuations in phenomena being tracked through time required the development of the theory of stochastic processes. Stochastic process models are mathematical, not deterministic models that permit movement away from the nomothetic nature of inferential statistics. Inferential statistics mute the importance of individual differences in predicting future behavior. Instead they propose that the relationships of human behavior can be summarized in simple mathematical terms by generalizing from aggregate behavior. Inferential statistics, specifically regression analysis and the theory of stochastic processes propose that the future is determined in part by the past. Sequences of observations evolve through time according to probabilistic laws. Thus the future evolution of any behavioral series can be predicted by knowledge of its past values (Kendall, 1973; Nelson, 1973). The process of prognosticating future events based on these derived models is called forecasting.

Classical time-series analysis is rarely explored in nursing research, but time as a factor is sometimes included in the guise of repeated measurements (RM)-ANOVA. Unfortunately, either the rigid assumptions (e.g., independence) of the RM-ANOVA are too rigid for use in most clinical paradigms or these assumptions are violated, and false conclusions are made when the model is applied in spite of the rigid requirements.

Time-series analysis techniques are basically idiographic. They provide the tools essential to analyzing unique behavioral fluctuations through time and a framework for predicting future changes in that individual behavior. Prediction to the individual from the individual has many implications to nursing practice. It allows the uniqueness of the individual concept to exist as a basis for nursing care and provides a framework for assessing change, not as a deviation from an aggregate mean, but as an alteration in a unique but consistent pattern. Beyond this, forecasting individual clinical behavior is an important goal for clinical nursing research.

Model Building

Theory development, testing, and clinical predictions are dependent on model building. Two major types of conceptual models are: explanatory (structural) and predictive. The two are not mutually exclusive or necessarily interdependent. Models vary in purpose, type, and utility. They are highly conscious summaries of actual or anticipated findings. In general, models force the scientist to state hypotheses clearly, explicitly, and definitely. They provide more constant bases for clinical decison

Bonnie Lou Metzger, PhD, RN, is a postdoctoral research associate at the University of Michigan, Ann Arbor, MI.

Samuel Schultz II, PhD, is the director of computing facilities, professor of nursing, Center for Nursing Research, the University of Michigan, Ann Arbor, MI.

From *Nursing Research,* November/December 1982, *31,* 375–377.

making, practice evaluation, and scientific critique. Models are paramorphic systems. They are analogues of real systems; they obey the same laws as the original. The advantage of the model is that it is accessible to the application of analysis and other mathematical tools, permitting manipulations not practical in the prototype system.

Time-Series Analysis

The characteristic feature of a time series is that observations occur in *temporal order,* for we are interested in the relationship of the variables' values from one data point to the next. This is a primary difference between time-series analysis and classical inferential statistics. In time-series data sets, successive values are not assumed or intended to be independent. The number of observations loses some of its predictive significance and the temporal internal structure of the data series becomes essential to precise estimates of future fluctuation.

Classical inferential statistics are based on the assumption that the amount of information in a random sample is most positively related to the size of the sample: the number of independent observations (Cohen, 1969). The power to detect differences and the error of estimates decreases with increased sample size. Thus the researcher's confidence in the estimates or predictions increases as the sample size (n) increases. In time-series analysis, however, observations are not independent, one from the other. They have highly correlated, successive values. A sample size of 10 does not provide 10 pieces of new information. The interrelatedness of each piece of data in a time series demands *dense data sets.* Many pieces of information are needed for a reasonable degree of prediction confidence to occur. Therefore, this analytical process depends on the availability of data, distributed much more densely over time than is sampled in most nursing research. This is a more involved and more costly venture than other nursing research methods. It may, however, be worth the extra effort, especially when used for idiopathic clinical prediction. As a point of reference, Land and others (1980) used a series of 50 observations as a minimum for time-series samples sizes.

Time-series analysis can be the most appropriate scientific technique for those interested in change occurring on any variable(s) for the same unit of analysis (cell, man, nation) over a series of time points (minutes, hours, days, months, years). Specifically a time series is a collection of data points X_t ($t = 1,2, \ldots ,T$) with the intervals between X_t and $X_t + {}_1$ being fixed and constant (Ostrom, 1978). Although gathering data at an exact point in time may be difficult in clinical settings, time-series analysis techniques are robust enough to handle data collected at "functionally" equidistant points, allowing for minor variations in times. It would not be essential to take blood pressures every morning at 6:00 A.M. exactly, if the question concerned blood pressure recordings immediately following awakening. The blood pressure can be taken when the subject awakens. The time the subject awakens one morning (7:00 A.M., 8:00 A.M.) is functionally equidistant from the awakening time the next morning. Another approach that assumes ordinally scaled time is a more restrictive class of models but may fit more paradigms in nursing research. Still another approach consists of defining sampling windows that set the limits for capturing data points from rare events processes, which later under certain known rules can be aggregated into functionally defined time processess.

The internal *structure* of a time series is a mixture of four components: trend, long-term movement; fluctuations about the trend of greater or less regularity; a seasonal component; and a residual, irregular, or random effect (Kendall, 1973).

These are the classical components of a time series, but this characteristic structure may not always be appropriate for short-term clinical settings. The discovery of the component patterns of past events allows us to develop predictive models from time series. Normally the components are mixed and contain both deterministic and stochastic elements. The seasonal/cyclic and trend components appear to be deterministic functions of time. Seasonal effects may vary somewhat, though generally there is a predictable degree of regularity to cyclic generators of seasonal components. Examples include the predictable diurnal variations seen in human body temperature and the seasonal variations observed in triacylglycerol and lipoprotein serum levels. Trends appear to be a function of permanent forces uniformly operating in the same direction, for example, hypertension and increased adiposity, both viewed as a function of increasing age.

Once the deterministic aspects of time series have been identified and extracted from the data, a stationary series is left. Stationary series are defined by a constant mean and the residual fluctuations that occur oscillate about that mean. The residual fluctuations may be entirely random. However, if these movements about the mean are not random, they become the basis for the development of precise stochastic predictive models. The major tool in identifying the stochastic predictive model is the *autocorrelation* technique. Autocorrelation determines the degree of association between X_t and X_{t+k}, where K represents different time lags, $0,1,2, \ldots ,N$ and $K < N$, where N is equal to the number of observations in the series (Vigderhous, 1977). A large autocorrelation

(r_k) implies high association for the observations at time points t and $t + k$. For example, high correlations for r_{12} and r_{24} suggest a yearly seasonal cycle when observations are made monthly. In the preceding example the observation made in October 1979 ($t = 0$) had the strongest relationship (autocorrelation coefficient) with observations made in October 1980 ($0 + k$, $k = 12$) and October 1981 ($0 + k$, $k = 24$). The autocorrelation function allows us to identify seasonal components, and suggests the type of stochastic probability model that will best replicate this particular time series.

Once a particular model type has been identified from the autocorrelation of sample data, the next advisable step is to determine if the selected model does provide an adequate description of the data. The recommended next analysis stage is the examination of the residuals. Residuals are the differences between the actual observations and the model fitted values. Significance tests have been and are being developed that use the autocorrelation of the residual values to determine the goodness of model fit (Chatfield, 1975).

Box and Jenkins (Nelson, 1973) have developed stochastic techniques that allow identification, estimation, and forecasting of time series. The *Box-Jenkins methodology* consists of matching original time series to a postulated general class of available models (Box and Jenkins, 1970).

The first step in developing the Box-Jenkins forecasting model is to isolate a tentative model from the autocorrelation of the original time series and the first differencing (residuals) of this original series (detrending). If no significant autocorrelation is present in the first regular difference, that series is considered stationary. Stationary residuals are considered random noise and do not contribute to final model development in the Box-Jenkins technology. If, however, the residuals are significantly correlated, they are classified as nonstationary time series and are used in the final model development.

This procedure uses past observations of a given time series to extrapolate a model and is called a univariate prediction procedure. Prediction can be made by taking observations on other variables (time series of other variables) into account. These multivariate models serve as a basis for causal or structural models, which both explain and predict.

Multivariate time-series analysis is similar in concept to other multivariate analysis techniques. We could be primarily interested in the relationship between two different variables (time series); cross-correlation is the principal technique used to examine the strength of association between two time series. Here we cross-correlate the two series of variables trying all combinations of time lag between them. On the other hand, our fundamental concern may be the effect of one time series on another. In this case, time-series regression techniques are the ones most commonly employed.

Once the model that best describes the sample data has been identified, the question to be answered is whether this model allows us to estimate X_{n+q} from the observed time series $X_1, X_2, \ldots, X_n$, where q represents the value of numbers of steps ahead. Ostrom stated that the "great advantage of time-series regression analysis is that it is possible to both explain the past and predict the future behavior of variables of interest" (1978). The achievement of these tasks is dependent on being able to correctly postulate a model and estimate its parameters.

Time-series regression analysis demonstrates the basic difference between time-series analysis techniques and classical inferential statistics. Time-series analysis is based on the fact that observed different data points in time are not independent from one another. For example, an individual's blood pressure at t_1 could be expected to be highly correlated with observed blood pressure at point t_2. Once the regression model has been fitted to the sample time-series data the residuals are most likely not independent but serially correlated or autocorrelated and the assumption of normality is violated. Since individual error terms are not independent of each other, naïve inferences concerning the goodness of fit of the regression model at this point in the analysis process often lead to type II errors and erroneous acceptance of false models.

Since autocorrelation of the residuals are expected in time-series regression analysis, the data management technique consists of several steps beyond deriving a regression equation. Once the equation is estimated, the residuals are obtained and used as a basis for autocorrelation. The results of the residual autocorrelation are the substructure for developing a second model: a model of the disturbance time-dependent process. Once the time-dependent process is identified, parameters can be estimated and used to strengthen the predictive model.

The primary focus of this article is the analysis of discrete time series. However, it is probable that nursing research problems may include the need to examine continuous time series. Continuous time series are different from discrete series in that data collection is not interrupted and frequency of wave form becomes as important as amplitude. In the discrete time series, data are collected at specific, approximately equal intervals, and the frequency of peaks and troughs in the series is controlled by the investigator. Scientific techniques, such as spectral density analysis, a modification of Fourier analysis, which expresses data with sine and cosine functions, are available to analyze both frequency (quantity) and amplitude in continuous time series, opening up another dimension to the scientist interested in describing, understanding, and predicting significant turning points across time.

Another time-based class of stochastic models is *Markov Chain models*. This class of models assumes a small discrete set of state-space, where each observation depends on only the previous observation and none before that. The probabilities of transition from one state to any other are defined according to theory or empirical data. Markov models can be useful for the initial phases of model building, especially where previous behavior beyond the single preceding observation can be assumed to be independent. Other stochastic models beyond the scope of this paper are queuing theory models, server models, random walk models, and computer simulated continuous and discrete (e.g., GPSS) models. All these hold promise as modeling systems not yet fully tapped for clinical nursing phenomena.

Time-series analysis is not a simple enterprise. There are many mathematical manipulations and steps involved in the development and testing of projection and predictive models. It is not within the scope of this article to examine all those steps. However, many of the phenomena of interest to nursing are intimately related to time. The appropriate way to examine and understand those phenomena are time-series analysis techniques. Time-series analysis techniques can provide a basis for computer-assisted clinical decision making. It is not unlikely that the microcomputer will become part of the basic equipment of each clinical unit. Not only will this computer be used to store and process individual patient data, but it will be programmed with general trends and cycles gathered from aggregate data. The inferences drawn from group data can be regressed on each client's individual data, permitting more accurate predictions of that person's behavior across time.

References

Box, G. E. P., and Jenkins, C. M. *Time Series Analysis: Forecasting and Control.* San Francisco, Holden-Day, 1970.

Chatfield, C. *The Analysis of Time Series: Theory and Practice.* London, Chapman and Hall, 1975.

Cohen, J. *Statistical Power Analysis for the Behavioral Sciences.* New York, Academic Press, 1969.

Kendall, M. G. *Time Series.* New York, HafnerPress, 1973.

Makridakis, S., and Wheelwright, S. C. *Interactive Forecasting: Univariate and Multivariate Methods.* San Francisco, Holden-Day, 1978.

Nelson, C. R. *Applied Time Series Analysis for Managerial Forecasting.* San Francisco, Holden-Day, 1973.

Ostrom, C. W. Jr. *Time Series Analysis: Regression Techniques.* Beverly Hills, Calif., Sage Publications, 1978.

Petrinovich, L. Probabilistic functionalism: A conception of research methods. *Am Psychol* 34:373–390, May 1979.

Vigderhous, G. Forecasting sociological phenomena: Application of Box-Jenkins methodology to sucide rates. In *Sociological Methodology: 1978,* ed. by K. F. Schuessler. San Francisco, Jossey-Bass Publishers, 1977, pp. 20–51.

The Crossover Design in Clinical Nursing Research

Susan L. Beck

The crossover design is one that can be both appropriate and advantageous in nursing research. A crossover, change-over, or counterbalanced design is one in which the effects of different treatments are compared on the same subject during different treatment periods (Hills & Armitage, 1979). In its simplest form, subjects are randomly assigned to two groups that differ solely on the order of treatment. The first group receives the treatment in the order AB, and the second group receives the reverse order, BA (Brown, 1980).

This simple version of the crossover design can be expanded in several ways. These expansions include the addition of baseline periods, more treatments, or repeated measurements within each period. It is important to distinguish the crossover design from other types of research designs. Lavori, Louis, Bailar, and Polansky (1983) have identified three types of experimental designs that are based on the number of groups and treatments.

In a parallel comparison, two or more groups of patients are treated separately but concurrently. Parallel studies include classical experimental designs in which subjects are randomly assigned to treatment and control groups, as well as quasi-experimental designs in which randomization is not possible.

In a self-controlled study design, patients serve as their own controls—before, during, or after treatment (Louis, Lavori, Bailar, & Polansky, 1984). This experimental design is similar to the crossover in that each patient is observed under different conditions; however, it differs in that no randomization is possible.

A comparison of these three designs, all of which might be considered to answer the same research question, must take into account the relative strengths and limitations of each design.

As randomization to treatment group enables the investigator to rule out many of the threats to internal validity, the parallel group and crossover designs allow the researcher to infer a causal relationship with greater confidence. Comparison between these two designs shows that the crossover design may have an advantage. There is less likelihood of the threats of imitation of treatment, compensatory equalization of treatment, compensatory rivalry, and resentful demoralization, as each group will receive all treatments. These threats should still be considered, however, as they might occur on the basis of the treatment order.

Advantages of the Crossover Design

The main advantages of the crossover design are increased control of variance and decreased requirements in sample size. These advantages are most easily explained by further comparison with the parallel group design.

In a parallel group design, if the groups differ on factors that might affect the outcome, the observed results may be affected by these confounding variables as well as by the treatment (Lavori, Louis, Bailar, & Polansky, 1983). Several approaches to controlling variance due to such factors can be considered—both in the design (i.e., randomization, blocking, inclusion criteria) and analysis (i.e., ANCOVA) of a study.

When there are many confounding variables, the crossover design provides an ideal way of utilizing one of the design approaches for control of variance—matching. Subjects are paired with themselves and the influence of patient characteristics can be eliminated. Although Lavori et al. (1983) claimed that this pairing represents the ultimate form of statistical adjustment for such characteristics, it seems more precise to view it as the ultimate form of design adjustment.

The increased control of variance from the crossover design contributes to its main advantage, a potential savings in sample size. Because the influence of many patient characteristics can be removed, the sample size required to detect a significant effect is much less. Louis et al. (1984) stated that a crossover design based on a small sample can provide the same statistical accuracy as that of a larger parallel study.

Susan L. Beck, PhD, RN, is a nurse researcher at University Hospital and research assistant professor at the College of Nursing, University of Utah Health Sciences Center.

From *Nursing Research,* September/October 1989, *38,* 291–293.

In a novel approach to evaluating the advantages of using the crossover design, Brown (1980) presented a method for assessing the cost efficiency of the crossover design. According to this model, the cost of the crossover versus the parallel group design depends on two ratios: the ratio of between-subject variance to within-subject variance and the ratio of the cost of treating a patient for one period relative to the cost of recruiting a patient into the study. If recruiting costs are high and the variation between subjects large, the crossover design is clearly the most advantageous type of design.

Disadvantages of the Crossover Design

One of the major disadvantages of the crossover design is the increased potential for dropouts due to the length of the study. This result is enhanced by the extent of the response burden and side effects associated with participation in the study. Each subject must receive two or more treatments in order to provide a complete data set. With a smaller sample size, the effect of dropouts is greater as each subject contributes a significant portion of the data. The dropout rate can also lead to an imbalance in the design as more subjects in one sequence might drop out than in another. Initial planning should project a sample size large enough to compensate for dropouts. However, the necessity of overprojecting serves to counteract the gains in sample size made by choosing this design in the first place.

Other disadvantages of the crossover design are inherent in its basic structure and result from the effects of order and time. The extent to which these effects can significantly confound the results of a study can be minimized by careful attention to specific elements of the research design and analysis.

Order effects may be manifested both by carryover and period effects. Carryover or residual effects occur when the effect of the first treatment continues into the second treatment period. More serious residual effects would occur if a treatment has a reverse effect or if there is a marked effect based on the order or treatment sequence (Brown, 1980). Adequate comparison of two treatments is based on the assumption of no or equal residual effects. Grizzle (1965) identified a statistical test to check the validity of this assumption at the $p = .10$ or .15 level of significance. Brown (1980) confirmed that this test is valid but questioned its usefulness in testing the assumption using the crossover data because it lacks power. Thus, the main protection against violations of this assumption is to allow an adequate interval in between treatments. With such a washout period, the effects of the first treatment will dissipate and most likely there will be no residual effects at all (Grizzle, 1965). Another possible approach is to collect baseline data before each treatment period, but this solution would add to the length and expense of the study.

In addition to residual effects, the investigator must also consider the effects of period. The crossover design is most appropriate in the study of a relatively stable condition. If a condition changes during the course of the study due to disease progression, effects of treatment, or the healing process, it becomes difficult to measure the effects of the intervention. The result of this instability may be reflected in a period effect that is actually due to a within-subject variability in the phenomenon.

Control and analysis of the effect of the order of the treatments can be used to minimize and evaluate both carryover and period effects. Subjects should be randomly assigned to the treatment sequence in order to protect against conscious and unconscious bias. If a fixed sequence were used, there would be no way to evaluate whether the order of treatment might be causing a significant effect in the study. If possible, blinding the investigator and subject to both the crossover point and treatment assignment can minimize the effect of knowledge of the treatment on the response to it. Unfortunately, such double blinding is much more difficult to achieve in nursing studies where interventions obviously differ; in a field such as pharmacy, two identical capsules can be used.

The effect of time in a crossover study also merits attention. The study should be balanced in terms of time allocated for each period. The crossover point should be time dependent rather than dependent on a condition or symptom. For example, each period might last seven days and each subject would cross over to the alternate treatment on the ninth day, following a one-day washout period. Such measures to protect against time imbalances serve to minimize the variance due to this element.

In addition to design controls, statistical analysis can assist in interpreting these effects. Both nonparametric (Koch, 1972) and parametric models (Grizzle, 1965) for analysis of crossover designs have been described. Additionally, Wallenstein and Fisher (1977) have presented a model for analysis of the cross over design with repeated measurements.

These models provide statistical means to evaluate the direct, carryover, period, and time effects. In the nonparametric method, test procedures for hypotheses concerning direct, residual, and period effects are formulated in terms of Wilcoxon statistics and may be readily applied to small sample data. Using parametric statistics. Grizzle (1965) provided a linear model to guide an analysis of variance (ANOVA) that includes the effect of period, as well as the direct and residual effects of treatment. Wallenstein and Fisher (1977) built upon this model to include the effect of time in a repeated-measures study. The ANOVA model would also allow evaluation of the interaction of these effects, an important estimate of all the order effects that may be present. A small interaction relative to the treatment effect allows the investigator to more confidently answer the research questions.

A great amount of difficulty can occur in interpreting the results of such an analysis. If there is a significant residual, period, or order effect, it is recommended that the second period be excluded from the data analysis. The study should then be analyzed as a two-group parallel study comparing treatment A and B within the first period. If there is a baseline period, the difference between the treatment and baseline might also be compared. Brown (1980) estimated that the sample size required to do such an analysis would be larger than that required in a parallel group study. This requirement would negate one of the main advantages of the crossover design—savings in sample size. Nonparametric analysis could be considered in this instance and would be appropriate in the small sample situation. However, the nonparametric approach is not as powerful and in some cases may result in a significant loss in the sensitivity, and even meaning, of the data.

Because of these limitations, attention to both design and analysis are critical to the success of a crossover study. The design is used most appropriately in studies of relatively stable conditions in which there may be a significant amount of between-subject variation that could confound the results of the investigation. The treatment effect must be transient or reversible so that subjects return to baseline. Obtaining repeated measurements at different time points must be feasible. The study should be planned to minimize dropout rates and allow adequate intervals to washout residual effects. The analysis must evaluate the possible effects of period, time, and order before an accurate assessment of the treatment effect is possible. Although some have recommended that the crossover design be avoided, it can be very effectively utilized in the study of clinical nursing problems if careful attention is given to these elements of design and analysis.

Variations of Crossover Design Applications

A review of the nursing research literature provided some examples of how variations of the crossover design have been used in clinical investigations. In most of these studies, the design was not specifically called a crossover design but only one in which patients served as their own controls.

An excellent example is provided by the study of Hathaway and Geden (1983) in which the effects of three exercise programs and a control on energy expenditure, heart rate, respiratory rate, and blood pressure were compared in 36 volunteers. Following a five-minute baseline period, subjects participated in a randomly ordered series of three exercise programs (passive, isometric, and active). A five-minute period of no activity was allowed between each program to control for possible carryover effects. Although a repeated measures ANOVA was used to analyze the data, it was not reported whether a test for order or residual effects was completed. The study found that heart rate and oxygen consumption significantly increased during active and isometric exercise.

Crossover designs have also been appropriately used in studies of temperature. Baker, Cerone, Gaze, and Knapp (1984) examined the effect of type of thermometer and length of time inserted on the oral temperature of afebrile subjects. Four randomly ordered treatment conditions were assigned to 24 subjects. The investigators found that readings from mercury-in-glass thermometers with insertion times of 2 minutes were essentially no different from readings obtained by electronic thermometers.

Temperature, blood pressure, and pulse are some examples of outcome variables that are often studied in nursing practice, that tend to vary between subjects, and that can be appropriately investigated with a crossover design. These examples only scratch the surface of phenomena of interest to nurse researchers that meet these criteria. It is of interest that the design was not labelled "crossover" in these studies. In fact, the term *crossover design* has rarely been used in nursing research. Nonetheless, it has been used and has many uses. It is also noteworthy that none of these studies reported statistical evaluation of carryover, period, time, or order effects. As knowledge of the crossover design and its applicability increases, so too will the skill of nurse researchers using and evaluating this design in studies of nursing practice.

References

Baker, N. C., Cerone, S. B., Gaze, N., & Knapp, T. R. (1984). The effect of type of thermometer and length of time inserted on oral temperature measurements of afebrile subjects. *Nursing Research, 33,* 109–111.

Brown, B. W. (1980). The crossover experiment for clinical trials. *Biometrics, 36*(1), 69–79.

Campbell, D. T., & Stanley, J. C. (1963). *Experimental and quasi-experimental designs for research.* Boston: Houghton Mifflin.

Cook, T. C., & Campbell, D. T. (1979). *Quasi-experimentation.* Chicago: Rand McNally.

Grizzle, J. E. (1965). The two-period changeover design and its use in clinical trials. *Biometrics, 21,* 467–480.

Hathaway, D., & Geden, E. A. (1983). Energy expenditure during leg exercise programs. *Nursing Research, 32,* 147–150.

Hills, M., & Armitage, P. (1979). The two-period crossover clinical trial. *British Journal of Clinical Pharmacology, 8*(1), 7–20.

Koch, G. C. (1972). The use of nonparametric methods in the statistical analysis of the two-period changeover design. *Biometrics, 28,* 577–584.

Lavori, P., Louis, T. A., Bailar, J. C., & Polansky, M. (1983). Designs for experiments—parallel comparisons of treatment. *New England Journal of Medicine, 309,* 1291–1299.

Louis, T. A., Lavori, P. W., Bailar, J. C., & Polansky, M. (1984). Crossover and self-controlled designs in clinical research. *New England Journal of Medicine, 310*(1), 24–31.

Wallenstein, S., & Fisher, A. C. (1977). The analysis of two-period repeated measurements crossover design with applications to clinical trials. *Biometrics, 33,* 261–269.

Regression Discontinuity Design: Alternative for Nursing Research

Jan R. Atwood ■ **Wendell Taylor**

The purpose of this article is to identify the regression discontinuity design as a scientifically advantageous research approach. The relationship of this design to causal claims is also described.

The regression discontinuity design is a quasi-experimental design especially applicable when ethical concerns preclude random assignment of subjects to treatment and control groups, but resources or other reasons prohibit putting everyone in the intervention group as in the classic A-B-A-B design (Campbell & Stanley, 1963). The little known regression discontinuity design is a pretest-posttest program comparison group strategy (Trochim, 1984).

The purpose of the regression discontinuity design is to evaluate the effects of a new treatment or intervention program. The components of the design are a preintervention (pretest) measure, cut-off criteria, and one or more postintervention measures. The pre-post measures assess some health care research variable, e.g., a patient's dependency on a caregiver. The cut-off criteria, decided upon by the researcher for theoretical or practical reasons, are used to determine who will receive the treatment and who will not. The intervention is given to those above or below the cut-off or between two or more cut-offs. Therefore, the groups are not equivalent but rather the source of design comparison is based on how the groups would have progressed had neither group received an intervention.

The unique characteristic of the regression discontinuity design is the method of assignment. The method of assignment is not random but systematic, with assignment to groups based solely on cut-off scores at preintervention. Systematic assignment is fully specifiable and can be a valuable alternative to randomization.

Jan R. Atwood, PhD, FAAN, is professor, Curriculum in Public Health Nursing and Health Behavior/Health Education Department and member, Lineberger Cancer Center, University of North Carolina, Chapel Hill, NC.

Wendell Taylor, PhD, MPH, is assistant professor, Center for Health Promotion Research and Development, School of Public Health, The University of Texas, Health Sciences Center at Houston.

From *Nursing Research,* September/October 1991, *40,* 312–315.

The following example illustrates the design. Two hundred and fifty individuals are receiving curative outpatient treatment for a particular illness. A new supportive nursing intervention program is available to increase patients' self-care ability and to decrease their dependency on their caregiver; but there are resources only for 125 of those 250 individuals to receive the nursing intervention. For whatever reason (political, ethical, administrative), random assignment of patients to experimental and control groups is not an option. Therefore, with the regression discontinuity design, the nursing intervention can be administered to the most severely ill individuals or any other subset of the group based on cut-off measures. In each case, the patients are assigned to the experimental group on the basis of a preintervention illness measure. Based on the preintervention illness measure, the new nursing intervention is administered to the 125 most severely ill patients or another subset of the group in order to maintain the integrity of the design in support of a causal claim. After administering the intervention, it can be determined if the data for individuals receiving the intervention show a statistical function that is different from what would have been expected without the intervention, i.e., a discontinuity in the regression line. Figures 1, 2, and 3 graphically illustrate the preceding example with the regression discontinuity design.

Figure 1 shows a Dependency on Caregiver Scale ranging from 1 to 40. The higher numbers on each axis indicate greater levels of dependency on the caregiver. Each dot represents one person's pretest and posttest scores on the scale. A group of individuals is given the Dependency on Caregiver Scale as a pretest. Then, in the absence of any interventions, program, or treatments, the same group of individuals is measured again later with the scale as a posttest. Figure 1 shows that individuals with lower pretest scores of dependency on caregiver also are the ones with the lower posttest scores of dependency on caregiver (see "a" in Figure 1). Correspondingly, the individuals with higher pretest dependency on caregiver scores have higher posttest scores (see "b" in Figure 1). This bivariate distribution, a strong positive relationship between the preintervention and

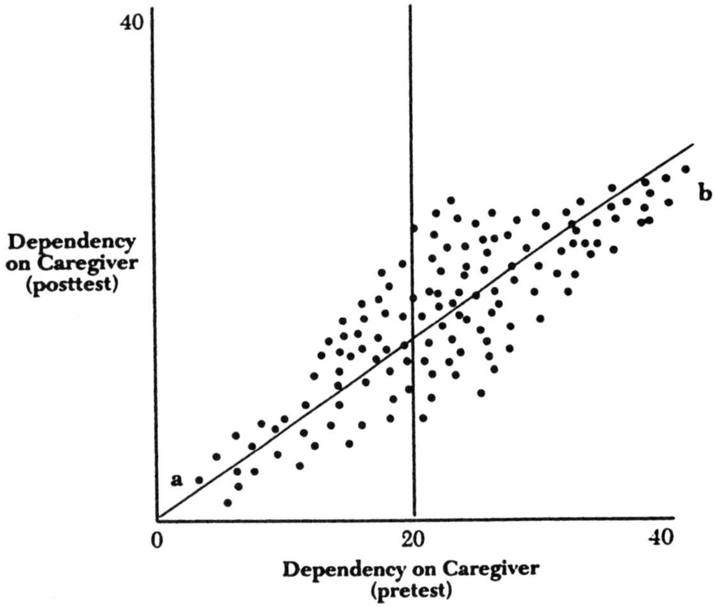

(adapted from Trochim, 1990)

FIGURE 1 No Intervention

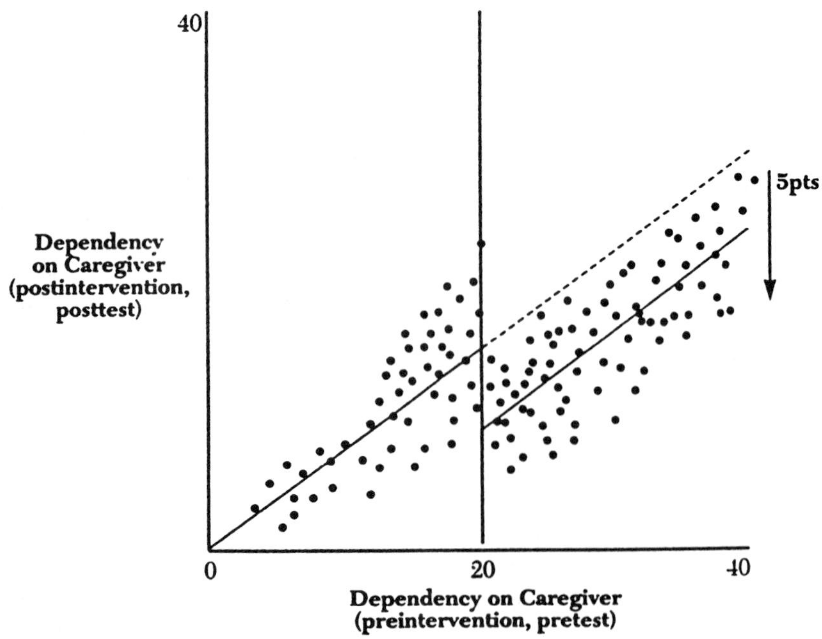

(adapted from Trochim, 1990)

FIGURE 2 Intervention with Constant Effect

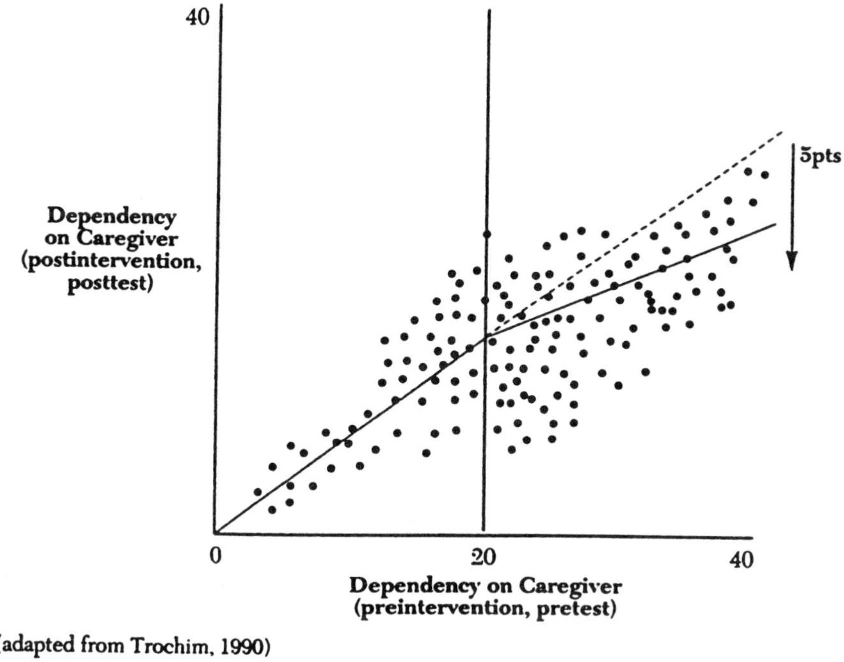

FIGURE 3 Intervention with Interaction Effect

postintervention measures, is best represented by a linear regression line.

Figure 2 indicates that scale point 20 on the Dependency on Caregiver Scale was used as the cut-off criterion to separate patients who will receive the intervention and those who did not receive it. In this example, those who initially scored above 20 on the scale, the patients scoring highest on the Dependency on Caregiver Scale, received the intervention. At scale point 20, there is a dashed line and a solid line. The solid line represents the Dependency on Caregiver scores for those individuals who received the treatment. The dashed line in Figure 2 represents the no intervention effect of Figure 1. In the case of Figure 2, the intervention has a uniformly beneficial effect on the treated group. This is evidenced by an average of a five-point decline in the Dependency Scale scores and the accompanying discontinuity in the regression line at scale point 20, hence, the name regression discontinuity design.

Figure 3 shows an interaction effect for the treated group rather than the constant effect seen in Figure 2. The intervention in Figure 3 reveals no effect for the treated individuals slightly above the cut-point of 20. On the other hand, the individuals with the highest dependency on caregiver scores in the treated group received the greatest benefit (five-point decline) from the intervention as evidenced by the discontinuity in the regression line. Based on the extent of the discontinuity, statistical analysis can identify to what extent the intervention had an effect in causing the regression discontinuity and whether the difference in the regression discontinuity line is statistically significant.

A general strategy to perform the analysis for significant difference follows. Set the intercept equal to zero by subtracting the cut-off score from each pretest score. Check for linearity in the bivariate slope of the distribution and create higher-order terms and interactions as indicated by the distribution. (Specifying this function carefully is basic for being able to detect significance in the discontinuity.) Then conduct multiple regression on the postintervention scores. Vertical discontinuity will be estimated by the regression coefficient for the dummy variable for intervention recipient versus nonrecipient. The significance of the main effects coefficient can be tested with a Student's *t*-test of the standard error of that coefficient or by viewing the .95 confidence interval around the beta. Efficiency can be built into the estimation procedure (Trochim, 1984, 1990).

To interpret the results, it is important to know the nature of the assignment variable, who received the program, and the nature of the outcome variable (Trochim, 1990).

In the preceding example, it is important to know that the cut-off score of 20 can only be achieved by scoring high enough on at least some of the Dependency on Caregiver Scale items to disrupt or notably rearrange the caregiver's usual living habits. Characteristics of the patients who received the intervention and those who did not would be described.

The preceding example considers only one cut-off score. More than one cut-off score could have been used if it made better conceptual and clinical sense. For instance, if scores of 15 and 30 identified major increments in lifestyle change for the caregiver, two cut-off scores could have been used with concomitant accommodations in the required sample size for robust regression analysis.

Causal Claims and Nursing Research

The regression discontinuity design is a strong alternative to a randomized experimental design for making causal claims. Causal claims are particularly relevant for health care research, in general, and nursing research, in particular (Given, Given, & Coyle, 1985; Medoff-Cooper, 1986; Miller, Wikoff, McMahon, Garrett, & Ringel, 1985; Verran & Reed, 1987). Enough is known in some areas of nursing science to support intervention studies, some of which appropriately have the quasi-experimental scientific base required for a regression discontinuity design. Regression discontinuity designs help establish causal claims for the effectiveness of nursing and other health care interventions. Definitionally, a cause-and-effect relationship implies perfect prediction, perfect explanation, and inevitability (Cook, 1990). Perceptually, the attributes of a causal claim are covariation, temporal order, contiguity, similarity, short causal chains, and absence of alternatives (Einhorn & Hogarth, 1985). Traditionally, from a research perspective, there are three conditions that are necessary to support a causal claim (Cook & Campbell, 1979; Cordray, 1986): (a) the suspected cause and the suspected effect must co-vary so that changes in one are accompanied by changes in the other; (b) the suspected cause must precede the suspected effect; and (c) to demonstrate a causal claim it is necessary to rule out plausible alternative explanations of the effect. The three conditions that are necessary to support a causal claim can be illustrated by the controversy surrounding the relationship between smoking and lung cancer. Clearly, the research has shown that as smoking rates increase the incidence rates for lung cancer increase (Doll & Peto, 1981). Thus, the requirement of condition one is met. Just as compelling, the research has demonstrated that smoking precedes the onset of lung cancer (Doll & Peto, 1981). Thus, the requirement of condition two is met. It is the requirement of condition three that fuels the controversy about the causal link between smoking and lung cancer. Unconvinced observers dispute the claims of a causal connection between smoking and lung cancer. These observers make the case for plausible alternative explanations to account for the association between smoking and lung cancer. For example, perhaps there is a genetic component that causes lung cancer and also predisposes a person to smoke. After all, there are people who smoke and do not get lung cancer. Conversely, there are people who do not smoke but do get lung cancer. This controversy highlights the importance of satisfying the requirement of all three conditions to support a causal claim.

The regression discontinuity design addresses condition three by ruling out alternative hypotheses. With experimental designs, there is random assignment of units to treatment conditions in an unbiased fashion with known probability of being in a particular group. The importance of random assignment is that the probability of substantial pretreatment difference between groups is small and specifiable. In contrast, with quasi-experimental designs, such as the regression discontinuity design, the assignment to groups is not done by formal randomization. There is no assurance that the comparison conditions are equivalent prior to treatment. This fact increases the ambiguity of the results. Accordingly, quasi-experimental designs are most vulnerable to the threat of plausible alternative explanations for whatever effects are found on the outcome measures. The regression discontinuity design addresses this issue by obtaining a clear statistical baseline curve, an unwavering criterion for assignment to the intervention, and a sample large enough to support the analysis. Therefore, given the prevalence of quasi-experimental designs and the corresponding difficulty in ruling out rival explanations, methods to strengthen causal claims such as the regression discontinuity design are particularly appropriate for health care research in areas of mature scientific knowledge.

The Importance of Causal Claims

Causal claims represent the core of the scientific method, inductive and deductive logic, and empirical observations. Philosophers and scientists from the earliest of recorded history to contemporary times have been concerned with causal claims. Epidemiologists, too, have expressed their concern with causal claims as other scientists and philosophers. For example, Weed (1986) wrote that " . . . the fundamental scientific problem for the epidemiologist remains: how to propose and test causal hypotheses . . . in brief, it requires that we examine the logic of causal inference" (p. 965). Similarly, psychologists, statisticians, and nurse scientists have been concerned with research designs and causal claims (e.g., Hinshaw, Gerber, Atwood, & Allen, 1983). In sum, causal claims are a basic explanatory form of science (Cook, 1990).

Advantages and Issues

The two major advantages of regression discontinuity design are ethical and analytical. The ethical advantage is that the treatment can be targeted to those who need it most or a selected subset of the group. The analytical advantage is that it is much easier to rule out alternative explanations. An alternative explanation must invoke another event or effect coincident with the intervention precisely at the cut-off causing the same kind of discontinuity in the regression line. The likelihood is small of another event occurring precisely at the cut-off. Another analytical advantage of the regression discontinuity design is that it is particularly suited for health care research. Health care research features continuous quantitative indicators (Trochim, 1990) such as quality of life, degree of illness, dependency on caregiver, and vital signs. These measures and others such as risk factors, self-care practices, and commitment to healthy lifestyles, are easily used to determine cut-off criteria.

There are several key assumptions or prerequisites to meet before it is appropriate to use the regression discontinuity design. These assumptions are: (a) there are no exceptions to the cut-off criterion for who gets the intervention, (b) the distribution of the pre-post intervention scores is a polynomial function, (c) the preintervention sample must be large enough to support a regression line estimation, (d) "both pretest groups must come from a single continuous pretest distribution . . . and naturally discontinuous groups must be used with caution" (Trochim, 1990, p. 132), and (e) all participants must be given the same standardized intervention (Trochim, 1990). For interested readers Trochim (1984, 1990) and Judd and Kenny (1981) detail extensively the function, adaptations, restrictions, and implementation of the regression discontinuity design. To use the design, all of the prerequisites must be met. Nevertheless, the regression discontinuity design remains a valuable alternative to a randomized design for many current clinical nursing or administrative intervention studies.

References

Campbell, D. T., & Stanley, J. C. (1963). *Experimental and quasi-experimental designs for research.* Chicago: Rand McNally.

Cook, T. D. (1990). The generalization of causal connections: Multiple theories in search of clear practice. In L. Sechrest, E. Perrin, J. Bunker (eds.), *AHCPR Conference Proceedings: Research Methodology: Strengthening Causal Interpretations of Nonexperimental Data* (pp. 9–31). Rockville, MD: Agency for Health Care Policy and Research.

Cook, T. D., & Campbell, D. T. (1979). *Quasi-experimentation.* Chicago: Rand-McNally.

Cordray, D. S. (1986). Quasi-experimental analysis: A mixture of methods and judgment. *New Directions for Program Evaluation, 31,* 9–28.

Doll, R., & Peto, R. (1981). *The Causes of cancer.* Oxford: Oxford University Press.

Einhorn, H. J., & Hogarth, R. M. (1985). Ambiguity and uncertainty in probabilistic inference. *Psychological Review, 92,* 433–461.

Given, C. W., Given, B. A., & Coyle, B. W. (1985). Prediction of patient attrition from experimental behavioral interventions. *Nursing Research, 34,* 293–298.

Hinshaw, A. S., Gerber, R. N., Atwood, J. R., & Allen, J. R. (1983). The use of predictive modeling to test nursing practice outcomes. *Nursing Research, 32,* 35–42.

Judd, C. M., & Kenny, D. A. (1981). *Estimating the effects of social interventions.* New York: Cambridge University Press.

Medoff-Cooper, B. (1986). Temperament in very low birthweight infants. *Nursing Research, 35,* 139–143.

Miller, P., Wikoff, R. L., McMahon, M., Garrett, M. J., & Ringel, K. (1985). Indicators of medical regime adherence for myocardial infarction patients. *Nursing Research, 34,* 268–272.

Trochim, W. (1984). *Research design for program evaluation: The regression-discontinuity approach.* Beverly Hills, CA: Sage.

Trochim, W. M. K. (1990). The Regression-Discontinuity Design. In L. Sechrest, E. Perrin, Bunker (Eds.), *AHCPR Conference Proceedings: Research Methodology: Strengthening Causal Interpretations of Nonexperimental Data* (pp. 119–139). Rockville, MD: Agency for Health Care Policy and Research.

Verran, J., & Reed, P. (1987). Replicated testing of one nursing technology model. *Nursing Research, 36,* 190–194.

Weed, D. L. (1986). On the logic of causal inference. *American Journal of Epidemiology, 123,* 965–979.

Case-Control Design: An Appropriate Strategy for Nursing Research

Barbara J. Polivka ■ Jennie T. Nickel

Nurse researchers have traditionally drawn upon observational designs in conducting research (e.g., ex post facto, cross-sectional, longitudinal), yet observational retrospective case-control designs have rarely been reported in nursing studies (Jacobsen & Meininger, 1985; Meininger, 1989). This lack of use contrasts sharply with that of epidemiology, where case-control designs have not only served as a central analytical strategy since the 1950s, but have detected such well-publicized associations as tobacco smoking and lung cancer (Wydner & Graham, 1950), tampon use and toxic shock syndrome (Davis, Chesney, Wand, & LaVenture et al., 1980), and aspirin use and Reye's syndrome (Halpin et al., 1982). The benefits and pitfalls of use of the design have been reported by epidemiologic researchers, who have also designed strategies to offset design weaknesses (Kleinbaum, Kupper, & Morgenstern, 1982; Schlesselman, 1982).

The case-control design represents a well-developed approach to research with considerable potential for use in nursing. The purpose of this article is to present the structure of the design and to elaborate on points that must be considered when conducting case-control studies. A case-control study conducted by the authors, both of whom are nurse researchers, will illustrate points made. Initially, a brief summary of the study will be provided, then the basic features of the case-control design will be presented with reference to this study.

Illustration: Risk Factors for Cerebral Palsy: A Multivariate Model

In brief, cerebral palsy (CP) is a nonprogressive complex of motor dysfunctions detectable among children one to two years of age with a prevalence of approximately 2.5 cases per 1,000 live births (Kiely, Lubin, & Kiely, 1984). The etiology of cerebral palsy is unclear. While increased risk for CP has consistently been associated with low birth weight and prematurity, these may represent concurrent features of an already dysfunctional pregnancy rather than etiological factors per se. Researchers have increasingly called for investigation of factors that may affect the development of the pregnancy *in utero*.

This case-control study assessed a spectrum of maternal and paternal factors, exposures, and behaviors that might be associated with increased risk for CP in the offspring. Cases included 112 preschool children with diagnosed CP who received services from one of three agencies for handicapped children in a Midwestern urban area. Two sets of controls also participated in the study: 87 preschool children who were family friends of the cases and 66 preschool children drawn randomly from state birth certificate records. Data were collected via structured telephone interviews and birth certificate record review. All procedures were approved by the university and agency human subjects review boards.

Data were analyzed through odds ratios and logistic regressions and a profile of risk factors for CP developed. Maternal urinary tract infections during pregnancy, maternal use of medication to prevent miscarriage, infant Apgar scores, and infant low birth weight/short gestational age were independently predictive of cerebral palsy risk in the final logistic regression model.

Barbara J. Polivka, PhD, RN, is a staff researcher at the Ohio Department of Mental Health, Columbus, OH.

Jennie T. Nickel, PhD, RN, is an assistant professor, Department of Family and Community, at the Ohio State University College of Nursing, Columbus, OH.

From *Nursing Research,* July/August 1992, *41,* 250–253.

Structure of the Case-Control Study

In contrast to experimental design strategies, retrospective case-control and prospective follow-up studies are observational in nature, focusing on assessing the effects of exposures and experiences in life situations. The case-control design is depicted in Figure 1 in relation to the prospective design, which is generally more familiar to researchers.

Retrospective case-control and prospective studies differ with respect to three major features: the point of sample selection, the temporal direction of data collection, and the capabilities for measurement of multiple exposures and multiple effects. The prospective study begins with individuals selected and/or categorized on

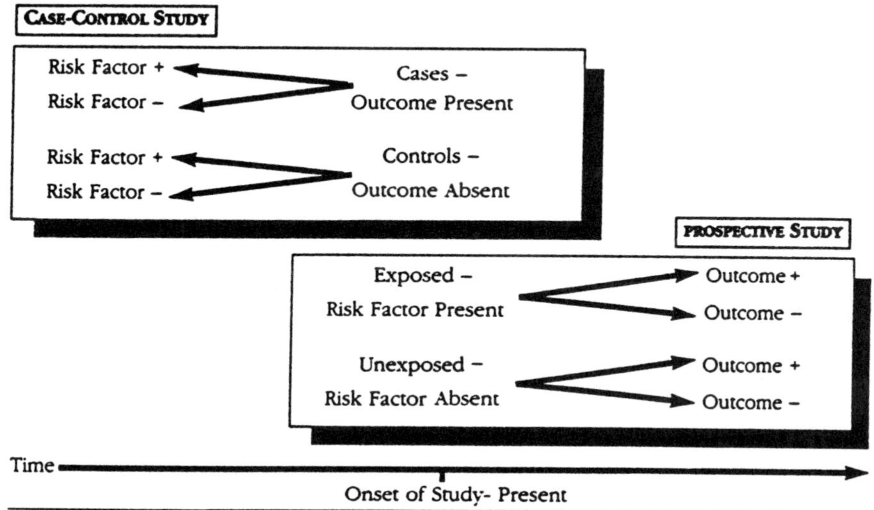

Note: Arrows within boxes indicate direction of time. In case-control box, arrows signify retrospective investigation; in prospective box, arrows signify longitudinal investigation.

FIGURE 1 Comparison of Structures of Case-Control and Prospective Studies

the basis of factors present and followed over time to see if the outcome occurs. The prospective approach thus allows for assessment of both multiple antecedent factors and multiple outcomes (e.g., associations of both heart disease and strokes with hypertension and family history).

In contrast, with the case-control study, the outcome has already occurred and the investigator retrospectively assesses past history of the exposure(s) or factor(s) hypothesized as antecedent. The outcome can be any illness or condition; the factor can be any exposure, attribute, or event hypothesized as related to the outcome (Kelsey, Thompson, & Evans, 1986; Schlesselman, 1982). The process of case-control selection generally limits the researcher to a single effect, but associations can be studied for single or multiple hypothesized antecedent factors. In the study described, CP was the outcome factor; multiple antecedent factors were assessed such as parental reproductive histories and parental illnesses during pregnancy.

Advantages

The unique design of the case-control study yields both advantages to the investigator and challenges to the maintenance of the integrity of the research. Clear advantages are provided in terms of time and resource requirements for the research, sample sizes, and appropriateness of this design for relatively infrequent or rare conditions. A prospective study of CP would require several thousand subjects to be followed for at least 2 years to detect a difference between exposed and unexposed individuals. This design was used by the nation's largest CP study, the National Collaborative Perinatal Project, which was initiated in the late 1960s and followed approximately 50,000 pregnancies, identifying 189 cases of CP (Nelson & Ellenberg, 1985). In comparison, the case-control study serving as the base of this report required 112 cases and an equal number of controls to detect a relative risk of 2.5 (assuming a 25% exposure frequency for the controls; alpha = .05; and beta = .10) (Schlesselman, 1982).

Disadvantages

Among the major disadvantages of the case-control design is the difficulty in distinguishing causation from correlation. Because data are assessed retrospectively, case-control studies identify factors associated with risk of the outcome and not necessarily a direct causal link (Breslow & Day, 1980). Another limitation is the reliance on data from existing records and/or recall. Data may be improperly recorded or omitted from records or individuals may not accurately recall exposure information. Other concerns with this design include vulnerability to bias, difficulty in determining and obtaining a suitable control group, and limited information that may be available on confounders. A confounder is a variable associated with both the outcome and the exposure. The effect of the confounder on the outcome occurs even in the absence of the exposure of interest (Schlesselman, 1982). Finally, unless population-based samples are used, it is not possible to calculate incidence rates for the outcome. Instead, odds ratios (ORs), which are an estimation of the relative outcome frequency in the sample, are generally estimated (Breslow & Day, 1980).

Potential Biases and Common Strategies for Control

Because the prospective design and controlled administration of the factor (i.e., intervention) so central to clinical trials are not possible for the case-control study, this design is vulnerable to a number of biases—that is, errors within the design, conduct, or analysis that can result in an erroneous estimate of the effect on risk of the outcome (Sackett, 1979; Schlesselman, 1982). A summary of the major biases and strategies directed toward their control is presented in Table 1. The CP study is reviewed below in reference to these potential biases. Features that were introduced into the CP study to counter potential biases are described.

Survivor bias presented threats to the study because prevalent (existing) cases were used rather than incident (new cases emerging from a pool of susceptibles). Infants with CP could have been lost through fetal wastage or neonatal death. The sample may thus represent survivors rather than all cases. *Selection* bias was countered by selecting cases from three different community agencies, assuring a wider range of socioeconomic levels and severity of symptoms than would be obtained from a single agency. Also, two types of controls were used—friends of case families and population controls randomly selected from birth certificate records. Effects of *nonparticipation* for cases and birth certificate controls were assessed by comparing information on birth records for participants and nonparticipants. The investigators were particularly concerned about under-representation of minority groups. African Americans were found to be equally willing to participate in the study but more likely than other groups to be categorized as unable to locate. The CP study is thus vulnerable to bias from reduced representation of this group.

Measurement bias was countered by using items from questionnaires from similar research and by pilot testing the procedures and interview guide. In addition to using interview information, birth certificate data were obtained and, for a sample of subjects, hospital records were reviewed for information such as birth weight and Apgar scores. It was not possible to collect and record interview data without knowledge of case/control status, but occupational exposure codes were assigned using a blinded system. Information on the strength and timing of exposures was obtained whenever possible.

With respect to *misclassification,* CP diagnosis was based on agency records. Ideally, the diagnosis would have been validated by a physician specializing in the field. To avoid misclassification of controls, respondents were asked about a history of CP diagnosis. The mother

TABLE 1 Design Biases and Control Strategies in Case-Control Studies

Bias	Description	Control Strategy
Survivor	Identification of cases after outcome onset may omit those who experience early death.	Restrict to incident cases.
Selection	Cases selected differ systematically from the population of cases; controls differ systematically from population of controls.	Randomly select cases from an inclusive frame. Use multiple sources for both cases and controls.
Nonparticipants	Potential subjects who are not located or those who choose not to participate differ substantively from participants.	Obtain information on significant variables for nonparticipants and compare to participants.
Measurement	Error in measuring relevant variables.	Select valid and reliable data collection tools. Use multiple sources for the same data and check congruence. Collect, record, and analyze without knowledge of case/control status.
Misclassification	Error in categorizing case/control status.	Validate the outcome and exposure data.
Recall	Time lapse may adversely affect subject provision of complete information on exposures. Cases may be more likely to ruminate over past events and thus overestimate exposures.	Limit time between exposures of interest and data collection. Use memory prompts within questionnaires. Verify interview data with clinical records.

of one birth certificate control revealed that her child had once been considered to have CP. This child was subsequently dropped from the study. Misclassification of exposures can result if a respondent denies an exposure when in fact there was an exposure, or vice versa. If the misclassification is experienced equally by chance among cases and controls, the result can be an underestimate of the magnitude of the association, rather than an error in direction (Schlesselman, 1982).

To minimize *recall* bias, the study was restricted to preschool children. Also, as noted earlier, birth certificate and hospital records were used to validate certain items, such as recalled birth weight, gestational age, and delivery complications.

Confounding

Since the design of the case-control study precludes random assignment to exposed and nonexposed groups, the investigator must work to identify and control for confounding effects of extraneous variables. At the outset, known confounders should be identified from the relevant research literature. Subject exclusion criteria may be based on these identified confounders. At a minimum, collection of data on the confounders must be incorporated into the research instruments. For major confounders, control may be achieved through matching of the cases and controls (Breslow & Day, 1980). In the analytical phase of the study, confounders may be assessed further through statistical means, and control achieved through stratification and/or use of multivariate statistical models. In the CP study, category matching (as opposed to one-to-one matching) was used to control for the potential confounders of child's age, sex, ethnic group, and mother's county of residence at the time of birth. Socioeconomic status was indirectly controlled through the use of a friend control group, since friends are generally of the same socioeconomic status. Because the primary goal of the CP study was the construction of a model explanatory of CP risk, rather than the testing of a single exposure or experience with risk, variables were assessed and entered into the model on the basis of explanatory power rather than for control of confounding.

Analysis

When the outcome of a case-control study is defined as dichotomous (either case or control categorization), the method of analysis is the odds ratio (OR) or logistic regression. The OR is the odds of an outcome factor in an *exposed* person relative to the odds of the outcome factor in an *unexposed* individual and serves as a measure of relative risk when the outcome is rare. An OR is derived from a 2 × 2 table and, in an unmatched or categorically matched design, is calculated as *ad*/*bc* (Table 2). (For one-to-one matched analyses, see Schlesselman, 1982.) The null hypothesis for the OR is that there is no association between the outcome and the exposure: H_o: OR = 1. An OR of one therefore indicates no difference in risk for the exposed as compared to nonexposed group. Statistical significance of the OR may be indicated through either a chi-square test or by use of confidence intervals (CI). A CI provides a range of plausible values and indicates the precision of estimate of effect (Kelsey et al., 1986). If the 95% CI contains one, the OR is not statistically significant; if the interval excludes one, the OR is significant at an alpha level of .05.

An odds ratio calculation from the CP study further illustrates these points. The factor of interest is history of premature birth (Table 2). There were 11 case and 4 control mothers who reported previously delivering a premature infant. The OR was calculated as 4.1 (95% CI of 1.26, 13.1), indicating that case mothers were 4.1 times as likely to report a history of premature birth as control mothers, $\chi^2 = 6.3$, $p = .012$. The CI indicates that odds ratios less than 1.26 or greater than 13.1 can be ruled out with 95% confidence.

Multivariate tests were conducted through the use of logistic regression. Logistic regression is a maximum likelihood estimation method used to control confounders and develop explanatory and predictive models. It is a type of log-linear model in which the dependent variable is dichotomous or categorical, and there are few assumptions regarding the distribution of the independent variables (Kelsey et al., 1986). The risk of developing the outcome is expressed as the following function of the predictor variables:

$$\text{Log odds of outcome} = a + b_1x_1 + \ldots + b_fx_f \qquad (1)$$

with *a* and *b* the estimated constants, *x* the individual's values for the predictor variables, and *r* equal to the number of regressor variables (Kelsey et al., 1986). Exponentiating the beta coefficient yields an estimate

TABLE 2 Two-by-Two Table for Calculating Odds Ratio

	Cases	Controls
(Exposed)	(a)	(b)
History of premature birth	11	4
(Nonexposed)	(c)	(d)
No history of premature birth	101	149

Odds Ratio = ad/bc

of the change in the OR associated with a unit change in a given predictor variable, holding the other variables constant.

For example, Table 3 illustrates the adjusted odds ratios for three predictor variables from the CP study: (a) maternal use of a medication for potential miscarriage, (b) maternal history of previous premature birth, and (c) maternal age at the time of birth. The regression coefficients, standard errors, adjusted OR, and 95% CI are included for each independent variable. Exponentiating the beta coefficients yielded odds ratios of 9.18 for medication for potential miscarriage (vs. no medication), 4.25 for history of premature birth (vs. no such history), and 0.95 per year maternal age. The adjusted OR for history of previous premature birth was essentially similar to the crude OR obtained through univariate analysis, indicating no evidence of confounding between these predictor variables. The 95% confidence intervals were calculated straightforwardly using the beta coefficient and the standard error (SE):

$$\text{Log of 95\% CI} = \text{Beta} \pm 1.96\ (\text{SE}) \qquad (2)$$

These calculated values were then exponentiated to yield the upper and lower limits of the 95% confidence intervals. For example, the 95% confidence intervals for the maternal age variable was calculated as:

$$-0.55 \pm 1.96\ (0.26) = -0.004, -0.106 \qquad (3)$$

Exponentiating these values yielded the 95% CI of 0.9 and 0.996. Because the CI did not include one, the OR was considered significant at the .05 alpha level, indicating that with each year increase in maternal age, there was a decrease in the odds of risk for CP by a factor of .95 (Kelsey et al., 1986; Homer & Lemeshow, 1989).

TABLE 3 Sample Logistic Regression Table with Odds Ratios and 95% Confidence Intervals

Variables	Beta	Standard Error	Odds Ratio	95% Confidence Interval
Intercept	0.986	.711		
Medication for miscarriage (Yes:No)	2.217	.780	9.18	1.99–42.33
History of premature birth (Yes:No)	1.447	.608	4.25	1.29–14.00
Maternal age (1 year)	−0.55	.026	0.95	0.90–0.996

Summary

The case-control design is a well-established research method in epidemiology and has considerable potential for nursing research. It is particularly appropriate for studying health or service outcomes that occur relatively infrequently and offers advantages in time, sample size, and resource requirements. While the retrospective observational nature of the design presents challenges in selection of subjects, avoidance of biases, and control confounding, the processes for managing these pitfalls are increasingly being explored. The analysis is straightforward and presents estimates of risk that are clearly interpretable by nurse researcher, policy makers, and other research consumers.

References

Breslow, N. E., & Day, N. E. (1980). *Statistical methods in cancer research: The analysis of case-control studies* (IARC Pub. 32). Lyons, France: International Agency for Research on Cancer.

Davis, J. P., Chesney, P. J., Wand, P. J., & LaVenture, M. (1980). Toxic shock syndrome. Epidemiologic features, recurrence, risk factors and prevention. *New England Journal of Medicine, 303,* 1429–1435.

Halpin, T. J., Holtzhauer, F. J., Campbell, R. J., Hall, L. J., Correa-Villaseñor, A., Lanese, R., Rice, J., & Hurwitz, E. S. (1982). Reye's Syndrome and medication use. *Journal of the American Medical Association, 248,* 687–691.

Homer, D. W., & Lemeshow, S. (1989). *Applied logistic regression.* New York: Wiley & Sons.

Jacobsen, B. S., & Meininger, J. C. (1985). The designs and methods of published nursing research: 1956–1983. *Nursing Research, 34,* 306–312.

Kelsey, J. L., Thompson, W. D., & Evans, A. S. (1986). *Methods in observational epidemiology.* New York: Oxford University Press.

Kiely, M., Lubin, R. A., & Kiely, J. L. (1984). Descriptive epidemiology of cerebral palsy. *Public Heath Review, 12,* 79–101.

Kleinbaum, D.G., Kupper, L. L., & Morgenstern, H. (1982). *Epidemiologic research: Principles and quantitative methods.* New York: Reinhold.

Meininger, J. C. (1989). Epidemiologic designs. In P. J. Brink & M. J. Wood (eds.), *Advanced design in nursing research* (pp. 201–222). Newbury Park, CA: Sage Publications.

Nelson, K. B., & Ellenberg, J. H. (1985). Antecedents of cerebral palsy: I. Univariate analysis of risks. *American Journal of Diseases in Children, 139,* 1031–1038.

Sackett, D. L. (1979). Bias in analytic research. *Journal of Chronic Diseases, 32,* 51–63.

Schlesselman, J. J. (1982). *Case-control studies: Design, conduct, analysis.* New York: Oxford University Press.

Wydner, E. L., & Graham, E. A. (1950). Tobacco smoking as a possible etiologic factor in bronchiogenic carcinoma. *Journal of the American Medical Association, 143,* 329–338.

A Mixed-Method Approach for Using Cross-Sectional Data for Longitudinal Inferences

Lauren S. Aaronson ■ Margaret J. Kingry

Longitudinal designs are best for studying patterns of behavior changes over the course of time, questions of a developmental nature, or the temporal sequencing of phenomena necessary for establishing causal relationships (Barnard, 1985; Polit & Hungler, 1987). Longitudinal designs minimize sources of error due to sampling variability. Therefore, small but real changes in behavior are detectable.

However, longitudinal studies are expensive and time-consuming. Advances in theory and instrumentation may lead to changes in research equipment or protocols. Many of the threats to the validity of experimental and quasi-experimental designs—such as repeated testing and changes in the external environment—also threaten longitudinal studies.

The long-term commitment required of subjects in longitudinal studies makes it more difficult to recruit subjects and increases the likelihood of subject mortality. This in turn often results in smaller sample sizes and less sample variability, limiting the ability to generalize findings. Further, results that might be considered substantively significant may not show statistical significance because of the decreased stability and larger effects or differences needed with smaller samples.

Cross-sectional designs are more cost-effective and easier to manage. The opportunity to increase the number of subjects often results in greater variability within the sample and may allow for more generalizability of findings. An important disadvantage of the cross-sectional design is the difficulty of establishing or identifying behavior patterns, changes over time, or causal relationships. Ideally, longitudinal designs are used for research problems such as these. Cross-sectional designs are used when questions asked can be answered at one point in time (e.g., descriptive studies). However, due to many potential and real constraints, cross-sectional data are sometimes used to make longitudinal inferences. It is important, therefore, to consider when and under what circumstances cross-sectional data can be used in this manner and when a mixed method that combines features of both approaches is preferable.

Cross-Sectional Survey Approaches

Babbie (1973) proposed three cross-sectional survey approaches that may provide data approximating longitudinal data. The first approach is to ask respondents to provide current data as well as information about the past. Ryder (1980) found both " . . . observations about the same unit as of two times and observations at two times concerning the same unit" (p. 195) legitimate for longitudinal inference. Moreover, this historical approach eliminates many problems associated with longitudinal designs such as expense, time, and sample attrition.

However, there are limitations to this approach. The most problematic is that subjects may have difficulty accurately recalling information. Selective retention and reporting of information and reconstruction of events after the fact also pose problems (Cahalan, 1968). Although the significance of the event moderates the effect, most investigations find underreporting is a function of time (NCHS, 1965, 1971).

Gutek (1978) specifically tested the assumption that attitudes are recalled less accurately over time. She hypothesized that patterns of relationships among attitudes about events that occurred at increasingly distant points in time would reflect increased error variance and yield lower correlations. Only 2 of 15 comparisons investigated substantiated the expected dissimilarities. Gutek concluded that although problems in recall or cognitive distortion may occur, retrospective data about events as much as 10 to 15 years in the past are no less accurate than retrospective data about events that occurred several months previous to data collection. Powers, Goudy, and Keith (1978) compared respondents' responses with their recollections 10 years later and found that retrospective and concurrent items were usable as estimates for the sample as a whole or for examining relationships

Lauren S. Aaronson, PhD, RN, is an assistant professor in the School of Nursing, University of Michigan, Ann Arbor.

Margaret J. Kingry, PhD, RN, is an assistant professor in the College of Nursing, Michigan State University, East Lansing.

From *Nursing Research,* May/June 1988, *37,* 187–189.

among variables. They cautioned, however, that the validity of retrospective accounts of specific individuals is more questionable because recall responses tend to present a more favorable picture of the respondent.

Another problem with the use of historical cross-sectional data is that all findings are from a single sample measured at one point in time, opposed to cross-sections of the population measured at different points in time. Consequently, specific cohort effects cannot be disentangled and the impact of external events that occurred at the referent time point may have unknown effects.

Process or change also can be approached with cross-sectional data through age or cohort comparisons. Babbie (1973) offered a specific example of the dilemma that this approach poses. If young and old people are sampled, and younger persons are found to be less religious, one could conclude either that there is a general decline in religiosity—believing young people hold more current values—or that as people grow older they tend to become more religious. Cross-sectional data cannot distinguish between these two plausible interpretations.

Another approach suggested by Babbie and used in many qualitative investigations is to seek answers to longitudinal questions with cross-sectional data by making logical interpretations of the data. For example, Hutchinson (1986, 1987) used the grounded theory method in collecting and analyzing interview and participant observation data in a study of chemically dependent nurses. From these data she identified a series of stages and phases of self-annihilation and self-integration processes that are experienced by chemically dependent nurses. Studies using causal modeling techniques also use the logical interpretation approach, often relying on assumptions about the temporal sequence of variables that are measured simultaneously.

Each of these three approaches has limitations and leaves open the question of whether findings are biased by or are completely an artifact of the design employed. Sorting out answers to these questions requires replication of a study using each design approach. There are, however, few large scale studies that directly compare the cross-sectional design approach with the longitudinal approach (Cook & Alexander, 1980; Hilton & Patrick, 1970).

Although the choice of design depends on the specific substantive questions to be studied, this procedural decision also has important substantive implications. For example, in an investigation of adolescent goal formation and attainment using both longitudinal and cross-sectional data, Cook and Alexander (1980) found the impact of social support and goal orientation greater in cross-sectional data and ascriptive and structural constraints such as race and socioeconomic status more pronounced in longitudinal data.

A Mixed-Method Approach

Although studies do not always simultaneously use both design approaches, sometimes when a cross-sectional design is adequate for most of the goals of a study, a small longitudinal study can be run to help assess the validity of inferences from the cross-sectional data that are related to change or time. This approach was used in a study of health behavior and beliefs during pregnancy (Aaronson, 1984). Although the study was primarily cross-sectional, repeated measures late in pregnancy were obtained on a subsample of subjects who originally participated in the study early in their pregnancies. By combining the two design methods, the efficiency of a cross-sectional design as well as the soundness of a longitudinal design were realized.

Allows Greater Confidence in Findings

The first advantage of the mixed-method approach is that greater confidence can be placed in the validity of cross-sectional findings about change or time-bound issues that are supported by longitudinal evidence.

Example Using Aaronson's (1984) data, attitude stability in relation to health behaviors was compared over the course of pregnancy. Eight attitudes were assessed for each of six health behaviors. The longitudinal sample ($N = 82$) comparisons were made using paired t tests; the cross-sectional sample ($N = 415$) comparisons, standard t tests. Only those women who fit the gestational distributions of the longitudinal sample at their first and second measurement periods were used for the cross-sectional sample comparisons. Although there are statistical probability hazards in performing multiple tests, the objective was to discover patterns in the findings—not isolated results. The study question was: Did inferences about gestational effects differ as a function of design factors?

That there were no statistically significant differences in demographic characteristics in the longitudinal sample ($N = 82$), the early pregnancy cross-sectional sample ($N = 71$), and the late pregnancy cross-sectional sample ($N = 267$) was established first. The cross-sectional analyses of attitude stability were then replicated with the longitudinal sample. Attitudes were found to be consistent, suggesting a fair amount of stability across the course of pregnancy, whether measured and tested with longitudinal or cross-sectional data.

The longitudinal comparisons suggested seven significant changes in women's attitudes or beliefs from early to late pregnancy: a decrease in perceptions of support from family for alcohol abstinence and for adhering to their prenatal diet, a decrease in perceptions of support from friends for that diet, an increase in perceptions of support from their health care provider for caffeine abstinence, an increase in the perceived costs associated with exercising, a decrease in beliefs about the efficacy of the prenatal diet, and a decrease in the beliefs about the consequences of that diet for the baby. Only two of these, decreased support from family for alcohol abstinence and decreased support from friends for diet, were detected in the cross-sectional comparisons. On the other hand, the cross-sectional comparisons suggested three other changes, a decrease in the perceived benefits of alcohol abstinence, a decrease in support from friends for alcohol abstinence, and a decrease in support from health care providers for exercising, none of which were confirmed by the longitudinal comparisons.

Thus, the general attitude stability suggested by the cross-sectional data was validated with the longitudinal data. Further, in instances of significant differences in the same direction with both approaches, the validity of inferences about attitude change that might be drawn from the cross-sectional findings also was strengthened.

Increases Ability to Detect Differences

A second advantage of the mixed-method approach is that differences that may not be evident in cross-sectional data may be detected with a longitudinal analysis. Longitudinal samples are less subject to random variation because subjects serve as their own control. Cross-sectional comparisons may not detect these differences simply because of the greater random variability inherent in cross-sectional samples.

Example Each of our findings using the longitudinal data is intuitively reasonable. The increase in perceived costs associated with exercising in late pregnancy may reflect greater difficulty and less pleasure in exercising at that time. The decrease in perceived support from family for alcohol abstinence may reflect their weariness with forgoing alcoholic beverages. The general decrease in beliefs about the impact of diet in late pregnancy (four of the seven significant findings involved diet) suggests a mistaken belief that diet is less crucial at this time. Data from the cross-sectional sample would not have showed this important substantive finding. Only one of the four findings from the longitudinal sample regarding diet was found in the cross-sectional sample. And, the increase in perceived support from providers for caffeine abstinence may be attributed to when these data were collected. In 1982, concern about caffeine during pregnancy was not as widely publicized as that about smoking and alcohol. The initial study questions about caffeine may have led the women to ask their provider about caffeine and the subsequent measures on the longitudinal sample may reflect these discussions.

Promotes Cautious Interpretation of Findings

A third advantage of the mixed-method approach is that the investigator is alerted to look carefully at findings that are significant in the cross-sectional data but are not confirmed by the longitudinal data. Both the larger cross-sectional sample size and the greater sample variability increase the likelihood that significant findings may occur merely by chance. To reject the null hypothesis based on these findings alone could result in committing a Type I error. In general, when findings regarding change or other time-bound issues from cross-sectional and longitudinal analyses are at odds, the greater control implicit in longitudinal designs leads to greater faith in findings from longitudinal data, and the greater potential for random variability in cross-sectional samples renders findings from those data more suspect. In the data discussed here, the three uncorroborated cross-sectional findings fell into this category. Because analyses with the longitudinal sample did not support these findings, we would hesitate to interpret them.

Conclusions

The overriding issue in selecting a design is identifying one that is most appropriate for the research question. If for practical reasons it is not always possible to conduct a full longitudinal study, a combined approach of imbedding a longitudinal subsample within a cross-sectional design is better than relying exclusively on evidence from cross-sectional data.

References

Aaronson, L. S. (1984). Health behavior in pregnancy: Testing a general model. (Doctoral dissertation, University of Washington, 1983.) *Dissertation Abstracts International, 44*-11A, 3498.

Babbie, E. R. (1973). *Survey research methods.* Belmont, CA: Wadsworth Publishing Company, Inc.

Barnard, K. E. (1985). Studying patterns of behavior. *MCN, 10,* 358.

Cahalan, D. (1968). Correlates of respondent accuracy in the Denver Validity Survey. *Public Opinion Quarterly, 32,* 607–621.

Cook, M. A., & Alexander, K. L. (1980). Design and substance in educational research: Adolescent attainments, a case in point. *Sociology of Education, 53,* 187–202.

Gutek, B. (1978). On the accuracy of retrospective attitudinal data. *Public Opinion Quarterly, 42,* 390–401.

Hilton, T. L., & Patrick, C. (1970). Cross-sectional versus longitudinal data: An empirical comparison of mean differences in academic growth. *Journal of Educational Measurement, 7,* 15–24.

Hutchinson, S. (1986). Chemically dependent nurses: The trajectory toward self-annihilation. *Nursing Research, 35,* 196–201.

Hutchinson, S. (1987). Toward self-integration: The recovery process of chemically dependent nurses. *Nursing Research, 36,* 339–343.

National Center for Health Statistics (1965). Health interview responses compared with medical records. *Vital and Health Statistics,* Washington, DC: US Government Printing Office. (PHS Publication No. 1000—Series 2—No. 8.)

National Center for Health Statistics (1971). Effect of some experimental interviewing techniques on reporting in the Health Interview Survey. *Vital and Health Statistics,* Washington, DC: US Government Printing Office. (No. 1000—Series 2—No. 41.)

Polit, D. F., & Hungler, B. P. (1987). *Nursing research—Principles and methods.* (3rd ed.). Philadelphia: J. P. Lippincott.

Powers, E. W., Goudy, W., & Keith, P. (1978). Congruence between panel and recall data in longitudinal research. *Public Opinion Quarterly, 42,* 380–389.

Ryder, N. B. (1980). Where do babies come from? In *Sociological theory and research* (pp. 189–202). New York: The Free Press.

Longitudinal Research Using Computerized Clinical Databases: Caveats and Constraints

Anne K. Wuerker

Computerized clinical databases are becoming commonplace, and although data collection in these systems is generally driven by fiscal and management concerns, valuable clinical data are obtained and stored in the process. These databases offer excellent opportunities for nurse researchers to explore clinical questions, in particular those that require information over time, without gathering new data. Some of the issues unique to research using these databases are described in this article.

Types of Clinical Databases

Probably the earliest clinical databases were psychiatric case registers, many of which have been maintained since the 1960s. There has been a recent surge of interest in exploring questions using these data, for example, Eaton et al. (1992) studied long-term outcomes in schizophrenia using psychiatric case register data from the United States, Australia, England, and Denmark. Historically psychiatric case registers recorded only inpatient admissions, but there are increasingly numbers of databases that include all mental health care in a given system. Some of these systems are primarily fiscal, such as records of Medicaid paid claims, as used by Hadley, McGurrin, Pulice, and Holohean (1990) to identify "heavy users" of the psychiatric system. Other systems are primarily clinical, for example, the Los Angeles County Department of Mental Health (LACDMH) data, which has information on every admission to any mental health service throughout the county since 1969. LACDMH data have been used to generate many articles in the past decade (e.g., Flaskerud & Hu, 1992; Takechui, Bui, & Kim, 1993; Wuerker and Keenan, 1997).

The types of clinical databases available for research have changed dramatically with the advent of managed care. One of the most important sources of data on more general medical care is from Health Maintenance Organizations (HMOs) (Durham, 1994). These data systems are becoming increasingly sophisticated, therefore fiscal data and service use in many areas are now more likely to be linked. Durham writes that this abundance of longitudinal data on a well-defined population offers a great opportunity for researchers. Most large medical systems also have some system of computerized data collection in place.

Other longitudinal data sets that might be of interest to nurse researchers include the Illinois Integrated Database on Children and Family Services (Goerge, Van Voorhis, & Lee, 1994), which documents all child contacts with foster care, child abuse and neglect, mental health, and other state services throughout the past decade, and the National Child Development Study in Great Britain, which has data on 17,000 children born in 1958. The latter data set, although not clinical, includes medical information from records at birth and from physical examinations and histories at ages 7, 11, and 16 years, as well as measures of mental health, scholastic ability, and academic achievement (Fox & Fogelman, 1990).

Research Issues in the Use of Computerized Clinical Data Sets

Since few clinical data systems were designed for research, the task of designing a study using available data can be a challenging one. Newer systems are more likely to include clinically relevant variables, but they are also likely to be less interesting in the extensiveness of the information over time. The questions must be framed in a way that they can be answered with the data; therefore, the researchers need to be very familiar with the data as collected. It is important to know how the data are collected and by whom. Familiarity with the clinical setting is vital for understanding the limitations of the data set and for clinically relevant interpretations.

Often familiarity with the clinical setting means being familiar with the system as well because terminology can be idiosyncratic. An example is a term such as unit of care, which may mean anything from a day of hospitalization to any encounter with a staff person. It may be necessary to spend time familiarizing oneself with the patterns of care and the data entry procedures

Anne K. Wuerker, MSN, PhD, is an assistant professor, School of Nursing, University of California, Los Angeles.

From *Nursing Research,* November/December 1997, *46,* 353–355.

used in the system. Of course, the more structured data sets such as the Illinois Integrated Database, which are designed to be research friendly, usually have adequate documentation.

The population must adequately represent the group of interest. For example, Thompson (1994) notes that no national databases have information on the psychiatric problems of minority elders and that even when data have been collected on this group specifically, samples are too small to allow meaningful analysis. Thus, when researchers wish to examine an issue in a subset of patients (e.g., patients with a particular illness, perhaps an uncommon one, patients in a given age group or a minority status), they must be very careful that adequate data on the subpopulation exists.

Obtaining Permission to Use the Data

Some large national data sets are in the public domain, but most research projects using clinical data will require the same steps in securing permission that are required for gathering data. The subjects do not ordinarily have to be recontacted, as presumably they already gave permission when the data were collected. However, as Colby and Phelps (1990) note, permission to use the data beyond the original intent has rarely been obtained explicitly. Human subjects committees will usually determine whether the use of the data represents a threat to confidentiality. Much depends on the nature of the research, whether linked records can result in confidentiality being breached, and whether names must be used or identifiers can be provided. If the risk to confidentiality is high, the subjects may have to be recontacted. Once the data are obtained, the same precautions must be followed as with new data collected (Goerge, Van Voorhis, & Lee, 1994).

Confidentiality is an emerging problem in computerized clinical data sets (Wedding, Topolski, & McGaha, 1995). As more systems are linked, they are a better source of data, but confidentiality becomes more difficult to guarantee and therefore access to the records may be denied. Mental health information is a case in point; confidentiality is normally carefully protected. However, records of psychiatric service use may be linked to records for general medical care, and confidentiality may thus be breached. On the other hand, mental health information is often not included in the medical record because of these issues (Durham, 1994), which may limit the research questions.

Structuring the Data

Although some clinical data sets are designed for research, most are not. The data may consist primarily of records of care, and it is up to the researcher to compile a workable data set from them.

Great care must be used with electronic data to check for accuracy and reliability. Because the data are often already assembled, it may be tempting to assume accuracy, but careful checking for duplications and errors is essential. Goerge, Van Voorhis, and Lee (1994) note that the multiple sources of data in integrated databases make it possible to detect and correct errors in many instances. For example, demographic data such as date of birth and education can be checked because of multiple entries for the same person. Data recorded as missing may be available in earlier records. Education level (highest grade attained), an example from the author's research, was reported as missing for most of a group of homeless mentally ill persons. However, their early records in the system contained that information.

One of the common problems in clinical data sets is redundant entries. The safest way to find these and other errors as well is to visually inspect a printout of all of the data. Because they are usually organized chronologically, duplications are detectable. A related problem is in dates of service. Researchers often have questions based on time intervals (e.g., how long the interval was between admissions or for how long a patient received care). Admissions to one service may occur before discharge from another, therefore intervals between episodes of care become meaningless unless the data are carefully scrutinized and redefined. Another problem can be in the definition of episode, which might vary with the system. Most data sets contain the information needed to define an interval of care, but the data may need to be converted from event data to episode data or from what Goerge, Van Voorhis, and Lee call summary records.

Codes used in clinical databases can be extremely complex. Once again, knowledge of the system is essential for deciding how to collapse codes. When considering the Diagnostic and Statistical Manual of Mental Disorders (DSM) codes for psychiatric diagnosis, for example, the investigator might need to know when DSM-III-R or DSM-IV was introduced in that particular setting. The same is true of the International Classification of Diseases, 9th revision (ICD-9), and the ICD-9-CM codes.

Analysis of Longitudinal Data

The advantage of computerized databases are that all episodes of care within the system are documented. Therefore, research questions are likely to involve care over time in some way. An important element in the decision about analytic methods is whether the sequential structure needs to be preserved. This decision must be based on substantive concerns because some research goals may require temporal ordering and some may not. For example, in one study it might be important to know how many times a child was admitted for emergency care for asthma, and in another, the pattern of follow-up care after each admission might be more important. Analytic strategies for sequential data are often different than those in which only frequencies are used.

Two examples of methods that work well for longitudinal data are cluster analysis and survival analysis. Cluster analysis is a method for grouping individual cases into a homogeneous group on the basis of some set of variables. For example, for each patient, admissions to various services for differing diagnoses or treatments can be treated as "scores" and then cluster analysis can be used to group patients according to their profiles. The basic reference for cluster analysis is Aldenderfer and Blashfield (1984); the overview of cluster analysis by Rapkin and Luke (1993) is very readable and informative.

Survival analysis is an appropriate strategy when the focus is in the timing of an event and the variables related to that. The event might be relapse, recovery, or length of time of remission. Standard statistical packages now include a variety of survival analysis routines, and several recent reports present clear and comprehensive explanations and examples (Griffin, 1993; Luke, 1993; Singer & Willet, 1991; Willet & Singer, 1993).

Analyses that preserve sequencing of the data range from simple contingency analysis examining probabilities of one thing occurring given the occurrence of another to complex methods comparing long sequences of events. An interesting discussion of the factors guiding a choice of methods for sequential analysis will be found in Abbott and Hrycak (1990); Gottman and Roy (1990) present a more elaborate discussion of analyzing sequential data.

The proliferation of computerized databases combined with more readily available statistical procedures for longitudinal analyses offers nurse researchers expanded opportunities to conduct interesting clinical research. There are clear limitations inherent in this type of research, but with careful planning, research using computerized databases can be productive and exciting. As funding for new studies continues to shrink, more researchers will turn to this rich source of clinical data.

References

Abbott, A., & Hrycak, A. (1990). Measuring resemblance in sequence data: An optimal matching of musicians' careers. *American Journal of Sociology, 96,* 144–185.

Aldenderfer, M. S., & Blashfield, R. K. (1984). *Cluster analysis.* Newbury Park, CA: Sage.

Colby, A., & Phelps, E. (1990). Archiving longitudinal data. In D. Magnusson & L. Bergman (eds.). *Data quality in longitudinal research* (pp. 249–262). Cambridge: Cambridge University Press.

Durham, M. L. (1994). Prospects and problems in using data from HMOs for the study of aging populations and their health care needs. *The Gerontologist, 4,* 481–485.

Eaton, W. W., Mortensen, P. B., Herrman, H., Freeman, H., Bilker, W., Burgess, P., & Wooff, K. (1992). Long-term course of hospitalization for schizophrenia: Part I. Risk for rehospitalization. *Schizophrenia Bulletin, 18,* 217–228.

Flaskerud, J., & Hu, L. (1992). Relationship of ethnicity to psychiatric diagnosis. *Journal of Nervous and Mental Diseases, 180,* 296–303.

Fox, J., & Fogelman, K. (1990). New possibilities for longitudinal studies of intergenerational factors in child health and development. In D. Magnusson & L. Bergman (eds.), *Data quality in longitudinal research* (pp. 233–248). Cambridge: Cambridge University Press.

Goerge, R., Van voorhis, J., & Lee, B. J. (1994). Illinois's Longitudinal and Relational Child and Family Research Database. *Social Science Computer Review, 12,* 351–365.

Gottman, J., & Roy, A. (1990). *Sequential analysis: A guide for behavioral researchers.* Cambridge, England: Cambridge University Press.

Griffin, W. A. (1993). Event history analysis of marital and family interaction: A practical introduction. *Journal of Family Psychology, 6,* 211–229.

Hadley, T. R., Mcgurrin, M. C., Pulice, R. T., & Holohean, E. J. (1990). Using fiscal data to identify heavy service users. *Psychiatric Quarterly, 61,* 41–48.

Luke, D. (1993). Charting the process of change: A primer on survival analysis. *American Journal of Community Psychology, 21,* 203–245.

Rapkin, B. D., & Luke, D. A. (1993). Cluster analysis in community research: Epistemology and practice. *American Journal of Community Psychology, 21,* 247–277.

Singer, J. D., & Willett, J. B. (1991). Modeling the days of our lives: Using survival analysis when designing and analyzing longitudinal studies of duration and timing of events. *Psychological Bulletin, 110,* 268–290.

Takechui, D. T., Bui, K. U., & Kim, L. (1993). The referral of minority adolescents to community mental health centers. *Journal of Health and Social Behavior, 34,* 153–164.

Thompson, J. (1994). National databases on minority elders. In American Psychiatric Association (eds.), *Ethnic minority elderly: A task force report of the American Psychiatric Association.* Washington, DC: APA.

Wedding, D., Topolski, J., & Mcgaha, A. (1995). Maintaining the confidentiality of computerized mental health outcome data. *Journal of Mental Health Administration, 22,* 237–244.

Willett, J. B., & Singer, J. D. (1993). Investigating onset, cessation, relapse, and recovery. Why you should, and how you can, use discrete-time survival analysis to examine event occurrence. *Journal of Consulting and Clinical Psychology, 61,* 952–965.

Wuerker, A. K., & Keenan, C. K. (1997). Patterns of psychiatric service use by homeless mentally ill clients. *Psychiatric Quarterly, 68,* 101–116.

Data Management Issues in Longitudinal Research

JoAnne M. Youngblut ■ Carol J. Loveland-Cherry ■ Mary Horan

Data management begins with the design of the study and includes such things as scheduling data collection, selecting a statistical package, deciding on the structure of the raw data, coding questionnaires, and entering and cleaning data preparatory to initiation of analysis. Although much has been written about various aspects of the research process, including design, instrumentation, sampling, attrition, and data analysis, little can be found about the practical aspects of data management, especially for longitudinal studies (Barhyte & Bacon, 1985).

Generally, researchers learn about data management issues and possible solutions by trial and error, by word of mouth from other researchers, or by problem solving using logic during the course of their study. The authors' premature infant project is illustrative of major data management issues. For this study, 120 families were recruited from two Level III neonatal intensive care units (NICUs). Data were collected in five waves over a period of 15 months from both parents in the home and from the baby's hospital record and outpatient clinic visits. The focus of the study is to investigate how parents' reactions to the premature birth of an infant affect family functioning and how their reactions and family functioning affect the infant's developmental progress.

Data Integrity

Maintaining the quality of study data is always of concern, but this is especially true in longitudinal studies. If data are to be collected on multiple instruments, from multiple respondents, at more than one time, and at more than one site, measures must be instituted to maintain consistency at the point of data collection and in subsequent coding and data entry. Consequently, several strategies were employed to enhance the quality of the data obtained.

JoAnne M. Youngblut, PhD, RN, is an assistant professor, Frances Payne Bolton School of Nursing, Case Western Reserve University, Cleveland, Ohio. At the time of the study, the author was a doctoral student at the University of Michigan, School of Nursing, Ann Arbor, MI.

Carol J. Loveland-Cherry, PhD, RN, is an assistant professor at the University of Michigan, Ann Arbor, MI.

Mary Horan, PhD, RN, is a professor and director of the Kirkhof School of Nursing, Grand Valley State University, Allendale, MI.

From *Nursing Research,* May/June 1990, *39,* 188–189.

First, interview forms were color coded by respondent and by interview time. Color coding helped the interviewer to sort forms for mothers and fathers while in the home and reminded her on which form each respondent's answers were to be recorded. Second, forms for each visit were collated ahead of time and placed in data collection packets to be distributed to interviewers at each site. Both of these measures made the interviewer's job easier and insured that a complete set of the correct forms were taken to each visit.

Finally, several record-keeping systems were implemented. Each site developed a system to keep track of when each family was to be seen so that family visits were performed according to study protocol. One of the sites used a tickler file similar to that used by community health nurses. Identifying data for each family were recorded on an index card, which was then placed in the file under the month during which the next visit would be done. The other site used a calendar to track visits. When a family was recruited to the study, all five of the family's visits were marked on the calendar during the appropriate months.

Flow sheets also were used for the data packets. These were marked when a packet was received, when it had been taken to the data entry firm, and when it was returned. Using the flow sheet made it easier to see the status of data coding and entry for each data collection period in a short amount of time.

Data Structure

Decisions about the best structure for the raw data need to be addressed early in a project. This allows computer column numbers to be printed on all instruments for direct data entry. There are several issues to consider, depending on the design of the study. One involves selecting a statistical package, another concerns defining the case, and a third involves handling the repeated observations.

Selecting a Package

If more than one program is available, the researcher should select a package that will meet most of the data analysis needs of the study. Doing so may save both time and money. This involves investigating differences among the packages and evaluating those differences. While almost all of the packages contain most of the statistical tests necessary for data analysis, some procedures are more complete or easier to use in one package and some packages have more options for a particular procedure or produce output that is easier to interpret. If a specific statistical procedure from another package is necessary, the raw data for the variables to be used can be written from the existing system file for one package (the file that the computer makes from the raw data and the instructions for reading the data) into a new data file and read into the other statistical package.

Familiarity of the project staff with the available packages is also important, as is the relative cost of performing specific analyses with each package. Finally, packages should be evaluated regarding the procedures necessary to perform data transformations. For some studies, the ease of creating new variables and recoding old ones may be the deciding factor.

Defining a Case

It is important to understand how statistical packages handle specific analysis procedures. For example, in the premature infant project, comparisons between mothers and fathers were planned using the paired *t* test. Some statistical packages will do paired comparisons across cases, while others expect paired comparisons to be within a case. Since the latter was true of the package selected for the study, the case was defined as the family rather than the individual.

Another reason for indexing the data by the family was the nature of the family and baby data. Data about family structure were collected from both parents together, rather than from each separately. In addition, there were data about the baby's hospital course, developmental progress, and the outpatient clinic visits that "belonged" to both parents. Indexing the data by the respondent would have required entering the family and baby data twice, at a significant increase in the cost of data entry.

While indexing the data by the family avoids the problems cited, it has its own problems. Defining the family as the case makes doing analysis with all parents, both mothers and fathers combined, more difficult. Some statistical packages have a routine to handle this while others do not. If the package chosen does not provide a solution, there are two ways to remedy this problem. When the variables for mothers and fathers are exactly the same and the data for those variables are in exactly the same column(s) on different lines in the raw data file, then writing a second setup file (the file containing the instructions for the program to read the data) defining the case as the individual is possible. If the data are in different columns or if some of the data will be the same for both parents (such as the family and baby data in the current study), two setup files (one to read the mothers' data and one to read the fathers' data) are necessary. The two resulting system files can be merged to produce one system file with all parents as the reference group and with the individual as the case.

Another way to deal with this problem is to modify the system file. Using this approach, one would subset the existing system file, first excluding the mothers' variables and then excluding the fathers' variables. Since mothers' and fathers' variables have different names in the original file, variables that mothers and fathers have in common must be renamed so that the same name is now used in both system files. In addition, a new variable indicating sex of respondent must be created in each file. The two resulting system files can then be merged to produce a system file of all parents.

Handling Repeated Measures

While data analysis can be accomplished on either a mainframe or a microcomputer, the mainframe was most practical for the authors' study because of the large number of variables in each wave. The following suggestions are made with the mainframe user in mind. Therefore, some aspects of the discussion may not be considered relevant for researchers who are using a microcomputer for data analysis.

There are three basic options to consider in handling repeated measures data. First, all the data for all data-collection points can be entered as a single case in one file. However, care must be taken if data entry and analysis are to begin before all data are collected. For example, since subject recruitment in the authors' project occurred over a two-year period, data collection for Time 1 overlapped with data collection for the other four time periods. In this case, the number of data records for each subject varied across subjects at any given time. Adjustments in the setup file or the raw data file must be made so that the computer correctly reads the data. In addition, since the cost of data analysis on a mainframe is often dependent on the number of variables in the system file to be analyzed, using such large files can appreciably increase the total cost of data analysis.

A second option is to enter each wave of data for each family as a case in the same file. In order to do this, the variables collected in each wave must be the same, although having a few more or a few less variables in a certain wave would not affect the result. This method is especially valuable when the number of observations will differ for different cases. For example, if the study design is to interview families every week during the first month of their infant's NICU stay, some families will be interviewed once, while others may be interviewed four times depending on their infant's length of stay. The disadvantage is that in order to do comparisons across time, the system file must be subsetted and the variables renamed as described above.

A final option is to put each wave of data in a separate file. This approach was most satisfactory for the authors' premature infant project because the number and types of variables collected at each time period were drastically different, making a single file impractical. Also, comparisons of variables across time were planned. Using a separate file for each wave makes such analysis easier. System files created for each wave of data can be merged as needed without subsetting the data and renaming variables. If a single file had been used, procedures similar to those described above for combining data on mothers and fathers would then have been necessary.

Summary

Much of the existing literature about the research process has neglected data management. While design, instrumentation, sampling, and analysis are important parts of the process, paying attention to the issues surrounding data management is crucial to the success of the study. Data entry and analysis are facilitated when the details of data structure and management are decided before data collection begins.

Reference

Barhyte, D. Y., & Bacon, L. D. (1985). Approaches to cleaning data sets: A technical comment. *Nursing Research, 34,* 62–64.

Strategies to Minimize Attrition in Longitudinal Studies

Barbara A. Given ■ Linda J. Keilman ■ Clare Collins ■ C. William Given

The experiences of individuals and families as they adjust to chronic diseases, physical and cognitive impairments, and the long-term effects of nursing interventions are examples of phenomena appropriately examined through longitudinal research designs. However, attrition of subjects poses a serious threat to the validity of findings from such research and little attention has been paid to practical methodological strategies to minimize it (Clinton & Beck, 1986; Flick, 1988).

In a longitudinal study with family caregivers of elderly with physical impairments, participants were asked to complete (a) five lengthy phone and home interviews and (b) a number of self-administered questionnaires. Criteria established for entry into the 12-month longitudinal study include (a) caregivers who were family members, (b) caregivers providing primary care for a patient 64 years or older, and (c) patients dependent in at least two activities of daily living or two instrumental activities of daily living. Throughout the course of study, a series of strategies were implemented to minimize the rate of attrition among a panel of 307 subjects. Excluding the event of death, attrition from the study was less than 4.5%. In this article, the strategies that were employed to minimize subject attrition are described.

Problem of Attrition

Two types of attrition, preinclusion and postinclusion, have been identified in longitudinal and experimental research (Flick, 1988). *Preinclusion attrition* occurs when potential subjects are not included in the sample due to selection bias on the part of either the researcher or the subjects. Preinclusion attrition is a problem only in studies using random sampling techniques (Flick). However, since the majority of descriptive longitudinal studies, including the care study, employ convenience samples, preinclusion attrition is an infrequent methodological issue.

Attrition occurs when subjects fail to complete the study following enrollment. Attrition jeopardizes the internal validity of the experiment (Howard, Krause, & Orlinsky, 1986). Postinclusion criteria jeopardize nonexperimental designs when subjects who drop out of the study differ from those who remain with respect to key study variables (Kish, 1965). To analyze data sets in which significant attrition has occurred, the assumption that nonrespondents do not differ significantly from respondents must be met (Kalton, 1983). Statistical techniques can be used to determine whether the remaining sample differs from the initial sample on key characteristics (Cook & Campbell, 1979). Although the impact of subject attrition lurks within nearly every longitudinal data set, the problem can be only incompletely addressed through the application of statistical techniques. Methodological strategies to prevent subject attrition need to be integrated into longitudinal research designs. The following strategies were designed and used to prevent attrition in the family caregiver study.

Strategies

Preparation of Data Collectors

Adequate preparation and supervision of data collectors is an important part of maintaining subject participation in longitudinal research studies. Data collectors must have skills that (a) enhance the desire of subjects to participate, (b) reflect knowledge and importance of the study, (c) demonstrate a high level of consideration and concern for others, (d) reflect excellent communication skills, and (e) demonstrate enthusiasm and commitment to the project. These skills may help to reduce subject reluctance and discomfort of ongoing participation and encourage accuracy and candor in their responses (Bradburn, 1983; Collins, Given, Given, & King, 1988). Protocol booklets

Barbara A. Given, PhD, FAAN, is a professor in the College of Nursing, Michigan State University, East Lansing, MI.

Linda J. Keilman, RN, MSN, is a graduate from the College of Nursing, Michigan State University, East Lansing, MI.

Clare Collins, PhD, RN, is an assistant professor in the College of Nursing, Michigan State University, East Lansing, MI.

C. William Given, PhD, is a professor in the Department of Family Practice, College of Human Medicine, Michigan State University, East Lansing, MI.

From *Nursing Research,* May/June 1990, *39,* 184–186.

were used that defined for interviewers the conditions for subjects' continued participation and strategies to maintain their commitment to the study. Frequent debriefing meetings with data collectors to discuss issues and problems helped to maintain interviewer consistency, enthusiasm, and commitment to the project.

Data collectors practiced interviewing in simulated situations, completed taped interviews, and critiqued their own interviewing techniques at regular intervals. Each data collector continued working closely with a senior member of the research team to receive feedback and to deal with problem situations needed to keep subjects engaged and involved in the study.

Data collection training occurred over a 4- to 6-week period in order to allow time for simulated interviews and for the careful training of the interviewers. Some interviewers require more practice and monitoring than others and some individuals may not become acceptable interviewers. To prevent false expectations, all prospective interviewers were informed that they would not be formally employed until they successfully completed the interviewer training.

Subject Bond with the Study

Participants in a longitudinal study need to bond with, and become committed to, active, involved participation in the study. At the onset of the caregiver study, a logo and theme were created and used to establish caregiver association with the project. The logo and theme were used on letters, envelopes, gifts, certificates, questionnaires, newsletters, and with all communication with study participants. Questions or concerns about the credibility of the study and any suspicions about data collectors were thus limited. Subject identification with the study served to establish the trust and credibility that was needed. Normative expectations were established that enabled caregivers to call and report when events occurred in their caregiving situation.

Communication with Subjects

Ongoing, open communication by the researchers with subjects enhances retention and active participation in a longitudinal study. Expectations of frequency, duration, and extent of participation should be clearly communicated to each subject at the beginning of the study. Sharing these expectations enables subjects to make an informed decision about participation. In the Family Caregiver Studies, data collectors reviewed with participants at the initial interview the duration of the study and the frequency with which they would be contacted.

Expectations of the research team related to the anticipated time involved and the type of contact (i.e., phone, home, or self-administered questionnaire) were shared with participants prior to each phase of data collection. Precontacting subjects by letter or newsletter ensured that the respondents were aware of their upcoming response role. Opportunities for questions and clarifications were given to participants at every contact point. Each mailed questionnaire included a cover letter and a deadline so participants were aware of expectations for completion of the mailed questionnaires.

Access and Continuity of Subject Contact with Data Collectors

Creation of a positive interpersonal environment and rapport between the data collectors and each subject is crucial to retention in longitudinal studies (Woodward, Chambers, & Smith, 1982). Where attrition is a major problem, lack of continuity of interviews may be the issue. In the caregiver study, data collectors were assigned a group of subjects at the beginning of the study and continued with those same individuals throughout the 12-month period. Continuity increased the likelihood of establishing trust between the subject and data collectors, which enhanced the quality and completeness of data collected. Subjects often called and asked for their data collector by name and sent personal letters or cards to them. Caregivers often prepared special treats and comforts to host the data collectors during in-home interviews. Empathetic listening skills promoted "story telling" by the research participant and gave data collectors a sense of the caregiver's overall role and situation. This continuity enhanced subsequent contacts and allowed subjects to build on and refine their accounts of caregiving since the last contact. The risks of such personal contact between caregiver and data collector are outlined in an article by Collins, Given, and Berry (1989) and may threaten the validity of a study.

Quarterly newsletters provided participants with current information about the phase of the study, publications and presentations, general information about family caregiving, and information about the members of the reseach staff. Access and availability of the research staff to participants was another method used to maintain involvement and prevent attrition. This approach gave participants access to the staff at the time, or for the situations, they deemed appropriate. A toll-free telephone number was established to enable participants to call the project staff during business hours. This toll-free number was printed on all materials mailed to the subjects. An open invitation to contact the research staff by letter or phone, with any questions, suggestions, concerns, change in interview time, status change, or problems related to the study was included with all regular study communications. Caregivers wrote letters and cards of a personal nature to the principal investigators and data collectors with important anecdotes about their caregiving situations.

Contacts from participants were responded to promptly. They were primarily to change appointments, clarify directions on the mailed sections of the questionnaire, question whether they could or should continue to participate with the study, or report a death or institutionalization of the care recipient. This ongoing access enabled the research team to stay current on subject situations. Research team members were also available to participants who had questions or concerns about the overall nature or progress of the study.

Respect for Subject's Time

Respect for time and schedules of participants helps to maximize retention. Flexibility in scheduling data-collection appointments should include evening and weekend hours to enable subjects to be interviewed at their convenience.

After interviews were scheduled at caregiver convenience, letters personally signed by data collectors were sent to participants confirming the date and time of the interview, nature of the interview (i.e., home phone, or self-administered questionnaire), and phone number to call if participants needed to change their appointment. A statement expressed appreciation of the participants' time and contribution in the past and awareness of time and energy for them to participate.

Follow-up by data collectors immediately after a missed appointment was used to convey a concern for missing the appointment and to reschedule.

Collaborative Effort between Participant and Researcher

Participants in research frequently express concern and hesitation about their ability to make contributions to a research study. An attempt should be made to assure participants of the adequacy of their skills and the importance, value, and contribution of their participation. Data collectors reminded subjects that they were the "experts" in caregiving and that information was needed to know what they did in their important work as family caregivers. During data collection, interviewers were instructed to give feedback to participants to validate the value/contribution and social usefulness of the information subjects were making to the project.

Expressions of Appreciation

Appreciation of extensive time and effort required in a longitudinal study and positive regard for each individual should be conveyed to participants. In the family caregiver research, participants could expect to spend 30–90 minutes at 3-month intervals for a phone interview or home visit in addition to the time required to complete the mailed, self-administered questionnaires. To demonstrate appreciation for the participant's involvement, gifts were given following completion of the initial interview, and at 6- and 12-month interviews. Gifts included coffee mugs, desk calendars, clocks, and ball-point pens with the logo and theme of the caregiver project embossed on them. Gifts were used instead of money or payment as an incentive. Money once spent is gone without any evidence of study participation, whereas a memento acknowledging participation and contribution remains for some time as recognition of their importance to the research study. Gifts were often prominently displayed. Thank-you notes with additional anecdotes were often received from study participants. Birthday cards with a simple expression of best wishes were sent to each caregiver during the week of his or her birthday. Sympathy cards were also sent to those caregivers who experienced the death of their care recipient during the longitudinal study. Numerous participants took this as an invitation to write and share with the research staff further information about the final stages of their caregiving.

At the completion of the study, a personalized certificate of appreciation for participation was mailed to every participant. A brief summary of the study was sent to each subject to terminate the relationship.

Importance of Using Strategies

In summary, attrition of participants from longitudinal studies seriously threatens the internal and external validity of the research. Retention of subjects in longitudinal studies is a major factor in the achievement of research goals. It is critical to report attrition in clinical studies and to explain how attrition rates affect the results. Retention strategies should be maximized and should be described in research reports.

References

Bradburn, N. M. (1983). Response effects. In P. H. Rossi, F. D. Wright & A. B. Anderson (eds.), *Handbook of survey research* (pp. 289–318). New York: Academic Press.

Clinton, J., & Beck, R. (1986). Time series designs in clinical nursing research: Human issues. *Nursing Research, 35,* 188–191.

Collins, C., Given, B., Given, C. W., & King, S. (1988). Interview training and supervision. *Nursing Research, 37,* 122–124.

Collins, C., Given, B., & Berry, D. (1989). Longitudinal studies as intervention. *Nursing Research, 38,* 251–253.

Cook, T. D., & Campbell, D. T. (1979). *Quasi-experimentation: Design and analysis issues for field settings.* Chicago: Rand-McNally.

Flick, S. N. (1988). Managing attrition in clinical research. *Clinical Psychology Review, 8,* 499–515.

Howard, K. I., Krause, M. S., & Orlinsky, D. E. (1986). The attrition dilemma: Toward a new strategy for psychotherapy research. *Journal of Consulting and Clinical Psychology, 54*(1), 106–110.

Kalton, G. (1983). *Introduction to survey sampling.* San Mateo, CA: Sage Publications.

Kish, L. (1965). *Survey sampling.* New York: John Wiley.

Woodward, C., Chambers, L., & Smith, K. (1982). *Guide to improved data collection in health and health care systems.* Ottawa, Ontario, Canada: Canadian Public Health Association.

Longitudinal Studies as Intervention

Clare Collins ■ **Barbara Given** ■ **Debra Berry**

Studies using longitudinal survey designs are increasingly prevalent in nursing research. Longitudinal or panel designs involve the use of time-ordered observations of individuals with the goal of studying the processes and causes of inter- and intraindividual change (Nesselroade & Baltes, 1979).

For over 2 years, we have been studying the changing situations of a panel of family caregivers of elderly relatives in the home. Our primary data-collection technique has been the use of intensive in-home or telephone interviews at five points in time during the 12 months participants were enrolled in the study. Throughout the course of the study, we have become increasingly aware of the unintended effects that study participation has had on family caregivers. Systematic study of the direct impact of participation in longitudinal surveys on the variables, which are the focus of such investigations, have been infrequent (Caserta, Lund, & Dimond, 1985; Rubin & Mitchell, 1978). Thus the purpose of this article is to describe participants' perceptions of how involvement in longitudinal research influenced their views of their caregiving situations and the strategies which they used to care for themselves and their elderly family member.

Potential Effects of Study Participation

An established principle of measurement states that the potential exists for an interaction to occur between the methods used to measure a phenomenon and the phenomenon itself. These interactions between the subject and factors existing in the experimental situation pose threats to the internal validity of the experiment (Cambell & Stanley, 1963). In experimental and quasi-experimental designs, instrument reactivity can occur in three ways. Instruments may directly affect subjects so that true measurements are distorted (Spector, 1981). For example, respondent attitudes can be influenced by filling out an attitude questionnaire prior to an experimental simulation. In addition, experimenter characteristics such as sex, age, and status, as well as behaviors such as empathy and hostility, can influence participant response (Rosenthal, 1966). Experimental designs such as the Solomon four-group design allow for the systematic examination of the degree to which methods of measurement influence the variables under investigation. However, such designs are both costly and unwieldy in studies that take place outside the laboratory context.

Investigations of effects of study participation in nonexperimental studies have focused largely on the issue of interviewer effects as sources of nonrandom error (Cannell, Oskenberg, & Converse, 1977; Collins, Given, Given, & King, 1988; Fowler & Mangione, 1986). The repeated measurement of a sample of individuals has the potential to alter the natural history of their growth and development and thereby obscure understanding of the natural course of a phenomenon (Nesselroade & Baltes, 1979). Some reactive effect of testing can be expected whenever the testing process itself is a stimulus to change rather than a passive record of behavior (Campbell & Stanley, 1963). For example, Rubin and Mitchell (1978) reported that couples who participated in a longitudinal study on the development of relationships between men and women tended to engage in more searching examinations of themselves and their relationships and to increase their level of self-disclosure with their partners. Caserta, Lund, and Dimond (1985) noted the potential for interviewers in a longitudinal study of bereaved elders to become incorporated into the social network that was the focus of the study. In longitudinal surveys that use clinicians as research interviewers, repeated interviewer contact with subjects increases the likelihood that situations requiring referral or other active interventions will occur (Clinton et al., 1986).

Clare Collins, PhD, RN, is an associate professor, College of Nursing, Michigan State University, East Lansing, MI.

Barbara Given, PhD, RN, FAAN, is a professor, College of Nursing, Michigan State University, East Lansing, MI.

Debra Berry, BS, RN, is a master's candidate at the College of Nursing, Michigan State University, East Lansing, MI.

From *Nursing Research,* July/August 1989, *38,* 251–253.

Method

The Family Care Study

Three hundred and eight family caregiver/patient dyads were identified in which the patient was 64 years of age or older and dependent in at least one activity of daily living. The caregivers were family members who provided the most care to the dependent relative. The family caregivers ranged in age from 25 to 84 years, with a mean age of 64. The average duration of caregiving was 5.2 years. Forty percent of the sample were spouse caregivers, 31% were adult children caring for elderly parents, and the remainder of the sample were inlaws or other relatives.

Family caregivers were interviewed five times during a 12-month period. Two of these interviews were conducted in the caregiver's home and lasted approximately 1½ hours. One interview was a phone interview that lasted approximately 1 hour. Participants provided information about patient and caregiver characteristics, caregiver involvement, informal and formal support, financial aspects of caregiving, caregiver mental and physical health, and reactions to providing care (Given, Collins, & King, 1988). During these three intensive interviews, caregivers were also asked to fill out questionnaires, which were mailed back to the interviewer. In addition, two brief phone calls to subjects were interspersed between the longer interviews to obtain information about health service utilization by patients and caregivers.

The interviewers were intensively trained in interview techniques and problem management. Only respondents who specifically requested information and referral were provided with these resources and any of these activities were recorded on interview assessment forms. Approximately 30% of the respondents had the same interviewer throughout the study; the remainder of the sample had two interviewers over the course of the study. Two hundred seventy-six caregivers completed the final measure of the study. Fifty caregivers of this group had experienced the death of their relative and were not asked to complete the questions on the effects of participation.

At the last measure, respondents who were still providing care in the home or had institutionalized their relative were asked to respond to four open-ended questions about the effects of study participation. Participants were asked how study participation had influenced how they thought or felt about being a caregiver, the way they provided care to their relative, and changes they had made in their lives during the past year as a result of participation. The survey was self-administered to promote self-disclosure and anonymity. Following each interview, data collectors were asked to record whether the subject requested information or referral and the type of information requested.

Development of Category System for Responses

Subject responses to the four questions were reviewed to develop a category system to summarize the major types of responses. After reviewing the open-ended comments, we concluded that the major impact of the study on participants was on how they coped with the strains of caregiving. A theoretical model of stress and coping developed by Pearlin and Schooler (1978) was selected to provide guidance in developing categories of participant responses. Using this model, four categories of potential effects of study participation on the process of coping with chronic life strains were developed. In their examination of the stress and coping process, Pearlin and Schooler make a distinction between coping resources and coping responses. Coping resources are inherent psychological attributes that people draw on to help them withstand events in their environment. For example, an individual's self-esteem may protect that individual from the diminishment of self that may accompany stressful experiences (Pearlin, Menaghan, Lieberman, & Mullan, 1981). In contrast, coping responses are specific responses to external life strains that prevent, avoid, or control emotional distress. Coping responses can function to assist individuals to directly solve problems, to control the meaning of the problem, or to control subjective distress resulting from a stressful situation (Pearlin & Schooler).

Four categories of potential effects of study participation on the experiences of family caregivers were identified from the responses to the open-ended questions about study participation. The first category of responses includes those that indicated that participants experienced a change in the coping resource of self-esteem as a result of study participation. For example, one respondent commented, "I now feel like I'm doing a really good job and have realized how much I actually do"; another stated, "I realize now that I can accept challenges that I did not know I was capable of accepting fully." The second category of responses included changes in coping responses that involved modifications in the problem-solving strategies used by participants as they provided care to their impaired relatives. The most frequently occurring strategy involved obtaining more assistance either for the caregiver or for the care of the relative. For example, one respondent reported, "I accept more help now from family and friends"; another stated, "I have found more time for myself by hiring a nurse's aide so that I can get away for a breather when I'm not responsible for my husband's care." Other caregivers reported that they had changed their strategies for handling patient problems such as, "I try not to argue or reason with him—more to ignore him and save my energy"; "I try to be more patient and use as many positive methods as possible to help us get through these trying years."

A third category of study effects involved changes in participants' subjective appraisals of their caregiving situations. Examples of responses coded in this category include, "I have become aware that I can't change my circumstances, but that I can change my way of dealing with them," or "Participation in this study has brought me an up-front awareness of my attitudes and has had an influence on how I have thought about the various issues confronting me."

The final category of responses involved effects of study participation that assisted the individual in controlling the meaning of the caregiving situations. Responses in this category involved the phenomena of social comparison (Pearlin & Schooler, 1978). Social comparisons involve a process of judging one's situation as better or worse than another person's or better or worse than one's own situation at another time. Caregivers provided comments such as, "Some of the questions made me aware of problems other caregivers face and I might be confronted with. I realize how fortunate I am at the moment"; "I still feel obligated and somewhat trapped by caregiving but I realize that many other people are in similar situations."

Results

Of the 226 participants who completed the open-ended questions, 52% (n = 117) identified at least one effect of study participation. Many respondents identified more than one effect, resulting in a total of 188 identified effects of study participation. The most frequently occurring response involved the effect on the caregiver's appraisal of themselves or their caregiving situation. In 42% (n = 78) of the responses, subjects described some change in how they viewed themselves or their situation as a result of participation in the longitudinal study. Changes in problem-solving strategies were reported in 34% of the responses (n = 64) and most frequently involved obtaining additional assistance for self or patient (n = 37) and changes in strategies to manage the patient (n = 27). Thirteen percent of the responses (n = 25) involved the process of social comparison. The least frequently occurring responses were those that indicated respondents had experienced some increase in self-esteem through their participation in the study (n = 21).

Two major categories of information were requested by study paticipants: a) further information about the study and b) information about community agencies or patient care. As might be expected, requests for information about the study were highest at the start of the study and tapered off markedly by the last longitudinal measure. At the first interview, 18 caregivers requested information about community agencies or patient care, 16 caregivers requested information at the second interview, and 15 requested information at the final longitudinal measure.

Summary and Conclusions

The results of this descriptive study support the premise that through the research process researchers actively influenced the experiences of many of the family caregivers in the study. Caregivers seem to have been stimulated to evaluate and change their appraisals of their caregiving situation and, at times, their use of external resources and patient management strategies.

We speculate that the predominant way subjects were influenced was through the opportunity to examine their experience relative to that of other caregivers as they completed the study instruments. Although it is possible that the effect was related to the specific behavior of the data collectors, we are reasonably confident that the structured interviewer training methods minimized this effect. Direct comments about interviewers were rare in responses to open-ended questions, and requests for information or help from interviewers were relatively infrequent, lending further support to the idea that interviewer effects were not a major influence on subjects.

Although Rubin and Mitchell (1978) aptly described the unintended effect of study participation on their respondents, which was akin to counseling, little attention has been paid to this phenomenon in recent years. What family caregivers experienced as participants in our study, but failed to experience in their social network or formal contacts with the health care system, was an opportunity to: (a) examine their experience as a caregiver in depth, (b) anticipate what the future might hold for them and (c) compare their personal experience to the experience of other families providing care to elderly members. Further study of which aspects of study participation influence respondents and the strength of the impact of participation in longitudinal research may also provide specific guidelines for clinical interventions with the families who participate in research.

References

Campbell, D., & Stanley, J. (1963). *Experimental and quasi-experimental designs for research.* Chicago: Rand McNally and Company.

Cannell, C., Oskenberg, L., & Converse, J. (1977). *Experiments in interviewing techniques: Fields experiments in health reporting 1971–77.* Hyattsville, MD: US Department of Health and Human Services, National Center for Health Services Research and Health Care Technology Assessment.

Caserta, M., Lund, D., & Dimond, M. (1985). Assessing interviewer effects in a longitudinal study of bereaved elderly adults. *Journal of Gerontology, 40,* 637–640.

Clinton, J., Beck, C., Radjenovic, D., Taylor, L., Westlake, S., & Wilson, S. (1986). Time-series designs in clinical nursing research: Human issues. *Nursing Research, 35,* 188–191.

Collins, C., Given, B., Given, C., & King, S. (1988). Interviewer training and supervision. *Nursing Research, 37,* 122–124.

Fowler, F., & Mangione, T. (1986). *Reducing interviewer effects on health survey data.* Hyattsville, MD: US Department of Health and Human Services, National Center for Health Services Research and Health Care Technology Assessment.

Given, B., Collins, C., & King, S. (1988, April). *Development of instruments to measure the experiences of family caregivers.* Symposium presented at Thirteenth Annual Conference of the Midwest Nursing Research Society, Wichita, KS.

Nesselroade, J., & Baltes, P. (1979). *Longitudinal research in the study of behavior and development.* New York: Academic Press.

Pearlin, L. I., Menaghan, E.G., Lieberman, M. A., & Mullan, J. T. (1981). The stress process. *Journal of Health and Social Behavior, 22,* 337–356.

Pearlin, L., & Schooler, C. (1978). The structure of coping. *Journal of Health and Social Behavior, 19,* 2–21.

Rosenthal, R. (1966). *Experimenter effects in behavioral research.* New York: Appleton-Century-Crofts.

Rubin, Z., & Mitchell, C. (1978, January). Couples research as couples counseling: Some unintended effects of studying close relationships. *American Psychologist 31*(1), 17–25.

Spector, P. (1981). *Research designs.* San Mateo, CA: Sage Publications.

Data Management: Cleaning and Checking

Beverly L. Roberts ■ **Mary K. Anthony** ■ **Elizabeth A. Madigan** ■ **Yan Chen**

In research, the validity of the conclusions reached depends partly on the accuracy of the data. Thus, identifying and correcting errors in data collection, coding, and data entry are essential aspects of the data management process that support the integrity of the conclusions from data analysis. With advances in personal computers, there are fewer problems than with the examination of sheets of numerals or punch cards but more problems related to software failure and human error in using computer technology. Barhyte and Bacon (1985) and Suter (1987) have identified potential problem areas in data management. This article extends their work.

Both random and systematic errors can occur during data collection and data management. Although random errors are fluctuations that are usually out of the control of the investigator, some can be discovered and corrected. Random errors may include typing in the wrong value during data entry or coding the variable with an erroneous value. Systematic errors are usually more easily discovered. These might include errors in coding or a misunderstanding about how data are to be collected and recorded. Errors in data collection are most likely to occur in uncontrolled settings, such as a hospital where there is a high degree of subject variability or a distracting environment, and with the use of complex measurement protocols. Data cleaning should begin during data collection because systematic errors in data collection, coding, or entry can be corrected before an enormous amount of data is collected. Data cleaning can not only help find and correct errors in the data but also can be used to assess and correct problems occurring in data collection and coding.

Beverly L. Roberts, PhD, FAAN, is an associate professor.

Mary K. Anthony, PhD, RN, is an assistant professor.

Elizabeth A. Madigan, MS, RN, is an assistant professor.

Yan Chen, BSN, RN, is a doctoral student.

All authors are from Frances Payne Bolton School of Nursing, Case Western Reserve University, Cleveland, OH.

From *Nursing Research,* November/December 1997, *46,* 350–352.

With large data sets, data cleaning is an iterative process with data collection, coding, and entry. Frequent cleaning of large data sets serves to establish the accuracy of the data. Data cleaning can help the investigator to determine the extent of error, where in the process the errors occurred, and whether the errors are systematic or random.

Data Coding Strategies

Strategies to minimize errors in the data collected should start at the beginning of a study. When data collection forms are being developed, data coding instructions should be included on the forms so that the person doing the coding does not have to go between a data collection form and a codebook. Providing this information on one sheet minimizes coding errors. Use of embedded coding instructions also facilitates data checking because data can be checked simultaneously with data entry.

If existing records, such as laboratory value sheets, are used for data collection, then the sequence of the data collection form should follow the sequence of the laboratory value sheet. This helps to minimize systematic errors in data collection. Another data collection point that is subject to error is where scales contain some items that are reverse coded. To minimize error, the item responses should all be placed in the same sequence. The reverse coding can be performed by computer after data entry. Data collection points that require calculations, such as the determination of mean blood pressure, can easily be performed by computer to avoid calculation errors on the part of the data collector.

There are coding schemes that also simplify later analysis. If a dichotomous variable is to be used, coding it as 0 and 1 will allow for use of the variable as a dummy code without having to recode the variable. When assigning variable names to items that make up a scale, using the same two or three letters to start the variable names will ensure that the items appear sequentially in the list of variable names in the statistical software.

To minimize error, coding should be performed by one person and checked by another. Once data collection has begun, data should be coded soon after collection so that errors or questions can be corrected or subjects can be remeasured.

Data Entry Strategies

Software packages such as Statistical Package for the Social Sciences (SPSS, Inc., Chicago, IL) can be used for data entry. With this software, a program can be written to fill in logical responses to questions and to skip items that are not relevant. For example, if a response to a question determines the response to other questions, the data on these subsequent questions can be automatically entered with the appropriate response. The cursor then moves to the next field. For example, the question "Does the person use any assistive devices to walk?" has possible answers of yes and no. If yes, then other questions are asked about the type of device; if no, then all of the questions about the device are filled in as not applicable. The other advantage of using this software is that ranges of data values can be identified while the file is set up, and, thus, entry of out-of-range data is prevented.

To identify errors, data should be entered twice into two separate files. These files can then be compared to identify inconsistencies. Moreover, random samples of subjects can be drawn and the data entered compared with that on the data collection form. If there are multiple instruments for data collection, random samples should be drawn for each instrument to ensure thorough checking. Additionally, each data collector's work should be checked.

Handheld computers can be used to enter data directly and to eliminate the need for a paper record. This method reduces the frequency with which data are manipulated and hence reduces the chance of error entering the data file. No matter what method is used to enter data into a computer file, this information must be checked for errors. If one data collector has a significant number of errors in the data file, the investigator should review with the data collector the procedures for data entry to determine whether the problem is related to computer use or inaccuracies in data collection. If data cleaning begins at the same time as data collection, systematic errors can be identified, and research personnel can be informed and trained to correct problems either during data collection, coding, or entry.

Another strategy for data entry is using optical scanning technology (Dennis, 1994). The technology for this purpose is different than optical scanners and optical character recognition (OCR) software that capture an entire page of information and allow editing of data. OCR software cannot identify areas on the page with the data of interest and transfer data into a computer file that can be used with statistical software. Specialty software packages for optical scanning are available that can be used to develop the data collection instrument and to place fields where data can be entered and scanned into a data file (Dennis, 1994). Either the subject or data collectors can record the data on the section of the questionnaire that is scanned. Although some investigators have either data collectors or subjects record the information on the instrument, they may have someone else transfer the data to the scannable portion of the data instrument. However, this latter method introduces possible transcription errors. Although this technology reduces introduction of errors into data files, it does not compensate for recording incorrect data or extraneous marks on the instrument that the scanner attempts to read (Gerber, Atwood, Hinshaw, & Erickson, 1986). Data cleaning strategies must be used to identify information that is beyond the range of what is expected or logically inconsistent.

Data Cleaning Strategies

Depending on the level of measurement of variables, measures of frequency, central tendency and dispersion, and minimum and maximum values can be used to identify errors (Suter, 1987). Frequencies can be used to locate out-of-limit values. For example, a variable may include the answers yes (coded as 0), no (coded as 1), or missing (coded as 9). If there are any values other than 0, 1, or 9 in the frequency table, the data collection form can be checked to determine whether the error was a coding error or an entry error. Identifying errors in interval level data requires different strategies. Means and standard deviations can be compared with the known normal range for a variable, and the standard deviation can be used to identify variables with larger-than-expected variation. For example, a variable with larger-than expected normal values may occur because the code for missing data (for example, 99) is defined as a valid value rather than a missing value. Some investigators do not use data codes for missing values but leave the data field blank when information is unavailable. This latter method does reduce the chance that missing codes are used in computing indexes. However, the reason for the missing data may be important, and hence, a code that provides this information may be appropriate. For example, in a hospitalized population, subjects may not be able to complete portions of the data collection (e.g., walking or getting up from a chair) because they are medically unable, refuse to do so, or are unavailable because of diagnostic tests or interventions.

Some variables may have known relationships between them. For example, creatinine normally is less than blood urea nitrogen (BUN). Hence, all subjects where creatinine is greater than BUN should be checked.

When a logical order is expected among related questions, consistency of the data among these questions should be checked. For example, the answer to the question, "Did the patient receive home care?" may be no (coded as 0) or yes (coded as 1). The subsequent question asked may be, "If yes, which home care services were received?" If the answer is yes, receipt of visiting nurse service is either yes or no. If the answer is no, receipt of visiting nurse service is not applicable. To check accuracy, the data for each question can be listed and consistency between the questions can be checked.

Another way to identify errors is to find outliers and check their data against the data collection form. Although not all outliers are errors, extreme values merit examination because they can be erroneous. Frequency distributions and scatter, box, and whisker plots can provide information about possible outliers. When errors are found, the raw data should be corrected, and the date on which the data were recorded and by whom should be noted.

Data should be checked for computed variables as well as for variables whose values are derived from raw data. For example, the total score computed from scale items can be erroneous if one of the scale items is omitted from the computation. Scales on which the answer for one item makes another item not applicable are also subject to error. If the computation command for this type of scale is not performed correctly, then both values might be included in the scale score. The computation commands can be created by one person and checked by another to ensure that the correct items are included and that the correct values are assigned to each item.

With the widespread use of personal computers for data entry and analysis, care should be taken to ensure that sufficient backup procedures are in place. One way to guarantee intact data files is to copy the raw data file into a data file for computation and analysis so that if there are computational errors or computer problems, the raw data remain unchanged. This is especially important when cases are being deleted or selected.

Personnel who know the data well are instrumental in identifying potential errors and can be essential in resolving errors. In addition, strategies to minimize error can be used at every step from the development of data collection forms through the initial analysis of the data. Multiple strategies used by various personnel help to ensure the validity of the data from which conclusions are drawn.

References

Barhyte, D. Y., & Bacon, L. D. (1985). Approaches to cleaning data sets: A technical comment. *Nursing Research, 34,* 62–64.

Dennis, K. E. (1994). Managing questionnaire data through optical scanning technology. *Nursing Research, 43,* 376–378.

Gerber, R. M., Atwood, J. R., Hinshaw, A. S., & Erickson, J. R. (1986). Optical scanning and computer technology in nursing research. *Computers in Nursing, 4,* 241–245.

Suter, W. N. (1987). Approaches to avoiding errors in data sets: A technical note. *Nursing Research, 36,* 262–263.

PART FOUR

Correlational Techniques

Regression Analyses: What to Report

Thomas R. Knapp

Regression analysis, in any of its variations or disguises (simultaneous, hierarchical, or stepwise regression; logistic regression; path analysis or structural equation modeling), is among the most frequently used statistical analyses in nursing research. Since regression analysis is so commonly employed, one would expect that journals would have ground rules regarding the type of information that is essential for reporting results and the type of information that is interesting but not essential. Alas, such is not the case. The purpose of this article is to provide a recommended minimum list of regression statistics that are necessary for a critical evaluation of study findings.

Simultaneous Regression Analysis

For a simultaneous regression (all independent variables entered at the same time in a single analysis), the reader needs to have at least the following information: (a) The number of independent variables and their names (the name of the dependent variable should appear in the title of the summary table); (b) The number of observations in the group upon which the analysis is based; (c) The numerical value of R^2 and, unless the number of observations is very large, the numerical value of adjusted R^2 (Prescott, 1987); (d) The unstandardized coefficients (the *a* intercept and the *b* coefficients) in the regression equation; beta weights (standardized regression coefficients) should also be provided, either in addition to or instead of the *b* weights, if the units for the independent variables are arbitrary; (e) If the data are sample data, some indication of the statistical significance of, or confidence intervals around, the R^2 and the regression coefficients. If statistical significance is emphasized, each result should be related to a single preselected alpha level (Slakter, Wu, & Suzuki-Slakter, 1991).

It is also desirable to include a paragraph or two devoted to the extent to which the assumptions for regression analyses have been satisfied. Anything else is nice, but not crucial. Means and standard deviations for the variables are helpful in giving the reader a feel for the data, as is the correlation matrix. However, for large numbers of independent variables, it is awkward, and often economically prohibitive, to include these in a journal article. Scatter plots and plots of residuals (Verran & Ferketich, 1987; Weissfeld & Butler, 1988) are better yet, but even more impractical.

Thomas R. Knapp, EdD, is professor of nursing and education, The Ohio State University, Columbus, OH.

From *Nursing Research,* May/June 1994, *43,* 187–189.

Hierarchical Regression Analysis

For a hierarchical regression (independent variables entered in an order predetermined by the researcher, based on theoretical considerations), the reader needs to know: (a) The number (and names) of independent variables at each stage of the regression; (b) The size of the group that has been studied; (c) The R^2, adjusted R^2, and R^2 change at each stage; (d) The unstandardized and/or standardized regression coefficients at each stage; (e) For sample data, the appropriate inferential statistics for the R^2's and the regression coefficients.

Stepwise Regression Analysis

For a stepwise regression (independent variables entered in an order determined by degree of statistical significance), the requirements are the same as for hierarchical regression. This technique is generally inappropriate because the order of entry is based entirely on statistical significance, and some theoretically meaningful variables may never enter the analysis. (See Aaronson [1989] for a critique of the stepwise approach.)

Logistic Regression Analysis

Logistic regression differs from ordinary regression primarily in the nature of the variables involved. The dependent variable is dichotomous rather than continuous, normally distributed, and homoscedastic. The independent variables are typically a mix of continuous and categorical. The analysis can be simultaneous, hierarchical, or stepwise. The reporting requirements are the same as for ordinary simultaneous, hierarchical, or stepwise regression. (See Yarandi and Simpson [1991] for a discussion and application of stepwise logistic regression in nursing research.) Relative risks and/or odds ratios are usually given as well. There are no obvious counterparts to R^2 and adjusted R^2, but a number of goodness-of-fit indices are routinely provided by statistical packages, such as SAS, SPSS, and SYSTAT, which have logistic regression procedures. Munro and Page (1993, pp. 237–238) give a good summary of one of the indices, the log likelihood.

Path Analysis and Structural Equation Modeling

When a path analysis or a structural equation modeling analysis is carried out, things get complicated. In path analysis there are single indicators of all constructs, variables are standardized, and unidirectional causality (recursive) is hypothesized. On the other hand, in structural equation modeling (using LISREL or EQS) there are multiple indicators for some or all constructs (yielding both a measurement model within construct and a structural model between constructs), variables may or may not be standardized, and either unidirectional (recursive) or reciprocal (nonrecursive) causality may be hypothesized (Aaronson, Frey, & Boyd, 1988; Boyd, Frey, & Aaronson, 1988; Mason-Hawkes & Holm, 1989.)

In either case, the following information should be provided at a minimum: (a) The path diagram (model to be tested), with hypothesized directions for all relationships but without the path coefficients, which can also serve as a substitute for a long list of individual hypotheses; (b) The number of constructs and the number of indicators for each of the constructs, with names; (c) The results of each regression that has been carried out (see the minimum list for simultaneous regression); (d) A table of direct and indirect effects for each regressor; (e) The path diagram with the obtained path coefficients for the hypothesized model (This diagram provides a summary of the initial test of that model); (f) The path diagram(s) with obtained path coefficients for any revised (better-fitting) model(s).

Example of a Report of Regression Analyses

An example appeared recently in an article entitled "Replication and Validation of Anticipated Turnover Model for Urban Registered Nurses" by Lucas, Atwood, and Hagaman (*NR 42.* 29–35). In that article, the authors reported the results of several regression analyses carried out to test a theoretical model of anticipated turnover (see the path diagram in Figure 1). The diagram has all of the hypothesized relationships indicated in accordance with the first recommendation for reporting the results for a path analysis or structural equation modeling analysis.

The number of constructs is not perfectly clear. A simple count of the names indicated in Figure 1 yields 6 (Stage 1) + 2 (Stage 2) + 2 (Stage 3) + 1 (Stage 4) + 1 (Stage 5) = 12. There also appears to be one indicator per construct, as is typical for path analysis.

However, the results for each analysis are not fully supplied, nor is the reader told what regression analyses were actually carried out. The rules for path analysis would postulate six regressions: (a) Group Cohesion (one of the two Stage 2 variables) on all of the Stage 1 variables (Age through Shift); (b) Job Stress (the other Stage 2 variable) on the same set of Stage 1 variables; (c) Organizational Job Satisfaction (one of the Stage 3 variables) on both of the Stage 2 variables and on all of the Stage 1 variables; (d) Professional Job Satisfaction (the other Stage 3 variable) on those same sets of Stage 2 and Stage 1 variables; (e) Anticipated Turnover (Stage 4) on Organiza-

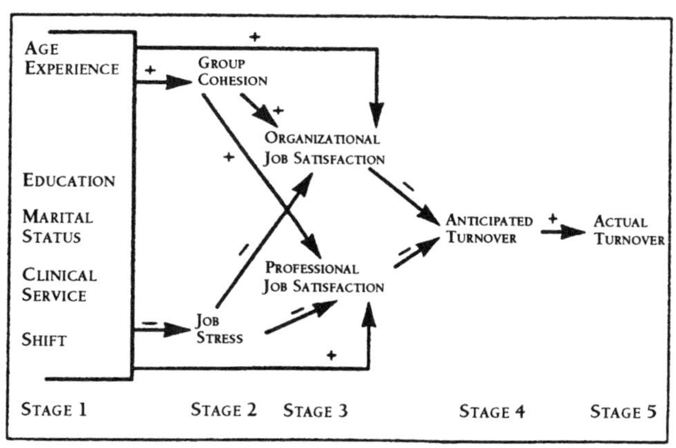

FIGURE 1 Theoretical Model of Anticipated Turnover for Urban RNs

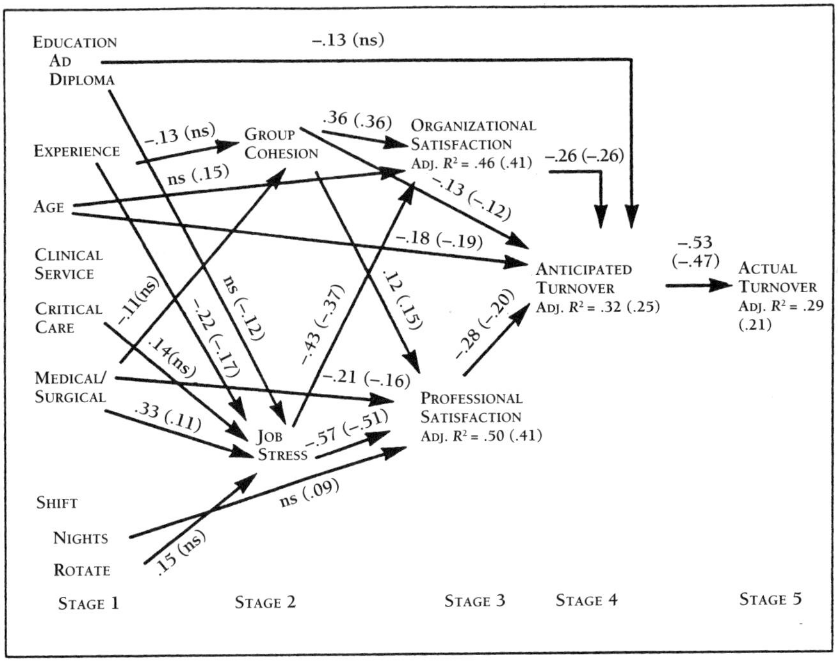

FIGURE 2 Direct Paths, Anticipated Turnover Model, Urban RNs

tional Job Satisfaction and Professional Job Satisfaction (Stage 3); (f) Actual Turnover (Stage 5) on Anticipated Turnover (Stage 4).

The adjusted R^2 values for these regressions, as well as the path coefficients, are provided in Figure 2. (The first coefficients are for the replication study, and the coefficients in parentheses are for the original study.) The unadjusted R^2 values are not provided, but they are undoubtedly very close to the adjusted R^2's because the sample sizes are large. The actual n's of 385 and 625 are provided in the text and in one of the tables.

The authors do not provide a separate tabulation of the direct effects and indirect effects, although some are referred to in the text. But, the authors do provide the total (= direct + indirect) effects, perhaps for economy of space. (See Table 1 and Table 2.) There may be one or

TABLE 1 Total Effects (Direct + Indirect) of Stage 1 and Stage 2 Variables on Job Satisfaction

	Predicted Variables			
	Organizational Job Satisfaction		*Professional Job Satisfaction*	
Predictor Variables	Replication	Original	Replication	Original
Stage 2 Variables				
Group cohesions	.36	.36	.12	.15
Job stress	−.43	−.37	−.57	−.51
Stage 1 Variables				
Age	—	.15	—	—
Hospital experience	.14	.06	.15	.09
Diploma education	—	.04	—	.06
Critical care	.06	—	−.08	—
Medical/surgical	−.18	−.04	−.41	−.22
Rotate shifts	−.06	—	−.09	—
Night shifts	—	—	—	.09

TABLE 2 Total Effects (Direct + Indirect) of Stage 1, Stage 2, and Stage 3 Variables on Anticipated Turnover

Predictor Variables	Replication Study	Original Study
Stage 3 Variables		
Organizational job satisfaction	−.26	−.26
Professional job satisfaction	−.28	−.20
Stage 2 Variables		
Group cohesion	−.25	−.24
Job stress	.27	.20
Stage 1 Variables		
Age	−.18	−.19
Associate degree education	−.13	—

more errors in Table 1 or Figure 2, however. For example, in Table 1, the total effect for (Hospital) Experience for the replication sample (.14) does not agree with the sum of the products of the appropriate path coefficients in Figure 2.

Although Figure 2 provides the principal results for a test of the hypothesized model, the numbers and names of some of the variables are different from those given in Figure 1. For example, Education (Figure 1) is now called Education AD and Diploma (Figure 2). The information for the Education variable, which originally consisted of four categories (Diploma, AD, BS, and MS), has been converted into three dummy variables. Two of the dummy variables (AD/non-AD and Diploma/non-Diploma) had an effect while the third did not, but the reader is not told this. Clinical Service and Shift have also been similarly converted. Marital Status has been dropped, since it bears no statistically significant relationship with any variables to the right of it, as pointed out in the text. This can be confusing to the reader. The names of the variables in Figure 1 and Figure 2 should be identical.

The authors provide in Figure 3 a revised model containing only those variables that were statistically significant in both the replication study and the original study. There is a minor problem with Figure 3: Education and Shift do not have any arrows emanating from them and should have been deleted.

The authors provide some additional information that is helpful (e.g., means and standard deviations for some of the Stage 1 variables) and some information that is not particularly helpful (e.g., a much-too-brief summary of a discriminant analysis that compares "leavers" with "stayers"). On balance, this article is much better than many other articles as far as the report of regression results is concerned.

Summary

In this article an attempt was made to provide some guidelines regarding what information to report in a regression analysis. An example taken from the nursing research literature was used to illustrate recommended practice. This writer holds no illusions that the suggestions provided here will be the last word on the subject, but it is hoped that they will help to alleviate some of the problems with the present situation, where it seems that just about anything goes.

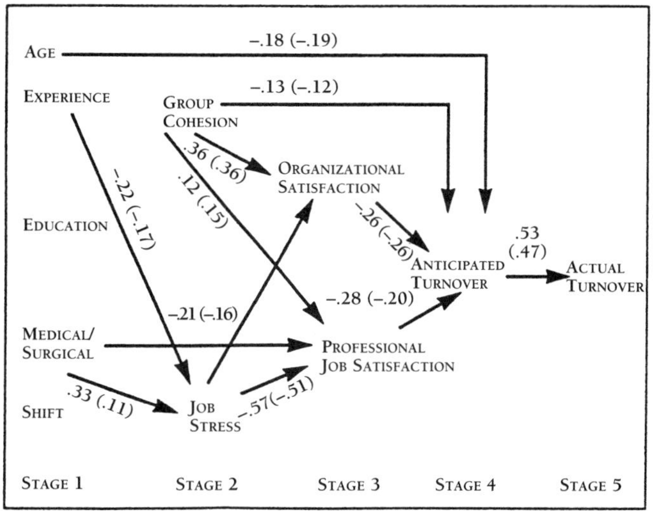

FIGURE 3 Replicated Test of Theoretical Model of Anticipated Turnover, Urban RNs

References

Aaronson, L. S. (1989). A cautionary note on the use of stepwise regression. *Nursing Research, 38,* 309–311.

Aaronson, L. S., Frey, M. A., & Boyd, C. J. (1988). Structural equation models and nursing research. Part II. *Nursing Research, 37,* 315–318.

Boyd, C. J., Frey, M. A., & Aaronson, L. S. (1988). Structural equation models and nursing research: Part I. *Nursing Research, 37,* 249–252.

Lucas, M. D., Atwood, J. R., & Hagaman, R. (1993). Replication and validation of Anticipated Turnover Model for urban registered nurses. *Nursing Research, 42,* 29–35.

Mason-Hawkes, J., & Holm, K. (1989). Causal modeling: A comparison of path analysis and LISREL. *Nursing Research, 38,* 312–314.

Munro, B. H., & Page, E. B. (1993). *Statistical methods for health care research* (2nd ed.). Philadelphia: Lippincott.

Prescott, P. A. (1987). Multiple regression analysis with small samples: Cautions and suggestions. *Nursing Research, 36,* 130–133.

Slakter, M. J., Wu, Y-W. B., & Suzuki-Slakter, N. S. (1991). *, ** and ***; Statistical nonsense at the .00000 level. *Nursing Research, 40,* 248–249.

Verran, J. A., & Ferketich, S. L. (1987). Testing linear model assumptions: Residual analysis. *Nursing Research, 36,* 127–130.

Weissfeld, L. A., & Butler, P. M. (1988). Use of regression diagnostics in nursing studies. *Nursing Research, 37,* 119–122.

Yarandi, H. N., & Simpson, S. H. (1991). The logistic regression model and the odds of testing HIV positive. *Nursing Research, 40,* 372–373.

Use of Regression Diagnostics in Nursing Studies

Lisa A. Weissfeld ■ Patricia M. Butler

Linear regression models are often used to analyze data in nursing studies. However, little attention is given to the impact that observations, singly or multiply, may have on the results obtained from a linear regression analysis. Aberrant observations can be easily missed in data analysis, where the use of the computer often causes the investigator to be less aware of all the observations in the data set. This is especially true for large data sets containing many observations or variables. In these settings, possible outlying or influential observations can easily go unnoticed in routine descriptive analyses.

The problems caused by influential observations can be greater in small samples in which a single observation is more likely to cause a substantially larger or smaller regression coefficient than would have resulted had the observation been omitted from the analysis. The impact of a single observation can manifest itself in yet another way by causing a variable to appear statistically significant in a regression analysis, indicating a supposed relationship, but deletion of the outlying observation causes the relationship to become nonsignificant. Single observations can also affect (a) clinical interpretations made on the basis of the size of regression coefficients and (b) their statistical significance. Thus, there is a need to use readily available measures to locate outlying observations in a data set.

The focus here is on the multiple linear regression model and regression diagnostics, that is, measures that can be used to locate outlying or influential observations in a regression analysis. The regression diagnostics discussed are currently available in statistical computing packages such as *SPSS-X* (1986), *BMDP* (Dixon et al., 1983), and *SAS* (1985). An example from a study examining nurses' continuing learning behavior illustrates the use and interpretation of these diagnostics and demonstrates the impact influential observations can have on results obtained from a standard regression analysis.

Lisa A. Weissfeld, PhD, is an assistant professor of biostatistics, Center for Nursing Research and Department of Biostatistics, University of Michigan, Ann Arbor.

Patricia M. Butler, PhD, RN, is an assistant professor of nursing in the Medical-Surgical Nursing Department, School of Nursing, University of Michigan, Ann Arbor.

From *Nursing Research,* March/April 1988, *37,* 119–122.

Linear Regression Model

The model considered is of the form:

$$Y = \alpha + \beta_1 x_1 + \beta_2 x_2 + \ldots + \beta_p x_p + \epsilon,$$

where α is the intercept term, β_1 denotes the regression coefficient (slope) associated with the *i*th independent variable of interest and ϵ is the underlying error term. This model is based on the following assumptions: Y is normally distributed with mean $\alpha + \beta_1 x_1 + \ldots + \beta_p x_p$ and variance σ^2, where σ^2 is the variance of the underlying error term ϵ. The error terms are assumed to be independent and normally distributed with mean 0 and variance σ^2, and $x_1, \ldots, x_p$ are fixed and measured without error.

Several items typically considered in fitting a linear regression model include the predicted values, residuals, estimates of α and $\beta_1, \ldots, \beta_p$, R^2, and test statistics. The predicted value, $\hat{Y}$, computed for each observation in the data set, is defined by

$$\hat{Y} = \hat{\alpha} + \hat{\beta}_1 x_1 + \ldots + \hat{\beta}_p \times_p,$$

where $\hat{\alpha}$, $\hat{\beta}_1, \ldots,$ and $\hat{\beta}_p$ denote the estimated values of $\alpha, \beta_1, \ldots,$ and β_p, respectively, as gleaned from the study data. These predicted values are then used to compute the residuals, e_i, which are defined as:

$$e_i = Y_i - \hat{Y}_i,$$

where e_i denotes the residual and Y_i and $\hat{Y}_i$ denote the observed and predicted values, respectively, for the *i*th observation. The residuals are assumed to be independent (uncorrelated) and normally distributed with mean 0 and common variance σ^2.

An estimate of σ^2, the underlying variance of error terms, is obtained by computing the mean square error (MSE), which is defined by

$$MSE = \Sigma e_i^2/(n - p - 1),$$

where p is the number of independent variables in the model. The MSE is also used to construct test statistics to investigate hypotheses related to the regression coefficients. The coefficient of multiple determination, R^2, also depends on the MSE.

The estimates of α and $\beta_1, \ldots, \beta_p$, labeled $\hat{\alpha}, \hat{\beta}_1, \ldots, \hat{\beta}_p$, are obtained using the method of least squares, i.e., the solution obtained when the sum of squares of the difference between the observed value Y_i and the predicted value $\hat{Y}_1$ is minimized. Points that have a large effect on the estimates of α and β may not be isolated by an analysis of the residuals only, as the least squares solution solves for α and $\beta_1, \ldots, \beta_p$ simultaneously using the sum of squares of all residuals. For this reason, residual analysis may not always be helpful and can be misleading when highly influential points are present in the data set. Currently, methods for locating outlying or influential observations in a regression analysis are available to assess varying types of possibly disparate observations, several of which will be discussed here.

Regression Diagnostics

Each observation is comprised of two parts: the observed value of Y_i, that is, the value of the dependent variable for the $_i$th observation in the data set, and the observed value of $x_{li}, \ldots, x_{pi}$, that is, the set of values for the independent variables. An observation can be an outlying or influential observation in a regression analysis with respect to: Y_i, any one or more of $x_{li}, \ldots, x_{pi}$ or both the value for the dependent variable, Y_i, and any of the independent variables $x_{li}, \ldots, x_{pi}$. Thus, methods for assessing the impact of Y_i and $x_{li}, \ldots, x_{pi}$ on the regression model separately and in combination have been developed.

The impact of an observation of the dependent, or Y, variable is typically measured through the size of the residual. This can be more accurately assessed by standardizing the residual so that all residuals under consideration have the same variance. One common standardization used is

$$R_i = e_i / MSE^{1/2},$$

where MSE is the estimated variance of the residuals, so that R_i has the form of a standard normal variate. Such residuals are readily available in statistical packages: denoted as ZRESID in the *SPSS-X* regression program, STUDENT RESIDUAL in the *SAS* program *PROC REG* and STANDARDIZED RESIDUAL in the *BMDP* regression routine 9R. These standardized residuals can be plotted and examined, using the same techniques that are used for unstandardized residuals (Verran & Ferketich, 1984).

There are other methods for flagging standardized residuals as possible outliers. The set of standardized residuals can be treated as a normal sample and the standard cutpoints of 1.96 or 2.58 can be used, that is, standardized residuals greater than 1.96 or less than −1.96 can be treated as possible outliers or influential observations. Another way of using standardized residuals to locate unduly large differences between observed and predicted values is to compute the sample quantiles of the residuals and flag all residuals above the 99th percentile and below the first percentile of the sample of standardized residuals. This method differs from using cutpoints from a normal table as the sample is used rather than an external cutpoint. In this case, if the 99th and first percentiles are used to flag observations, approximately 2% of the residuals will be flagged as influential. Finally, all values that are less than 3.5Q1 or greater than 3.5Q3, where Q1 is the 25th percentile and Q3 is the 75th percentile of the sample of residuals, can also be treated as influential observations (Belsley, Kuh & Welsch, 1980). Any of these techniques can be used to provide standards for judging when the value of a regression diagnostic indicates that an observation is influential.

To assess the impact of outlying observations in the set of xs, or independent variables, a diagnostic, called the hat matrix diagonal, designed to measure the distance between observations for the set of independent variables and thus the impact that the set of independent variables has in determining the predicted value $\hat{Y}$, is available (Hoaglin & Welsch, 1978). It measures the relative contribution that each set of xs, that is, each observation, makes in the estimation of the regression parameters. The values of the hat matrix diagonals, h_i, should be approximately equal across all observations in the data set when the observations have an equal influence on the parameter estimates. Observations in the regression model with hat matrix elements larger than $2(P + 1)/N$, where P is the number of independent variables in the model and N is the number of observations, are called leverage points. These points play an important role in data analysis because the presence of leverage points in a data set affects the residual plots obtained from a linear regression analysis. Leverage points may cause the residual plots to appear as if the residuals are normally distributed when, in fact, this may not be the case. This can result in misinterpretations of the residual plots (Cook & Weisberg, 1980). Once again, one can look at percentiles or points outside the range determined by 3.5Q1 and 3.5Q3 as possible outliers or use the $2(P + 1)/N$ cutpoint. The hat matrix diagnostic is available in the *SPSS-X* regression routine under the label LEVER and in *SAS*'s *PROC REG* routine under the label HAT DIAG.

A third measure combines the residual diagnostic and hat matrix diagonal so that the impact of outlying independent or dependent variables can be assessed simultaneously. This measure, defined as

$$D_i = \frac{e_i^2 \cdot h_i}{(p \text{ MSE } (1 - h_i)^2)}$$

is called Cook's D or Cook's distance measure (Cook, 1977). Notice that this measure depends on both the size of the standardized residual,

$$e_i / \sqrt{MSE}$$

and the size of the hat matrix diagonal, h_i. Thus, an observation will be flagged by this diagnostic if it has either a large residual value, a large hat matrix value, or both. This diagnostic has the advantage of looking at the impact of values for both the independent and dependent variables simultaneously. Observations with a Cook's D above 0.2 are often flagged as influential; however, the approach based on looking for gaps in the sample or points well outside the interquartile range can also be used to highlight possible outlying observations. This diagnostic is available in *SPSS-X* with the label COOK, *SAS* with the COOK'S D, and *BMDP* with the label COOK'S DISTANCE.

Example

Results from a linear regression analysis based on the continuing learning study illustrate the use of the regression diagnostic described in this article. The study had a twofold purpose: (a) to discover whether different hospital nursing departments had structures that facilitate the diffusion of innovations to the practicing nurse, and (b) to examine the relationship of nurses' continuing learning behaviors to nurses' knowledge of an innovation. Only the second is discussed here.

One hundred nurses each from six hospitals were sent questionnaires that contained information for a Knowledge score, Professional and Nonprofessional Learning scores, and background characteristics. The questionnaire was developed for a study completed by Butler (1986). Content validity was established by two groups of experts for the items in the Knowledge and Continuing Learning scores. Fourteen learning behaviors—nine professional and five nonprofessional—made up the two learning scores. Professional learning behaviors included such activities as number of professional journal subscriptions, professional journal articles read, number of in-hospital and out-of-hospital committee memberships, hours spent in the nursing/medical library, and hours of professional conferences and workshops attended. The nonprofessional learning behaviors included number of days per week the newspaper was read, hours of use of the public library, office and committee memberships held in nonprofessional organizations, and nonprofessional conferences and workshops attended. Questionnaires were returned by 354 of the 600 nurses (59%). For illustrative purposes, in this article, the subset consisting of 127 nurses with associate degrees in nursing was used.

Table 1 presents some descriptive statistics for the variables considered. Variables are Professional Learning score, Nonprofessional Learning score, day shift, a dummy variable with the value 1 indicating the nurse works the day shift, current position, a dummy variable indicating part- or full-time work, and highest degree, a variable indicating one of three educational levels: associate degree, bachelor's degree, master's degree. These variables were considered because they resulted in the most parsimonious regression model. The large standard deviations, disagreement between the mean and median, as shown in Table 1, and gaps in some of the values of the Professional and Nonprofessional Learning scores indicate there may be problems with these variables in an analysis.

The following regression model will serve as an example of the use of the diagnostic previously described: Professional = −3.91 + .0899 · Nonprofessional + 1.68 · highest degree + 2.22 · day shift + 2.53 · current position.

Table 2 lists the five largest values of each of the diagnostics considered along with the observation number associated with the extreme value. Any observation that appeared as extreme in two or more of the diagnostics was flagged. Each value for these flagged observations is given in Table 3. Note that although observation 84 had a large value for the hat matrix diagonal element, its standardized residual was not one of the largest in the data set, as its value was only −1.46. Thus, this observation would not be flagged when looking at the residuals alone. Note that COOK'S D flags both observations 84 and 116 as two of the most influential observations in the data set.

TABLE 1 Summary Statistics for Variables Included in Analyses: Mean, Median, and Standard Deviation

Variable	Mean	Median	Standard Deviation
Professional score	−0.2174	−.8911	4.14
Nonprofessional score	−0.3336	−.7344	5.25
Day shift	0.528	1	0.501
Current position	0.1890	0	0.393
Highest degree	1.22	1	0.576

TABLE 2 Five Most Extreme Values of the Standardized Residual, Hat Matrix Diagonal, and Cook's D

Standardized Residual		Hat Matrix Diagonal		Cook's D	
Value	*Observation Number*	*Value*	*Observation Number*	*Value*	*Observation Number*
2.8754	52	.1066	70	.109	52
2.4414	53	.5050	84	.040	59
2.3089	71	.1066	104	.433	84
2.2603	94	.1331	106	.133	106
4.3711	116	.1074	111	.440	116

Table 4 presents results from the above regression model when possible outliers were removed from the regression. In this example, only one outlier was removed at a time with the following observation being considered for removal: observation 84 because of the large COOK'S D and hat matrix diagonal element, observation 116 because of the large standardized residual and large COOK'S D, observation 106 because of the large hat matrix diagonal, and observation 52 because of the large standardized residual. Results obtained from removing these observations one at a time illustrate the impact that each one had on the results of the regression analysis. The impact of observations 52 and 106 on the regression analysis was not large enough to affect results of the analysis and is not presented in Table 4.

Results given in Table 4 indicate that observations 84 and 116 had an effect on results obtained from the analysis. In each case inferences drawn from the model changed when either of these observations was deleted from the analysis. Results for observation 84 indicate that the Nonprofessional Learning score was not related to the Professional Learning score when this observation was included in the analysis. When this observation was deleted from the data set, the inference changed with the Nonprofessional Learning Score related to the Professional Learning score. The value of the coefficient for nonprofessional learning doubled when observation 84 was deleted so that the inclusion of this observation in the data analysis could result in inaccurate inferences for the model. Observation 116 had a similar impact on results obtained from the analysis with the relationship between the variable highest degree and professional learning becoming nonsignificant when this observation was omitted in the analysis. Thus, a different conclusion could be drawn solely on the basis of a single observation. When both observations 84 and 116 were deleted from the data set, the combined effect of each observation was seen with highest degree becoming nonsignificant and Nonprofessional Learning score becoming significant.

Conclusion

This article has presented some of the commonly available methods for assessing the impact of observations in a linear regression analysis. The example presented demonstrates the importance of careful data screening and the use of diagnostics in a regression analysis. The use of these methods is necessary for the analysis of both large and small data sets. Although large or outlying values are less likely to affect an analysis of a large data set, they are also harder to locate. The need for this type of analysis is important in small data sets because the impact of a possible outlier is much greater. It is up to the

TABLE 3 Data Points Flagged as Possible Outliers

Observation Number	Professional	Nonprofessional	Day Shift	Current Position	Highest Degree
84	−0.0808	38.8494	1	0	1
116	18.8669	−1.1669	3	1	0
52	14.7542	0.4965	2	1	1
106	−0.9972	5.0311	3	1	1

TABLE 4 Regression Results When Influential Observations Are Deleted

Observation Deleted	Regression Coefficient Estimates			
	None	*84*	*116*	*84 & 116*
Intercept	−3.91*	−3.70*	−2.96*	−2.71*
Nonprofessional learning score	0.09	0.18*	0.09	0.20*
Day shift	2.22*	1.99*	1.96*	1.69*
Current position	2.53*	2.77*	2.77*	3.04*
Highest degree	1.68*	1.64*	0.85	0.80

*$p<.05$

investigator to decide how to report the results of an analysis that is affected by outliers. One approach is to report both sets of analyses, with the outliers removed for any tables in a paper and a discussion in the text indicating the impact that outlying observations have on the reported results.

References

Belsley, D., Kuh, E., & Welsch, R. (1980). *Regression diagnostics: Identifying influential data and sources of collinearity.* New York: John Wiley & Sons, Inc.

Butler, P. W. M. (1986). Hospital embedding-diffusion mechanisms and nurses' knowledge of an innovation. *Dissertation Abstracts International, 47*(6), 2368B. (University Microfilm No. 86-21, 256).

Cook, R. D. (1977). Detection of influential observations in linear regression. *Technometrics, 19,* 15–18.

Cook, R. D., & Weisberg, S. (1980). *Residuals and influence in regression.* New York: Chapman & Hall.

Dixon, W. J., Brown, M., Engelman, L., Frane, J., Hill, M., Jennrich, R., & Toporek, J. (1983). *BMDP* (Statistical Software). Berkeley, CA: University of California Press.

Hoaglin, D. C., & Welsch, R. E. (1978). The hat matrix in regression and anova. *The American Statistician, 32*(1), 17–22.

SAS user's guide (Statistics version, 5th ed.). (1985). Cary, NC: SAS Institute, Inc.

SPSS-X user's guide (1986). New York: McGraw-Hill Book Co.

Verran, J. A., & Ferketich, S. L. (1984). Residual analysis for statistical assumptions of regression equations. *Western Journal of Nursing Research, 6*(1), 27–40.

Multiple Regression Analysis with Small Samples: Cautions and Suggestions

Patricia A. Prescott

Correlational techniques such as multiple regression have great appeal to nurse researchers, as they are appropriate for many multivariate research questions and can be used for both descriptive and inferential purposes. Despite the versatility of multiple regression, its limitations should be considered and its findings examined in light of these potential concerns. This article discusses limitations of multiple regression when used with small samples and illustrates use of a suggested procedure for dealing with problems of instability and inconsistency of findings. Inconsistency refers to the degree to which variables different from the original set of significant predictors appear as significant in repeated analyses. Instability, on the other hand, refers to the degree to which predictors that remain consistent from one analysis to another change in statistical magnitude and/or sign.

Limitations of Multiple Regression

Techniques based on correlational procedures such as multiple regression maximize chance associations in a data set and often produce findings that vary substantially across samples (Mosteller & Tukey, 1977). This problem is particularly acute in studies using many predictor variables and small samples. Clinical studies are often of this type, exploring the effect of many variables on a criterion variable using a small number of patients or clients.

There is no common definition of what constitutes a small sample, and the needed sample size depends on a number of factors, including the reliability of the estimate desired, the accuracy of the estimate, and the relative variance of the variable under consideration (Levy & Lemeshow, 1980). Despite these sources of variability, Thorndike's (1978) rule of thumb for a rough estimate of the minimal sample size for multivariate analysis (10 subjects per variable plus 50 additional subjects) indicates that a minimally adequate sample of 100 subjects would be needed in a study with five variables (p. 184). Using this criterion, many clinical studies examine multiple factors with small samples that maximize the likelihood of chance association among predictors.

Selected Nursing Studies

Twenty studies reporting findings based on multiple regression analysis and clearly identifying the number of predictor variables were located in a review of 1983 and 1984 issues of *Nursing Research, Western Journal of Nursing Research*, and *Research in Nursing and Health*. Of these studies, 12 samples maintained a ratio of at least 10 subjects per predictor variable. However, only 4 of the 12 studies used samples that met Thorndike's criterion for a minimally adequate multivariate sample. The remaining 8 studies neither met Thorndike's criterion nor the commonly used criterion of 10 subjects per predictor; they used samples ranging from a low of $N = 8$ with two predictors to a high of $N = 299$ with 36 predictors. None of the 20 studies explicitly addressed the issues of stability and consistency of their findings, and no examples of cross-classification or jackknife analysis were located.

The instability of findings resulting from studies of this type can be estimated empirically (Willson & Reynolds, 1982). The expected decrease in explained variance from any one sample to the true population value, or the expected shrinkage, can be estimated by subtracting the obtained R^2 from the adjusted R^2, which reflects the estimate of true population values. Adjusted R^2 is commonly available as part of available statistical output for frequently used statistical libraries such as SPSS. In addition, it can be calculated as follows: Adjusted $R^2 = 1 - (1 - R^2)(N - 1)/(N - K - 1)$ where N = number of observations, K = number of predictors, R^2 = observed squared multiple correlation (Willson & Reynolds, 1982, p. 135).

Using this formula to examine shrinkage in clinical studies with small samples from the field of clinical neuropsychology, Willson and Reynolds reported substantial decreases in explained variance. Of the 17 R^2s obtained

Patricia A. Prescott, PhD, RN, is a professor and chair, Graduate Department of Psycho Physiological Nursing, School of Nursing, University of Maryland, Baltimore, MD.

From *Nursing Research,* March/April 1987, *36,* 130–133.

from the studies they reviewed, 12 were initially significant. After correcting for shrinkage, however, only 8 remained significant, indicating that a substantial amount of the explained variance was sample-specific and can be attributed to chance correlation. These findings raise concerns about both the consistency and the stability of findings and suggest that researchers should examine both aspects of their findings. Findings that are not consistent and stable have limited external validity, which should be acknowledged.

Approaches for Assessing Consistency and Stability

Two approaches for addressing the instability of findings from multiple regression are cross-validation and jackknife procedures (Mosteller & Tukey, 1977; Willson & Reynolds, 1982). Both involve an examination of the consistency and stability of predictors across more than one sample. Although there are a number of ways to use these approaches, cross-validation involves developing a predictive equation with data from one sample or one randomly selected half sample, and examining the adequacy of that equation with the second sample or the other half sample. The jackknife approach involves performing the analysis with the entire sample. Subsequently, the sample is divided into multiple randomly generated subsamples, and the analysis is repeated for each of the slightly reduced bodies of data obtained by deleting one subsample from each replication of the analysis. Predictors common to each replication then define a reduced set of independent variables to be used in a final multiple regression analysis based on the entire sample. In both approaches results are examined for consistency in both the significant predictors and the explained variance in the criterion. Also the stability of predictors is examined by magnitude and sign of beta weights.

Both techniques can approximate within the context of a single study what would be obtained by replicating a study with independently drawn samples. However, when the sample size is insufficient for subdivisions into halves, a second independently drawn sample may be necessary for cross-validation.

Example of Jackknife Analysis

Findings from a study of predictors of vacancy, stability, and turnover rates of 1,044 registered nurses working on 90 patient care units in 15 hospitals were examined for consistency and stability. The study, reported in more detail elsewhere (Prescott, 1986), evaluated 33 predictor variables using multiple regression analysis and three criterion variables. Results based on the entire sample of the 90 patient care units indicated that 52% of the variance in vacancy rates, 56% of stability rate variability, and 42% of the variance in relative turnover rates were accounted for by seven predictor variables (Table 1).

TABLE 1 Variables Predictive of Vacancy, Stability, and Turnover Rates of Registered Nurses ($N = 69$) (Initial Regressions)

	DEPENDENT VARIABLES		
	Vacancy Rates[a]	**Stability Rates[a]**	**Turnover Rates[a]**
Predictors	1. Working conditions adequacy*	1. Years experience of staff nurses*	1. Proportion of nurses in first position*
	2. Independence of nursing practice*	2. Head nurse years of experience*	2. Staff job satisfaction estimated by head nurse*
	3. Primary nursing organization*	3. Proportion of nurses working full time*	3. Staff/patient ratio, day shift*
	4. Nonsurgical units*	4. Staff job satisfaction estimated by head nurse*	4. Working conditions adequacy*
	5. Nonmedical units	5. Working conditions adequacy*	5. Proportion staff working full time*
	6. Staff/patient ratio	6. BS preparation of head nurse	6. Staff/patient ratio, night shift*
	7. Fringe benefits of nurses working less than 20 hr/wk	7. Staff/patient ratio	7. Primary nursing organization

*$p<.05$.

[a] R^2 for all predictors of vacancy rates was .52; R^2 for all predictors of stability rates, .56; R^2 for all predictors of turnover rates, .42.

NOTE: Of 90 units entered into analysis, after listwise deletion for missing data, 69 units remained.

TABLE 2 **Common Predictors of Vacancy, Stability, and Turnover Rates of Registered Nurses (*N* = 90) (Final Regression Following Jackknife Analysis)**

	DEPENDENT VARIABLES		
	Vacancy Rates[a]	**Stability Rates**[a]	**Turnover Rates**[a]
Predictors	1. Working conditions adequacy*	1. Years experience of staff nurses*	1. Proportion of nurses in first position*
	2. Independence of nursing practice*	2. Head nurse years of experience*	2. Proportion of staff working full time*
	3. Primary nursing organization*	3. Proportion of nurses working full time*	3. Staff job satisfaction estimated by head nurse*
		4. Proportion of nurses in first position*	4. Staff/patient ratio, day shift*
		5. BS preparation of head nurse	
		6. Staff job satisfaction estimated by head nurse	
		7. Working conditions adequacy	

*$p<.05$.

[a]R^2 for vacancy rates was .31; R^2 for stability rates, .54; R^2 for turnover rates, .23.

The choice of approaches for examining the consistency and stability of these findings was made largely on the basis of sample size ($N = 69$ after deletion of missing data). Use of cross-validation procedures with random halves was attempted. However, use of the technique was considered inappropriate, as the resulting sample sizes after listwise deletion for missing data were too small for multiple regression analysis $n_1 = 29$; $n_2 = 40$), and the results were largely uninterpretable. Thus, since selection of a second independently drawn sample for cross-validation was beyond the scope of available resources, a jackknife procedure was chosen.

Jackknifing was performed by forming subsamples that eliminated six patient care units (one hospital) from each replication of the multiple regression. Due to listwise deletion of missing data, 13 equations predicting stability, 12 predicting turnover, and 13 predicting vacancy rates were obtained from a total sample based on a possible 14 equations from the 15 hospitals.

Resulting equations were examined to identify predictors common to all solutions. Beta weights of all common predictors were plotted to examine their stability, and predictors common to all equations were entered into a final multiple regression analysis using the entire sample of 90 patient care units. Findings indicated that predictors common to all equations explained 31% of the variability in vacancy rates, 54% of the variance in stability, and 23% of the variance in turnover, compared with the original solution, which accounted for 52% of vacancy rate, 56% of stability rate, and 42% of turnover rate variability.

Comparison of Tables 1 and 2 shows that 3 of the 7 vacancy predictors, 6 of the 7 stability predictors, and 4 of the 7 turnover predictors are common to all equations. Without regard for the substance of the consistent predictors, it is clear that variables predictive of stability rates are considerably more consistent than predictors of either turnover or vacancy rates.

Examination of the direction and magnitude of the beta weights of consistent predictors revealed that consistent predictors of registered nurse stability rates were more stable in both size and direction than were predictors of registered nurse vacancy and turnover rates, which, while consistent or found in each jackknife solution, varied widely. Table 3 shows that some beta weights not only changed in magnitude from equation to equation but also changed in sign, making an interpretation of their impact on the criterion variable extremely difficult.

When the shrinkage for each of the three criterion variables was determined by comparing the obtained and adjusted R^2s, the expected shrinkage was 5% for vacancy, 5% for stability, and 7% for turnover rates.[1] This means that the expected relationship among predictors and the criterion variables in the population is estimated to be less than that obtained with this sample of 90 patient care units.

[1]Vacancy rate: Adjusted $R^2 = 1 - (1 - .52)(69 - 1)/(69 - 7 - 1) = .47$.
Stability rate: Adjusted $R^2 = 1 - (1 - .56)(69 - 1)/(69 - 7 - 1) = .51$.
Turnover rate: Adjusted $R^2 = 1 - (1 - .42)(69 - 1)/(69 - 7 - 1) = .35$.

TABLE 3 **Descriptive Statistics for Beta Weights of Consistent Predictors of Stability, Turnover, and Vacancy**

Criterion Variables	Predictors	Mean	SD	Standard Error	Range	
					Minimum	*Maximum*
1. Stability						
	Staff nurse months of experience	0.020	0.022	0.006	−0.030	0.033
	Head nurse years of experience	0.011	0.002	0.001	0.010	0.015
	Proportion of nurses working full time	−5.651	0.949	0.263	−7.185	3.791
	Staff job satisfaction estimated by head nurse	0.016	0.022	0.006	−0.026	0.043
	Working conditions adequacy	0.170	0.040	0.012	0.087	0.227
	BS preparation of head nurse	0.991	0.296	0.082	0.304	1.367
	Proportion of nurses in first position	3.410	0.621	0.173	2.593	4.261
2. Relative Turnover						
	Proportion of nurses working full time	−38.493	10.954	3.162	−54.260	−12.784
	Staff job satisfaction estimated by head nurse	−0.385	0.124	0.036	−0.572	−0.118
	Proportion of nurses in first position	6.706	5.566	1.607	−0.408	18.068
	Staff/patient ratio	−18.180	5.197	1.500	−25.427	8.303
3. Vacancy						
	Working conditions adequacy	1.057	0.431	0.125	0.427	1.890
	Independence of nursing practice	2.213	34.740	10.030	−44.470	56.166
	Primary nursing organization	−10.238	2.247	0.649	−6.150	12.010

Discussion

The degree to which the findings described here are typical is unknown, as few studies report the easily obtained adjusted R^2 or use jackknife or cross-validation procedures to assess the consistency of findings from multiple regression analysis. Of the 20 nursing studies reviewed, none used these techniques. This situation is not unique to nursing research. A recent review of multidisciplinary studies from the field of employee turnover, for example, produced only one study using these procedures. Bluedorn (1982) used a cross-validation procedure, developing a model with data from one questionnaire administration and testing it with data from a subsequent testing. The originally obtained R^2 was .12; that obtained with the cross-validation sample, $R^2 = .03$. No examples of studies using jackknife procedures were located, nor were studies that systematically examined the magnitude and sign of obtained beta weights.

Verran and Ferketich (1984) identified the assumptions of regression analysis and the consequences of violating these assumptions as a part of their argument for analysis of residuals. Although analysis of residuals is an important step in examining the adequacy of theoretical models, such procedures may produce misleading results if findings are basically unstable, inconsistent, and idiosyncratic to a particular sample. Thus, prior to engaging in sophisticated model testing procedures or using data transformations to correct for violated assumptions of multiple regression, it would seem prudent to examine the consistency and stability of obtained predictors.

The ideal approach to examining the generalizability of research findings is undoubtedly independent replication with numerous samples; however, individual researchers seldom have the resources or the inclination to repeat their research. Cross-validation and jackknifing procedures offer the researcher replication methods within the context of a single study. As such, they have limitations when compared with replication across studies. Nevertheless, recognition that findings based on correlational techniques and small samples capitalize on chance association should encourage researchers to temper enthusiasm for their findings with an examination of their consistency and stability. At the very least, researchers using multiple regression procedures should obtain and report an adjusted R^2 to alert readers to the amount of shrinkage to be expected under given circumstances.

To the degree that a study is based on a highly homogenous sample, cross-validation and jackknife procedures using randomly drawn subsamples will not result in substantially different findings. However, given the imprecision in much of the current measurement and the many sources of variability that threaten the statistical conclusion and external validity of many clinical nursing studies, it is likely that subsample analysis will be helpful in identifying findings based on chance correlation. This information may help to explain inconsistencies in findings among studies and thereby contribute both to theory development and testing and to more appropriate generalizability of findings.

References

Bluedorn, A. (1982). A unified model of turnover from organization. *Human Relations, 35,* 135–153.

Levy, P., & Lemeshow, S. (1980). *Sampling for health professionals.* Belmont, CA: Wadsworth, Inc.

Mosteller, F., & Tukey, J. (1977). *Data analysis and regression.* Menlo Park, CA: Addison-Wesley Publishing Co.

Prescott, P. A. (1986). Vacancy, stability, and turnover of registered nurses in hospitals. *Research in Nursing and Health, 9,* 51–60.

Thorndike, R. (1978). *Correlational procedures for research.* New York: Gardner Press, Inc.

Verran, J., & Ferketich, S. (1984). Regression analysis for statistical assumptions of regression equations. *Western Journal of Nursing Research, 6*(1), 27–39.

Willson, V. L., & Reynolds, C. R. (1982). Methodological and statistical problems in determining membership in clinical populations. *Clinical Neuropsychology, 4,* 134–138.

The Rough and Ready Jackknife

Barbara Resnick

The "jackknife" was first introduced by Quenouille in 1949 as a nonparametric device for estimating bias (Miller, 1964, 1968, 1974). Quenouille and Durbin continued to study the properties of the jackknife procedure and apply it to different situations. But it was Tukey who named the procedure the jackknife, using the metaphor of a Boy Scout's jackknife as a rough-and-ready tool to be used in any situation or emergency (Miller, 1964). Moreover, it was Tukey who later proposed the general use of the jackknife technique not only to reduce bias but to: (a) obtain approximate confidence intervals in problems in which standard statistical procedures could not be done; (b) consider the stability of an analysis; and (c) validate findings when a sample size is too small to do a cross-validation.

The Jackknife Estimator

The jackknife procedure is done by first dividing the data into an arbitrary number of equal-sized groups of size k, with $k = 1$. Estimates are then obtained by omitting each subset in turn and forming N "new" samples. Calculating the particular statistic of interest to each of the new samples results in a set of estimates, called pseudovalues. For example, in the case of a simple statistic, the mean, the jackknife estimator would be calculated by first deriving the mean from the scores 3, 2, 1, 5, and 4 (mean of 3). By omitting one score in turn, five new groups would be formed with four scores per group. The mean of each of these new groups is the pseudovalue (Table 1). The mean of these estimates or pseudovalues becomes the jackknife estimator (Dalgleish, 1994; Miller, 1974; Prescott, 1987). The subset approach allows the researcher to evaluate the properties of average scores without the need to assume distribution forms, and without the fear of being misled by biased results (Adams, Gray & Watkins, 1971; Chant & Dalgleish, 1992).

When calculating the jackknife estimator, a decision needs to be made regarding how to break the sample down into subgroups. While no clear guidelines exist regarding this decision, Miller (1968) suggested that a k equal to 5 was not as powerful as a k equal to 1. Others have indicated that the decision regarding the size of k needs to be made based on the research, and on computation time and effort (Fenwick, 1979). For example, in a large study it might be necessary to have a k larger than 1 because of computation time in the development of the jackknife estimator.

Use of the Jackknife

Bias Reduction

Bias refers to the difference between the true, but unknown, value for the population, and its estimate based on data from the sample. Therefore, bias is indirectly proportional to the validity of the estimate. The smaller the bias, the greater the validity of the estimate. When data are not normally distributed, the results are likely to be biased. Quenouille initially conceived the jackknife to reduce bias and was able to support this through subsequent work (Miller, 1974). The jackknife estimators tended to eliminate biases, particularly if the biases were inversely proportional to sample size (Mantel, 1967). With the reduction in bias, there is likely to be only a modest increase in estimator variance; in some cases, the jackknife may reduce variance (Fenwick, 1979).

While the jackknife eliminates bias in some cases (i.e. when the biases are inversely proportional to sample size), it may not do so in all situations. For example, if an estimator has a bias inversely proportional to the root of the sample size, the bias will not be eliminated but merely halved (Mantel, 1967). Additionally, for some nonlinear estimators, such as when a researcher attempts to estimate the maximum number in the population, the jackknife may actually increase bias (Fenwick, 1979).

Adams et al. (1971) investigated the effectiveness of first- and second-order jackknife estimators as tools for

Barbara Resnick, MSN, CRNP, is a geriatric nurse practitioner, University of Maryland, Division of Family Medicine, Baltimore, MD, and a doctoral candidate, School of Nursing, University of Maryland, Baltimore, MD.

From *Nursing Research,* May/June 1996, *45,* 185–188.

TABLE 1 Calculation of Jackknife Statistics of Five-Score Group

Sample Group	All 5 scores (3,2,1,5,4)	Omit "3" (2,1,5,4)	Omit "2" (3,1,5,4)	Omit "1" (3,2,5,4)	Omit "5" (3,2,1,4)	Omit "4" (3,2,1,5)
Jackknife Statistics (means)	3	3	3.25	3.5	2.5	2.75

bias reduction. They demonstrated also that the jackknife procedure can be used to remove bias when the order of the bias from the original estimator is known. They also found that the second-order jackknife estimator (calculated by omitting $2k$ per group) was actually more robust than the first-order estimator (omitting k). They suggested using the second-order estimator to reduce bias. However, the researcher should proceed with caution. As noted earlier, variance may increase when the bias is reduced.

Significance Testing

Tukey extended the use of the jackknife method to that of significance testing (Miller, 1964). He noted that the individual estimators calculated from the sample by omitting the subset could themselves be useful and suggested that these calculated numbers, or pseudovalues, be treated as approximately independent normal distributions. Therefore, the pseudovalues can be used as a sample mean. Using the pseudovalues, the researcher can apply significance tests in situations in which the usual assumptions for such tests are not satisfied, and for which significance tests are not usually available (Chant & Dalgleish, 1992; Crask & Perreault, 1977; Dalgleish, 1994; Fenwick, 1979).

Stability of the Analysis

After continued use of the jackknife procedure, Miller (1974) stated that the jackknife is not a device for correcting outliers. However, he also presented an example where observation of the pseudovalues helped identify intersample differences that could alter the results of the analysis. Fenwick (1979) suggested that use of pseudovalues in this way offers direct evidence of the stability of the analysis. Prescott (1987), in a study of predictors for nursing turnover, demonstrated that examination of the magnitude and sign of the beta weights (the pseudovalues) was a good indicator of the stability of the findings. Additionally, inspection of the pseudovalues can help the researcher identify data points that do not fit with the rest of the sample. For example, in looking at Table 1, the pseudovalues indicate that when Score 5 was omitted from the sample, there was a decrease in the mean score. Therefore, it was possible that the high score (5) in this dataset might have an impact on the study results. Further, this might indicate that the findings from this small sample might not be stable across samples.

Validation

The jackknife estimator offers a way to provide evidence for the stability of statistical findings when the sample is not large enough to do a cross-validation. It has been suggested that, particularly in statistical methods using multiple regression, the researcher may find strong relationships simply by capitalizing on chance and the relationships that exist within the sample (Crask & Perreault, 1977). The smaller the sample size, the greater the chance that the results in the sample will not generalize to the population of interest. Therefore the jackknife procedure, by evaluating the stability of the statistic of interest, provides some measure of the consistency or stability of the findings.

Application of the Jackknife to Statistical Tests

Overall, the jackknife estimate can be applied to any statistic that is a function of n independent and identically distributed variables (Efron, 1979; Efron & Gong, 1983). Additionally, the jackknife is useful in any research situation in which the analysis and test statistics assume a normal distribution but the data seriously violate the assumptions. Specifically, the jackknife estimator has been suggested as useful when using multiple regression with a sample that does not meet the 10:1 subject-to-indicator ratio suggested for a reliable prediction equation (Prescott, 1987; Stevens, 1992). The following example demonstrates how the jackknife procedure can be useful when a researcher only has a small number of subjects, such as from a pilot study, or when considering a subset of particular patients from a larger database.

The data for this analysis came from a pilot study of 251 older adult participants in a rehabilitation program. Since prior research (Daly, Adelman & Resnick, 1992) has indicated different outcomes in stroke patients and orthopedic patients in terms of functional ability (i.e., orthopedic patients have higher functional ability than stroke patients after completing a rehabilitation program), it was decided to evaluate the small group of 18 stroke patients separately. All subjects in the study participated in 180 minutes of therapy per day. The program consisted of 90 minutes of occupational therapy and 90 minutes of physical therapy. When appropriate, speech therapy sessions were also given.

In the analysis of the larger dataset, based on the bivariate correlations obtained (Table 2), the following variables were entered into the regression equation: admission Barthel index measures (Mahoney & Barthel, 1965), gender, race, marital status, age, number of minutes of occupational therapy and physical therapy, and admission standing balance. For purposes of example, the same variables were used in the analysis of the small 18-person sample.

Normally the use of eight predictors in a sample size of 18 is strongly discouraged, as it is likely that the findings would be neither reliable nor generalizable (Stevens, 1992). However, the jackknife procedure provides the option of using the eight predictors in the small sample, by testing the stability of the findings. In each analysis, Barthel index scores on admission were entered first to control for admission functional ability. All other predictors were entered into the equation using the forward method.

Based on the histogram and normal probability plot for the equation using these eight predictors, the residuals follow a normal distribution. Therefore the assumptions for the multiple regression model were met. The analysis was evaluated for outliers and influential data points. Although there were five outliers, only one was slightly significant ($p = .057$). Because of the small sample size, this was left in the analysis.

TABLE 2 Beta Weights for Discharge Function Regressed on Eight Predictors

Predictor	Beta Weights
Barthel index	.79*
Gender	.67*
Race	.06
Marital status	−.07
Standing balance	.20
Age	.08
Minutes in occupational therapy	1.16
Minutes in physical therapy	−.95

*$p < .05$.

Table 2 includes the beta weights for each predictor. The Barthel index (beta weight = .79, $p < .05$) and gender (beta weight = .67, $p < .05$) were the only statistically significant predictors of discharge function. Because of the small sample size, the jackknife procedure was used to decrease bias, and evaluate the stability and significance of the findings. While it has been suggested that data that are not normally distributed be transformed before use of the jackknife, it was not possible to correct the skewness of these data and so they were left unchanged.

Calculations of the mean pseudovalues/jackknife estimator for three predictors can be found in Table 3. There is generally no statistical software that will calculate the pseudovalues, or jackknife estimator for all types of statistics. However, for discriminant analysis the SAS DISCRIM program (SAS/STAT User's Guide, 1985) will compute the pseudovalues and jackknife estimator. This analysis was done using the SPSS for Windows™ statistical program to compute the regression analyses; hand calculations were done to obtain the jackknife estimators and *t* values.

Step 1: A series of 18 multiple regression procedures were done omitting one case for each equation.

Step 2: The new beta weights were used to calculate pseudovalues as defined by Tukey (Dalgleish, 1994).

Step 3: The standard error of the jackknife was calculated using the pseudovalues to determine the standard deviation.

Step 4: A *t* value was calculated by dividing each jackknife coefficient by the corresponding standard error. The degrees of freedom of the *t* value were based on the number of pseudovalues minus 1.

As seen in Table 3, the jackknife estimators were quite close to the original beta weights (with no case excluded) for the three variables. Additionally, gender and Barthel index were statistically significant, while race was not. Therefore, the researcher concluded that these beta weights are stable against changes in the sample composition.

Problems With Use of the Jackknife

While the jackknife procedure is useful for purposes of cross-validation, it is essential to remember that, ideally, generalizability of research findings must be examined by replication studies with numerous samples. The jackknife procedure, like the trusty Boy Scout knife, can be dangerous if not used appropriately. Specifically, there has been little or no success in the use of the jackknife estimator in time-series analyses or when used with some nonlinear estimators (Miller, 1964). Moreover, the jack-

TABLE 3 Jackknifed Beta Weights and Pseudovalues

Case Omitted	Barthel Index	Pseudo Value Barthel Index	Gender	Pseudo Value Gender	Race	Pseudo Value Race
0	.79		.67		.06	
1	.83	.11	.66	.84	.05	.23
2	.81	.45	.66	.84	.06	.06
3	.79	.79	.66	.84	.04	.40
4	.89	−.91	.72	−.18	.15	−1.47
5	.82	.28	.78	−1.20	−.03	1.59
6	.78	.96	.64	1.18	.14	−1.30
7	.80	.62	.68	.50	.08	−.28
8	.65	3.17	.75	−.69	.06	.06
9	.77	1.13	.71	−.01	.05	.23
10	.78	.96	.63	1.35	.07	−.11
11	.87	−.57	.64	1.18	.08	−.28
12	.74	1.64	.54	2.88	−.03	1.59
13	.80	.62	.65	1.01	.06	.06
14	.71	2.15	.73	−.35	−.00	1.11
15	.89	−.91	.67	.67	.07	−.11
16	.80	.62	.62	1.52	.06	.06
17	.76	1.30	.66	.84	.07	−.11
18	.88	−.74	.63	1.35	.12	−.96
Mean pseudovalue		.65		.70		.04
Standard error		.25		.22		.19
t value		2.60*		3.18*		.21

*$p<.05$.

knife does not do well with interval estimation on the median. Alternatives, such as the bootstrap, are suggested in these cases (Dalgleish, 1994; Efron & Gong, 1983). In regard to use of the jackknife with combined odds ratio, the jackknife estimator seems to underestimate the true odds ratio when its value increases. This can be a problem when there are a large number of contingency tables with only a few observations (Pigeot, 1991).

The literature on use of the jackknife technique alludes to other problems that may alter the effectiveness of jackknifing. The three most commonly addressed issues are: (a) the size of the omitted subset; (b) whether it is necessary to transform the data to facilitate a move toward a more normally distributed sample; and (c) whether the data should be transformed before or after jackknifing is done. In regard to size of the subset, Mosteller and Tukey (1968) suggested that the size of the omitted subset be adjusted to ensure the estimation process yields a number of different pseudovalues. However, further use of the jackknifing procedure will help determine how subset size can alter tests of significance.

Miller (1974) and Arvesen and Schmitz (1970) strongly advocate the use of variance stabilizing transformations in conjunction with the jackknife to test significance and stability of the findings. No consensus seems to exist in terms of *when* to transform. But continued use of the jackknife procedure will result in a greater understanding of the impact of these different options.

The jackknife estimator seems to be true to its name, a rough and ready tool that can help make more intensive use of a sample. However, it is important to remember that the usefulness of the findings still depends on the representativeness of the sample, and that the jackknife procedure cannot replace replication studies. The jackknife can be a helpful tool when doing pilot studies, or in studying a small sample. Additionally, as in the example given, the jackknife procedure is one that can be used to examine subsets of a larger database of interest.

References

Adams, J., Gray, H., & Watkins, T. (1971). An asymptotic characterization of bias reduction by jackknifing. *The Annals of Mathematical Statistics, 42,* 1606–1612.

Arvesen, J., & Schmitz, T. (1970). Robust procedures for variance component problems using the jackknife. *Biometrics, 26,* 677–684.

Chant, D., & Dalgleish, L. (1992). A SAS macro for jackknifing the results of discriminant analyses. *Multivariate Behavioral Research, 27,* 323–333.

Crask, M., & Perreault, W. (1977). Validation of discriminant analysis in marketing research. *Journal of Marketing Research, 14,* 60–68.

Dalgleish, L. (1994). Discriminant analysis: Statistical inference using the jackknife and bootstrap procedures. *Psychological Bulletin, 116,* 498–508.

Daly, M., Adelman, A., & Resnick, B. (1992). The supportive care unit-inpatient geriatric rehabilitation. *Maryland Medical Journal, 41*(6), 5–15.

Efron, B. (1979). The 1977 Rietz lecture; Bootstrap methods: Another look at the jackknife. *The Annals of Statistics, 7*(1), 1–26.

Efron, B., & Gong, G. (1983). A leisurely look at the bootstrap, the jackknife, and cross-validation. *The American Statistician, 37*(1), 36–48.

Fenwick, I. (1979). Techniques in market measurement: The jackknife. *Journal of Marketing Research, 16,* 410–414.

Mahoney, R., & Barthel, D. (1965). Functional evaluation: The Barthel index. *Maryland State Medical Journal, 14,* 61–65.

Mantel, N. (1967). Queries and notes: Assumption-free estimators using U statistics and a relationship to the jackknife method. *Biometrics, 23,* 567–570.

Miller, R. (1964). A trustworthy jackknife. *The Annals of Mathematical Statistics, 35,* 1594–1604.

Miller, R. (1968). Jackknifing variances. *The Annals of Mathematical Statistics, 39,* 567–582.

Miller, R. (1974). The jackknife—a review. *Biometrika. 61,* 1–15.

Mosteller, F., & Tukey, J. (1968). Data analysis, including statistics. In G. Lindzey and E. Aronson (eds.), *Handbook of social psychology* (pp. 38–41). Reading, MA: Addison-Wesley.

Pigeot, I. (1991). A jackknife estimator of combined odds ratio. *Biometrics, 47,* 373–381.

Prescott, P. (1987). Multiple regression analysis with small samples: Cautions and suggestions. *Nursing Research, 36,* 130–133.

SAS Institute Inc. (1985). *SAS User's Guide.* Cary, NC: SAS Institute.

Stevens, J. (1992). *Applied multivariate statistics for the social services.* Hillsdale, NJ: Erlbaum.

The Logistic Regression Model and the Odds of Testing HIV Positive

Hossein N. Yarandi ■ Sharleen H. Simpson

Regression methods have become an integral component of any data analysis concerned with describing the relationship between a dependent variable and one or more independent variables. Sometimes, the dependent variable is discrete and takes on only two or more values. In this situation, the logistic regression model can be used to describe the relationship between a dependent variable and a set of independent variables. What distinguishes a logistic regression model from the linear regression model is that the dependent variable in logistic regression is binary or dichotomous (Hosmer & Lemeshow, 1989; Draper & Smith, 1981; Kleinbaum & Kupper, 1978). The analysis and interpretation of logistic regression, however, is quite similar to the procedures of multiple regression (Cox, 1970). An illustration of the logistic model is presented below.

Multiple Logistic Regression Model

If $x_1, x_2, \ldots, x_k$ are a collection of independent variables and y is a binary random variable (the values of y are usually 0 or 1 with probability of success = p if a value 0 occurs), then the multiple logistic regression model is given by

$$\ln\left(\frac{p}{1-p}\right) = \beta_0 + \beta_1 x_1 + \beta_2 x_2 + \ldots + \beta_k x_k \qquad (1)$$

or, equivalently, if we solve for probability, p, then the model can be expressed in the form

$$p = \frac{e^{\beta_0 + \beta_1 x_1 + \beta_2 x_2 + \ldots + \beta_k x_k}}{1 + e^{\beta_0 + \beta_1 x_1 + \beta_2 x_2 + \ldots + \beta_k x_k}} \qquad (2)$$

$$\text{By definition, odds} = \frac{p}{1-p} \qquad (3)$$

$$\text{Therefore, probability} = p = \left(\frac{\text{odds}}{1+\text{odds}}\right) \qquad (4)$$

Computing the odds is a commonly used technique of interpreting probabilities (Fleiss, 1981). For example, if we say that the odds are 4 to 1 that one team will defeat another in a game, this expression means the favored team has a probability of 4/(1 + 4) = .80 of winning the game.

We see that p must always lie between 0 and 1, but the odds may vary from 0 to infinity (∞). When p = 0, .5, or 1, the odds are 0, 1, or ∞, respectively. Taking the natural logarithm of the odds {ln(odds)} will cure this asymmetry.

$$\text{Therefore, } \ln(\text{odds}) = \ln \frac{p}{1-p} \qquad (5)$$

According to (5), when p = 0, .5, or 1, the ln(odds) are −∞, 0, or +∞, respectively. The term *logit* is sometimes used instead of ln(odds). The ratio of two odds is known as the odds ratio (or relative risk when the data is retrospective). For the multiple logistic regression model in (1), the odds ratio relating to a dichotomous independent variable, x_i, which is coded as 1 if present and 0 if absent, is estimated by

$$\text{Estimated Odds Ratio} = \hat{OR} = e^{\hat{\beta}_i} \qquad (6)$$

Relationship (6) expresses the odds of x = 1 divided by the odds of x = 0 after controlling for all other variables in the logistic regression model (Hosmer & Lemeshow, 1989).

Application of the Logistic Regression Model

In April of 1985, a site for anonymous HIV antibody testing was established with a grant from the United States Department of Health and Human Services to the State of Florida. This program began under the auspices of the local Health and Rehabilitation Service (HRS) county public health unit. The clients utilizing this test site were self-diagnosed as at risk. As part of the testing procedure, individuals were first interviewed and then administered screening tests. Everyone was subsequently informed of the results in person and given further posttest counseling, as required by Florida statute. Referrals were made as necessary. Complete anonymity was maintained; only

Hossein N. Yarandi, PhD, is associate professor, College of Nursing and Biostatistics Unit, University of Florida, Gainesville, FL.

Sharleen H. Simpson, PhD, is assistant professor, College of Nursing, University of Florida, Gainesville, FL.

From *Nursing Research,* November/December 1991, *40,* 372–373.

a coded numbering system was used to identify the interview schedules and test results. The administered questionnaire included information about demographic characteristics, risk factors for AIDS, physical symptoms, and results of the HIV testing. A detailed description of demographic and sexual behavior is presented elsewhere (Simpson, Yarandi, Davis & Belcuore, 1990).

A stepwise logistic regression procedure on 559 questionnaires was used to calculate the risk of being HIV positive. The dependent variable is the result of the HIV testing (HIV = 1 if positive and HIV = 0 if negative). The independent variables are anal intercourse (as a percent of total sexual intercourse), number of short-term partners in the last 10 years, having an HIV positive partner (1 if yes and 0 if no), history of syphilis (1 if present and 0 if absent), history of gonorrhea (1 if present and 0 if absent), history of hepatitis (1 if present and 0 if absent), intravenous drug use (1 if yes and 0 if no), use of nonintravenous drugs (1 if yes and 0 if no), presence of a tattoo (1 if present and 0 if absent), and gender (1 if male and 0 if female).

The best fitting model relating the prevalence of HIV seropositivity to the risk factors is presented in Table 1 using the SAS/STAT software. All the estimated coefficients are statistically significant at the 0.10 level of significance.

Knowing the estimated logistic coefficients (Table 1) and using equation (2), it is possible to compute the whole range of probabilities of testing HIV positive under different conditions. For example, an individual male who lives in north central Florida and has had 20 short-term partners in the last 10 years and no other risk factors, has a 4.8% chance of testing HIV positive. This probability is obtained by plugging the estimated coefficients from Table 1 into equation (2) for a male individual (Gender = 1) as follows:

$$p = \frac{e^{-5.0423+0.0293(0)+0.0015(20)+1.2769(0)+2.0626(0)+0.9557(0)+1.1612(0)+2.0224(1)}}{1+e^{-5.0423+0.0293(0)+0.0015(20)+1.2769(0)+2.0626(0)+0.9557(0)+1.1612(0)+2.0224(1)}}$$

$$\text{then, } p = \frac{e^{-2.9899}}{1+e^{-2.9899}}$$

knowing that e = 2.71828, we will have,

$$p = \frac{(2.71828)^{-2.9899}}{1+(2.71828)^{-2.9899}} = \frac{0.0502926}{1.0502926} = .0478843, \text{ or almost } 4.8\%$$

The same procedure can be followed to calculate the following probabilities. For example, an individual male who has engaged in anal intercourse 50% of the time, had 20 short-term partners in the last 10 years, and had no other risk factors, has a 17.9% chance of testing HIV positive. On the other hand, an individual male who has engaged in anal intercourse 100% of the time, had 20 short-term partners in the last 10 years, and had no other risk factors, has a 48.5% chance of testing HIV positive. Similarly, if an individual male had 20 short-term partners, engaged in anal intercourse 100% of the time, had both hepatitis and syphilis, and used both intravenous and nonintravenous drugs, his chance of testing HIV positive would be 99.5%.

According to the logistic regression equation (Table 1), an individual female who has had 20 short-term partners in the last 10 years and had no other risk factors, has a 0.66% chance of testing HIV positive. If she had 20 short-term partners in the last 10 years and used intravenous and nonintravenous drugs, her chance of testing positive would rise to 5.2%. Her chance of testing HIV positive would be 60.9% if she had 20 short-term partners, had used intravenous and nonintravenous drugs, and had a history of both syphilis and hepatitis.

Using the estimated regression coefficients (Table 1) and equation (6), one can compute the odds ratio (or relative risk) of testing HIV positive, given the presence of a specific risk factor (if the risk factor is coded as 0 or 1). For example, for a male, the odds in favor of being HIV positive are 7.56 times as large as those for a female after controlling for all other independent variables in the model. For an individual with a history of hepatitis, the odds in favor of being HIV positive are 7.87 times as large as those for an individual with no history of hepatitis after controlling for all other inde-

TABLE 1 Results of a Stepwise Logistic Regression Model to the Data for the Dependent Variable HIV

Risk Factor (x_i)	Regression Coefficient ($\hat{\beta}i$)	Standard Error ($s_{\hat{\beta}i}$)	Chi Square (χ^2)	*P*-value
Intercept	–5.042	0.559	81.39	0.0001
Anal Intercourse	0.029	0.005	28.35	0.0001
Short-Term Partner	0.00	0.001	2.90	0.0887
Syphilis	1.277	0.602	4.49	0.0162
Hepatitis	2.063	0.983	4.40	0.0358
IV Drug User	0.956	0.514	3.46	0.0629
Other Drugs	1.161	0.354	10.77	0.0010
Gender	2.022	0.569	12.64	0.0004

pendent variables in the model. In comparison, an individual using intravenous drugs is 2.60 times as likely to test HIV positive as an intravenous drug-free individual after controlling for all other independent variables in the model.

In summary, logistic regression is based on the assumption that the logarithm of the odds of belonging to one population is a linear function of several predictors (independent variables) in the model. The use of a logistic regression model provides a fast and effective way to obtain the estimate of probability of belonging to a specific population and the estimate of odds ratio (or relative risk) of having a specific problem or condition.

References

Cox, D. R. (1970). *The Analysis of binary data.* London: Metheun.

Draper, N. R., & Smith, H. (1981). *Applied regression analysis.* New York: Wiley.

Fleiss, J. L. (1981). *Statistical methods for rates and proportions.* New York: Wiley.

Hosmer, D. W., & Lemeshow, S. (1989). *Applied logistic regression.* New York: Wiley.

Kleinbaum, D. G., & Kupper, L. L. (1978). *Applied regression analysis and other multivariate methods.* Belmont, CA: Wadsworth.

SAS Institute Inc. (1987). *SAS/STAT guide for personal computers: Version 6 edition.* Cary, NC: SAS Institute.

Simpson, S. H., Yarandi, H. Y., Davis, R. C., & Belcuore, T. R. (1990). Sexual behavior and demographic characteristics of individuals tested for human immunodeficiency virus infection in north central Florida. *Florida Journal of Public Health, II,* 30–36.

Contextual Regression Analysis

William L. Holzemer ■ Bonnie Mowinski Jennings ■ Donald B. Chambers ■ Steven M. Paul

Although the extent of their active involvement may vary, individuals participate in many groups. Psychological studies can explore individual issues and sociological investigations can examine group dynamics, but the researcher who is concerned with the effects of both groups and individuals is left to grapple with the problem of aggregate data.

The use of aggregate data has been discouraged, based on the assumption that, because the data can misrepresent the individual, all interpretations are suspect. As Borgatta and Jackson (1980) pointed out, this guidance is excessively cautious. Furthermore, analyzing the effects of the social milieu on individual behavior remains important to behavioral scientists (Firebaugh, 1980).

Contextual regression analysis is a statistical strategy that can be used to investigate the relationships of both individual and group characteristics with an outcome variable (Boyd & Iversen, 1979; Burstein, 1980a, 1980b; Lazarsfeld & Menzel, 1961). Its primary purpose is to determine the presence of a contextual effect, that is, whether group membership contributes to the explanation of the variance in an outcome measure after the effects of individual characteristics have been taken into account. Effects, as used here, refer to this concept of explained variance and do not imply causal relationships. The purpose of this paper, then, is to provide an overview of this statistical technique.

William L. Holzemer, PhD, FAAN, is professor and coordinator, Quality Assurance Program, and director, Office of Research, School of Nursing, University of California, San Francisco.

Bonnie Mowinski Jennings, DNSc, RN, is a lieutenant colonel in the U. S. Army Nurse Corps currently assigned as a nurse researcher, Health Care Studies Division, U.S. Army Health Services Command, Fort Sam Houston, TX.

Donald B. Chambers, MEd, is data analyst and computer laboratory manager in the Office of Research, School of Nursing, University of California, San Francisco.

Steven M. Paul, PhD, is statistician in the Office of Research, School of Nursing, University of California, San Francisco.

From *Nursing Research,* March/April 1989, *38,* 124–125.

The Statistical Strategy

Contextual analysis has a long social science history, especially in the study of organizational behavior and in large-scale evaluations of educational programs. The utility of contextual analysis is that it affords a way to combine variables aggregated at different levels, permitting the investigator to examine different units of analysis.

The general logic behind this multilevel analysis of variation is to examine the effects of specified group-level variables while controlling for the effects of specified individual-level variables, and vice versa. A *contextual* (program, organizational, or environmental) effect is present if group-level variables account for a significant proportion of variation in the dependent measure after controlling for the effects due to individual characteristics. In contrast, an *individual* effect is present if additional variance in the dependent measure is attributable to individual-level variables after controlling for the group effects. In distinguishing between covariance analysis and contextual analysis, Firebaugh (1980) stated, "Covariance analysis asks: how large is the total impact of the group? Contextual analysis asks: what characteristics of the groups have an effect?" (p.21).

All tenets common to traditional multiple regression analysis apply to contextual regression. For example, linear model assumptions must be met (Verran & Ferketich, 1987) and at least a 10:1 ratio of subjects to independent variables must be achieved (Marascuilo & Levin, 1982). Unique to contextual regression, however, is the process of assigning select variables to sets representing both the individual and the group. Actual respondent scores are used to represent individual variables; the group variables are comprised of scores reflecting both general attributes of the group (e.g., average daily hospital census, average number of faculty) and mean scores for relevant indicants (e.g., mean years of work experience).

Both hierarchical and stepwise multiple regression are used in the analysis. Sets of variables measured at either the individual or group level are entered into the analysis in a predetermined or hierarchical order. Conversely, variables within sets enter the regression in a stepwise fashion according to the amount of variance each accounts for in the dependent variable. Two independent studies using contextual regression analysis are summarized to demonstrate this statistical procedure.

Two Exemplars

Faculty Productivity

In the educational setting, it is often difficult to determine whether individual traits or the scholarly milieu has more influence on faculty productivity. Consequently, to unravel this phenomenon, 241 faculty representing 25 doctoral programs in nursing were surveyed to address the following question: What are the contextual effects of individual faculty and program characteristics on individual faculty productivity? (Holzemer & Chambers, 1986).

Faculty productivity was the dependent measure throughout the contextual analysis; 24 independent variables were used as predictors. Individual faculty data were represented by eight variables such as academic rank, percentage of time spent teaching, and percentage of time spent in research. Group-level data represented various nursing programs and included 16 variables, some of which were aggregated over individual faculty members within the programs (e.g., mean percentage of time faculty at each program spent conducting research), and others were constant for all faculty within the program (e.g., number of students enrolled in the program). To determine whether individual faculty characteristics or group (contextual) effects were better predictors of faculty productivity, two multiple regression analyses were performed.

In the first regression, when program-level variables preceded individual-level variables in the equation, five variables accounted for a total of 40% of the variation in faculty productivity. Although 14% of this variance was accounted for by group variables, a large individual effect of the faculty member was demonstrated. More specifically, an additional 26% of the variance in productivity was attributed to three individual-level variables. They were in hierarchical progression, academic rank (9% explained variation), respondent's age (6% explained variation), and the percentage of time a faculty member spent on research and other scholarly work (12% explained variation).

In the second regression, individual variables preceded group variables in the analysis in order to discern whether a contextual effect could be detected. A total of eight variables entered the equation; together they accounted for 43% of the variation in faculty productivity. Five individual-level variables accounted for 36% of the variance in productivity. Once the effects of the individual variables were accounted for, three program variables collectively accounted for an additional 7% of the variation in individual faculty productivity. Consequently, a small but significant contextual effect of the doctoral program was indicated. Faculty who worked in a productive environment and who perceived the environment more positively were more productive.

Head Nurses' Mental Health

A second example of contextual regression analysis is found in an investigation of 300 head nurses representing 37 army health care facilities. An exploratory question of the larger study was concerned with whether individual characteristics of head nurses or features of the hospital environments in which the head nurses worked were better predictors of the head nurses' mental health (Jennings, 1988). Variables were divided into two sets for this analysis—one representing the individual, and the other representing the group or hospital.

The nine variables used to reflect individual characteristics in this analysis were selected according to those indicants most strongly correlated with the outcome measure. These included demographic features such as years of head nurse experience and total hours worked per week, as well as measures of constructs central to the study such as social support and work stress. Group characteristics were represented by 12 variables, two of which were unique to each institution (e.g., hospital census, total staff supervised) and the remainder of which represented mean scores for each hospital on select variables.

The individual variables were entered as a set preceding the group or hospital variables in order to partial the effects of the individual indicants. No group effects were detected, however. Although five of the individual variables entered the equation in hierarchical progression and accounted for 37% of the variance in head nurses' mental health (work stress 18%, nonwork stress 11%, years of head nurse experience 5%, locus of control 2%, and social support 1%), no additional variance could be attributed to group characteristics. Consequently, a contextual effect was not found for this group of head nurses. It is also interesting to note that when the sets were reversed and group-level variables were given the opportunity to enter first, again only individual variables entered the regression.

That is not to suggest the group (i.e., environment or hospital setting) had no effect on mental health. Rather, the particular variables used in this analysis did not represent the group attributes that affected head nurses' mental health. Because organizational climate does influence individuals, identifying which group characteristics affect mental health of head nurses remains an important question to pursue.

Conclusion

Of the two studies summarized in this report, one demonstrated a small contextual effect—faculty who worked in a productive environment and who perceived the environment more positively were more productive—but the other did not find evidence of a contextual effect. Perhaps these findings support the claim by Borgatta and Jackson (1980) that contextual effects have " . . . had more claims for existence than evidence" (p. 11).

Nevertheless, the effects of groups and environments on individuals are vital concerns. Although variable selection and other idiosyncracies may complicate the actual testing of a contextual effect, contextual regression analysis remains an important method for dealing with aggregate data and multiple units of analysis.

References

Borgatta, E. F., & Jackson, D. J. (1980). Aggregate data analysis. An overview. In E. F. Borgatta & D. J. Jackson (eds.), *Aggregate data. Analysis and interpretation* (pp. 7–11). Beverly Hills, CA: Sage.

Boyd, L. H., & Iversen, G. R. (1979). *Contextual analysis: Concepts and statistical techniques.* Belmont, CA: Wadsworth.

Burstein, L. (1980a). The analysis of multilevel data in educational research and evaluation. *Review of Research in Education, 8,* 158–231.

Burstein, L. (1980b). The role of levels of analysis in specification of education effects. In R. Dreeben & J. A. Thomas (eds.), *The analysis of educational productivity, Volume I: Issues in microanalysis* (pp. 119–191). Cambridge, MA: Ballinger.

Firebaugh, G. (1980). Assessing group effects. A comparison of two methods. In E. F. Borgatta & D. J. Jackson (eds.), *Aggregate data. Analysis and interpretation* (pp. 13–24). Beverly Hills, CA: Sage.

Holzemer, W. L., & Chambers, D. B. (1986). Healthy nursing doctoral programs: Relationship between perceptions of the academic environment and productivity of faculty and alumni. *Research in Nursing and Health, 9*(4), 299–307.

Jennings, B. M. (1988). Stress, social support, and locus of control: Effect on head nurses' mental health (Doctoral dissertation, University of California, San Francisco, 1988). *Dissertation Abstracts International, 48,* 3249-B.

Lazarsfeld, P. F., & Menzel, H. (1961). On the relation between individual and collective properties. In A. Etzioni (ed.), *Complex orgnizations: A sociological reader* (pp. 422–440). New York: Holt, Rinehart & Winston.

Marascuilo, L. A., & Levin, J. R. (1982). *Multivariate statistics in the social sciences: A researcher's guide.* Pacific Grove, CA: Brooks/Cole.

Verran, J. A., & Ferketich, S. L. (1987). Testing linear model assumptions: Residual analysis. *Nursing Research, 36,* 127–130.

Theoretical and Methodological Differentiation of Moderation and Mediation

Patricia Lindley ■ Susan Noble Walker

Many of the causal models tested in nursing research involve the presence of one or more third variables, which may be crucial in explaining when, how, and why human phenomena occur. Confusion often arises when the terms *moderating* and *mediating* have been used interchangeably in describing third variables. Moderation and mediation represent different relationships among three or more variables in a proposed theory. Because theoretical clarity is critical to the specification of any causal model, the purpose of this article is to differentiate the moderator and mediator functions in causal models.

For ease in presentation and discussion, the examples of causal models are limited to one predictor variable (X), one third variable (Z), and one outcome or criterion variable (Y). It is recognized that specification of the causal model must be theoretically driven and assumptions necessary for the particular statistical analysis must be met.

The Moderator Function

A moderator is a third variable (Z) that influences the relationship between a predictor variable (X) and an outcome variable (Y). The moderator may be either a categorical or a continuous variable. It may act to reduce the magnitude and/or to reverse the direction of the relationship between the predictor and outcome variables. The moderator effect can be described as an interaction between a predictor variable and a moderator variable, such that the relationship between the predictor and an outcome variable differs depending upon the level of the moderator; the effect of X on Y is *conditional* upon the level of Z.

Patricia Lindley, PhD, RN, CS, ANP, is an assistant professor, University of Nebraska Medical Center, College of Nursing, Omaha, NE.

Susan Noble Walker, EdD, RN, FAAN, is a professor and chair, Gerontological, Psychosocial and Community Health Nursing, University of Nebraska Medical Center, College of Nursing, Omaha, NE.

From *Nursing Research,* September/October 1993, *42,* 276–279.

A causal model involving the moderator function is depicted by the path diagram in Figure 1. Note that, as antecedents of the outcome variable, the moderator and predictor variables are at the same level in the causal model. According to Baron and Kenny (1986), a moderator effect is present whenever the interaction (Path C) is significant; main effects (Paths A and/or B) may or may not be significant and are not essential to establishing moderation. However, it is desirable that the moderator variable not be correlated with either the predictor or the outcome variable if the interaction term is to be clearly interpreted.

An example of a moderator model with continuous variables is provided by the relationships among hardiness (X), social network (Z), and mental health (Y) illustrated in Figure 2. Social network is not significantly correlated either with hardiness or with mental health, yet it plays a vital role in the relationship between them. A moderator effect is seen by the significant path from the interaction of hardiness and social network to mental health in the path diagram in Figure 2, and by the significant change in R^2 when the interaction term enters the hierarchical regression (see Table 1).

Figure 3 shows how the effect of hardiness on mental health differs depending upon the size of the social network. The larger the individual's social network, the greater is the relationship between hardiness and mental health. When the social network is small, the relationship is nonsignificant. A significant *positive* relationship of X to Y at either high (as in the example in Figure 3) or low levels of Z is accompanied by a significant *positive* partial regression coefficient for the interaction product term (as in the example in Figure 2). In contrast, a significant *negative* relationship of X to Y at either high or low levels of Z would be accompanied by a significant *negative* partial regression coefficient for the interaction product term.

For comparison, an example of a causal model that does not involve moderation is presented in Figure 4. Note that the path from the interaction of social support and self-esteem to helpfulness of coping is nonsignificant. As shown later, self-esteem actually serves a mediator function when correctly modeled for the given data.

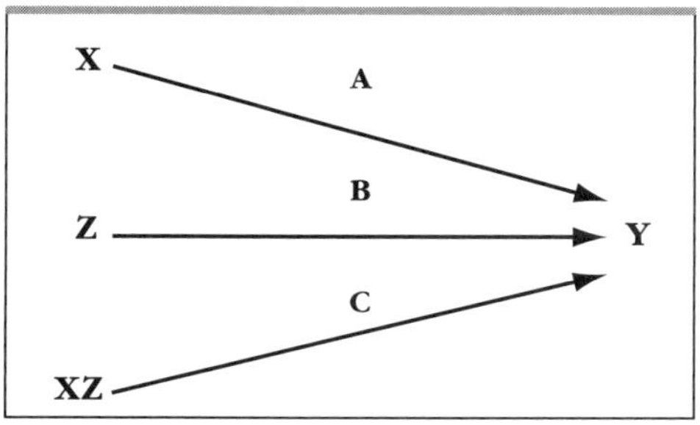

FIGURE 1 Moderator Model

Data analysis procedures for testing moderational hypotheses will vary depending upon the level of measurement of the predictor and the moderator variables. Procedures recommended and discussed in detail in other sources (Aiken & West, 1991; Baron & Kenny, 1986) are summarized in Table 2.

Aiken and West (1991) provide detailed description and discussion concerning the estimation, testing, and probing of interactions in regression models. Of particular value and interest to nursing researchers is their explanation of a procedure for centering continuous predictor and moderator variables in regression analyses. Centering involves subtracting the sample mean of the variable from the variable, thus creating a centered variable in deviation score form with a mean of zero. When uncentered variables are multiplied to form interaction terms, the correlation between the first order terms and the interaction term results in high multicollinearity when entered in regression (Cohen & Cohen, 1983; Pedhazur, 1982). The use of centered variables in regression analyses greatly lessens this problem and yields interpretable regression coefficients for both the first order and the interaction terms.

The Mediator Function

Similar to a moderator, a mediator is a third variable (Z) that influences the relationship between a predictor variable (X) and an outcome variable (Y). More specifically, the mediator represents a process or mechanism, often intrinsic to an individual, that accounts for the relationship between a predictor variable and an outcome variable. The mediator specifies how or why the relationship occurs (Baron & Kenny, 1986).

TABLE 1 Mental Health Regressed on Hardiness and Social Network

Predictor Variables	Cumulative R^2	R^2 Change	Significance of Change
Hardiness	.09	.09	.01
Social Network	.10	.01	.46
Hardiness × Social Network	.16	.06	.04

A minimum of three variables are needed to depict a causal model involving mediation, as illustrated in Figure 5. The predictor is an antecedent variable that precedes both the mediator and the outcome variables. The mediator is a consequence of the predictor variable and an antecedent to the outcome variable. The outcome variable is the consequence of both the predictor and the mediator variables.

To test for mediation, three regression equations are necessary. First, the outcome variable is regressed on the predictor variable (Step 1 in Figure 5). If this relationship is significant, then second and third equations are analyzed (Step 2 in Figure 5). In the second equation, the mediator is regressed on the predictor variable (Path A). The third equation involves regressing the outcome variable simultaneously on the predictor (Path C_2) and mediator (Path B) variables. According to Baron and Kenny, the mediator function is substantiated by three findings: (a) Path A is statistically significant; (b) Path B is statistically significant; and (c) after statistically controlling for Paths A and B, a previously significant relationship between the predictor variable and the outcome variable (Path C_1 in Step 1) becomes nonsignificant (Path C_2 in

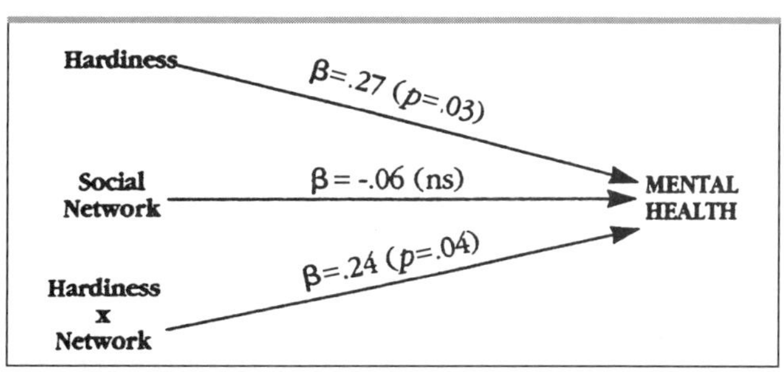

FIGURE 2 Example of Moderator Model

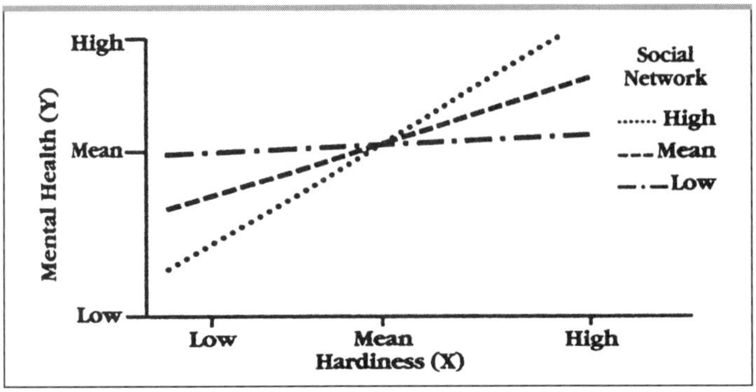

FIGURE 3 Effect of Hardiness on Mental Health Moderated by Social Network

Step 2). The strongest case of mediation occurs when Path C_2 in Step 2 becomes zero, suggesting that one dominant mediator is operating in the causal model.

An example of a mediator model is depicted by the path diagram in Figure 6. Social support (X) influences the helpfulness of coping (Y) through self-esteem (Z). In Step 1, there is a significant path from social support to helpfulness of coping when self-esteem is not included in the model. In Step 2, the mediator function of self-esteem is substantiated first by the reduction of the path coefficient from .32 to .15, and second by the change from a significant p of .03 to a nonsignificant p in the path from social support to the helpfulness of coping.

Mediator variables may produce either additive or suppressive influences on the relationship between predictor and outcome variables (Wheaton, 1985). To detect which type of influence is occurring, it is necessary to calculate direct, indirect, and total effects within the causal model. Readers unfamiliar with the calculation of effects are referred to Cohen and Cohen (1983) and Pedhazur (1982). An additive influence is evidenced by an increase in the total effect on the outcome variable, while a suppressive influence is evidenced by a decrease in the total effect on the outcome variable.

For comparison, an example of a model that does not involve mediation is presented in Figure 7. Note that the path coefficient from hardiness to mental health is unchanged when social support is entered as a mediator in the model, and that the other two path coefficients are nonsignificant. As shown earlier, social support actually serves a moderator function when correctly modeled for the given data. Table 3 provides a summary of the distinctions between moderator and mediator functions as described above.

Additional Comments

The testing of a causal model becomes more complex when both moderator and mediator functions are influencing the relationship between a predictor variable and an outcome variable. Baron and Kenny (1986) provide a detailed description of analyses testing for mediated moderation and moderated mediation.

One major and often overlooked source of error in testing causal models occurs when there is a reciprocal causal path (i.e., feedback) from the outcome variable to the predictor and/or third variable (Y to X or Y to Z). Such a model cannot be analyzed using the ordinary least squares (OLS) regression techniques described above.

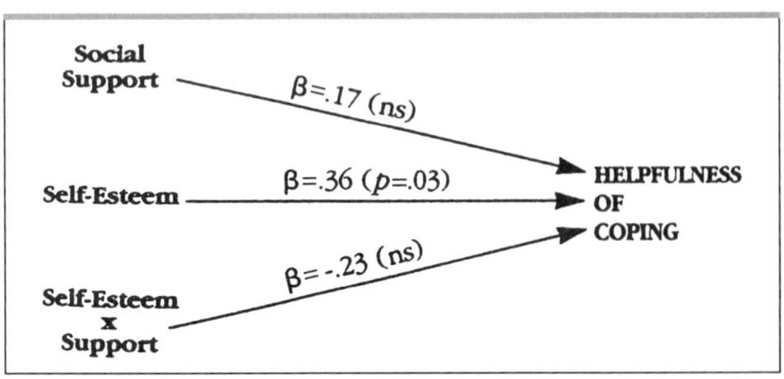

FIGURE 4 Example of Nonmoderator Model

TABLE 2 Statistical Analysis According to Level of Measurement of Predictor and Moderator Variables

Predictor Variable	Moderator Variable: *Categorical*	Moderator Variable: *Continuous*
Categorical (Dichotomous)	2 × 2 ANOVA	Hierarchical multiple regression of outcome on predictor, centered moderator, and interaction terms (and higher order terms if predictor/outcome relation is curvilinear)
Continuous	Separate regressions for each level of the moderator; *t*-test for differences between groups' unstandardized regression coefficients *OR* Hierarchical multiple regression of outcome on centered predictor, dummy-coded moderator, and interaction terms.	Hierarchical multiple regression of outcome on centered predictor, centered moderator, and interaction terms (and higher order terms if predictor/outcome relation is curvilinear)

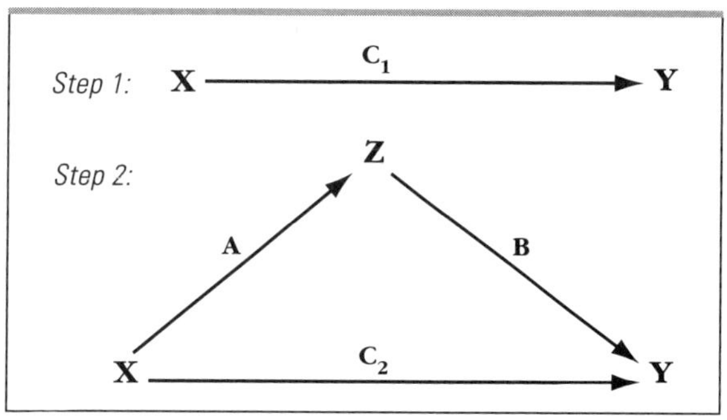

FIGURE 5 Mediator Model

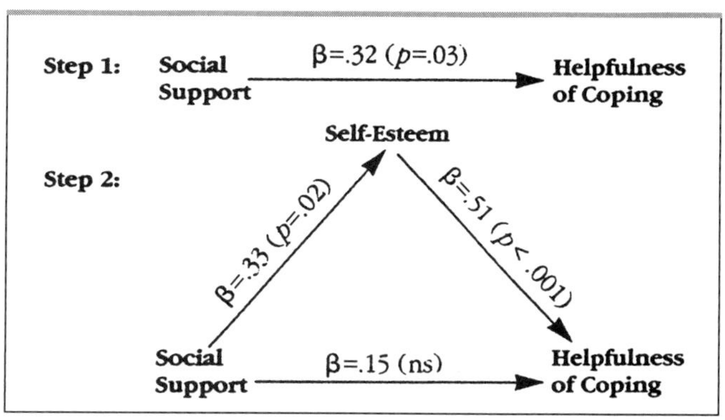

FIGURE 6 Example of Mediator Model

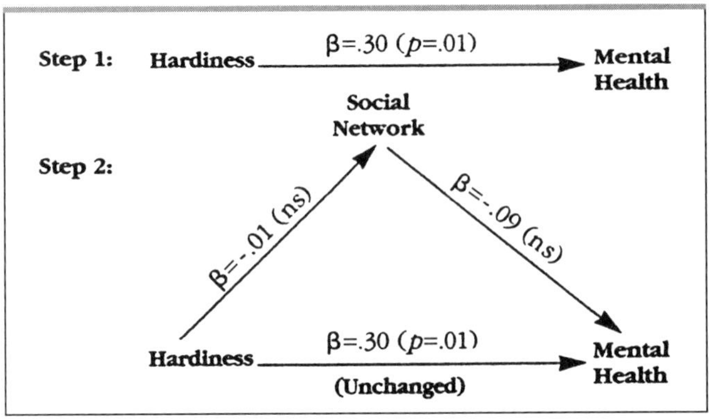

FIGURE 7 Example of Nonmediator Model

This potential problem may be avoided by employing an analysis of nonrecursive models using linear structural equation techniques as described by Bollen (1989).

Clarification of the moderator and mediator functions of third variables in causal models is critical for theoretical and methodological reasons. Failure to substantiate a hypothesized moderator or mediator function, which was originally derived from theoretical literature, may suggest a reanalysis of the theory. Inaccurate specification and/or incomplete testing of a moderator or mediator function may result in erroneous or missed results and inappropriate conclusions about the complex multivariate relationships so often encountered in nursing research.

TABLE 3 Comparison of Moderator and Mediator Functions

Moderator	Mediator
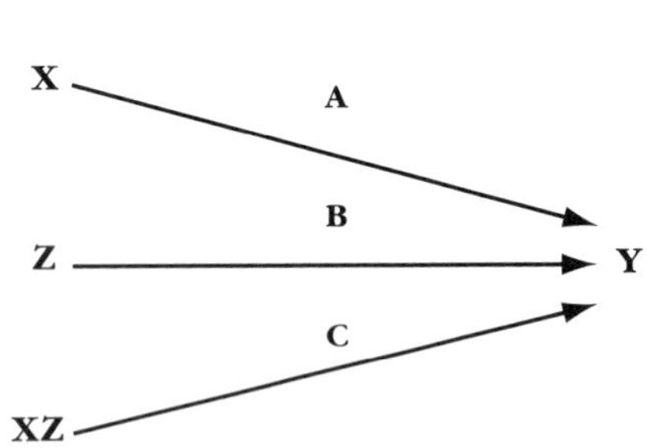	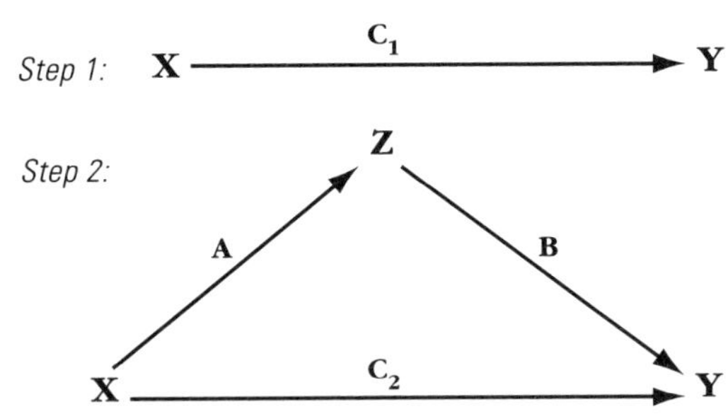
X and Z are antecedents of Y	Z is a consequence of X and an antecedent of Y; Y is a consequence of X and Z
Direction and/or strength of the influence of X on Y is a function of Z	Z is a process or mechanism through which X influences Y
Consider moderation when the relationship of X to Y is strong, weak, or inconsistent	Consider mediation when the relationship of X to Y is strong
Occurs when Path C is significant (and ideally Z is not related to X and to Y)	Occurs when Paths A and B are significant and when Path C_2 becomes nonsignificant
Specifies when or under what conditions X influences Y	Specifies how or why X influences Y

References

Aiken, L. S., & West, S. G. (1991). *Multiple regression: Testing and interpreting interactions.* Newbury Park, CA: Sage.

Baron, R. M., & Kenny, D. A. (1986). The moderator-mediator variable distinction in social psychological research: Conceptual, strategic, and statistical considerations. *Journal of Personality and Social Psychology, 51,* 1173–1182.

Bollen, K. A. (1989). *Structural equations with latent variables.* New York: Wiley.

Cohen, J., & Cohen, P. (1983). *Applied multiple regression/correlation analysis for the behavioral sciences* (2nd ed.). Hillsdale, NJ: Erlbaum.

Pedhazur, E. J. (1982). *Multiple regression in behavioral research* (2nd ed.). New York: Holt, Rinehart & Winston.

Wheaton, B. (1985). Models for the stress-buffering functions of coping resources. *Journal of Health and Social Behavior, 26,* 352–364.

Testing Linear Model Assumptions: Residual Analysis

Joyce A. Verran ■ **Sandra L. Ferketich**

Analysis of data involves a variety of methods. Classical statistical approaches include procedures that confirm hypothesized relationships. Recent advances in the analysis of research data emphasize the search for possible models that describe the universe of interest. This orientation views the empirical world as offering significant information to the researcher willing to explore the data.

Exploratory data analysis techniques are newer and less widely used by nurse scientists. These techniques are designed to assist in detecting different types of underlying data structures. Exploratory analytic methods are used with flexibility and the unexpected in mind but without restrictive model assumptions as prerequisites (Hartwig & Dearing, 1979). One such exploratory method is residual analysis. Although there are a variety of uses for this technique, the purpose of this article is to describe residual analysis as a method for building a more stable mathematical linear model.

In the context of the linear model, residual analysis may be viewed as a technique of exploratory data analysis initiated to examine the efficacy of the specified model. Inherent in the equation that defines the model is a set of mathematical assumptions. This set of assumptions forms the critical underpinnings of the model and the analysis procedures. If these assumptions are violated, the statistical techniques used to confirm the model may be so inappropriate that results are uninterpretable or are interpreted incorrectly.

Assumptions of the Linear Model

In the strictest sense, the assumptions of a linear regression model are stated about the error terms of the equation. In the early 1960s a body of literature developed that proposed the observable residuals from the sample regression could and should be used to examine for assumption violations (Anscombe & Tukey, 1963).

For the linear model, the usual set of underlying assumptions, as specified by Graybill (1976) and Neter and Wasserman (1974), are:

1. The residual mean is zero.

2. The residual variance is equal at all points of the predicted dependent variable.

3. The residuals are normally distributed.

4. The residuals indicate the independent variables have a fixed distribution.

5. The residuals show no evidence of departure from linearity.

6. The residuals are independent. In addition to these assumptions, the independent variables in an equation are assumed to be measured without error.

A model may depart from its mathematical assumptions in a variety of ways. Although regression analysis is a robust procedure, each of these departures, or combination of violations, has an impact on the stability of the final model. For example, regression coefficients (parameter estimates) may be unstable or the explained variance (R^2) may be biased (Belsley, Kuh, & Welsch, 1980; Hey, 1974). In addition, tests of significance, such as F tests, may be inaccurate. Thus, the researcher cannot have confidence in the stability of the results of the analysis.

Types of Residual Analysis

Residuals may be analyzed in two ways to assess for model violations. First, statistical tests that examine for specific assumption violations have been developed. Second, graphs may be used to examine for unusual or unexpected patterns. A judicious combination of these two methods is perhaps the best approach to analysis of residuals. It may seem that the two methods are mutually exclusive; however, they complement each other. For example, a graphic approach may demonstrate a curvilinear relationship that would not have been apparent if a linear summary measure of association, such as a Pearson cor-

Joyce A. Verran, PhD, RN, is an assistant professor and division coordinator, Medical–Surgical Nursing, College of Nursing, University of Arizona, Tucson, AZ.

Sandra L. Ferketich, PhD, RN, is an assistant professor and coordinator of the Parent–Child Program, Department of Physiological Nursing, School of Nursing, University of California, San Francisco, CA.

From *Nursing Research,* March/April 1987, *36,* 127–130.

relation coefficient, had been used. Alternatively, the subjective interpretation of a graph can be confirmed by the use of the appropriate summary statistic. In other words, the tandem use of graphs and statistics provides a base for the researcher not easily obtained when there is exclusive use of one approach.

Residual Analysis Procedure

This article suggests an approach to residual analysis that uses both graphs and summary statistics.

The flowchart in Figure 1 summarizes a pattern of examination for model assumptions. The order of examination is based on a natural flow of the analysis procedures and not on any ranking of importance. The *yes* or *no* beside the arrowed lines indicates the answer to the question posed in each of the boxes. Table 1 summarizes graphic and mathematic approaches useful in obtaining an answer to the posed questions in boxes 1 through 6.

Although the flowchart is self-explanatory, two portions require particular attention. The questions regarding zero mean and independence are crucial, and no acceptance of violations of these assumptions can be tolerated. The flowchart shows closed loops that permit no progress in the analysis of the model until these violations have been corrected.

Zero Mean

Examination for zero mean is accomplished by obtaining the summary statistics of the mean and its 95% confidence interval for the unstandardized residuals. If the confidence interval crosses zero, one can assume with

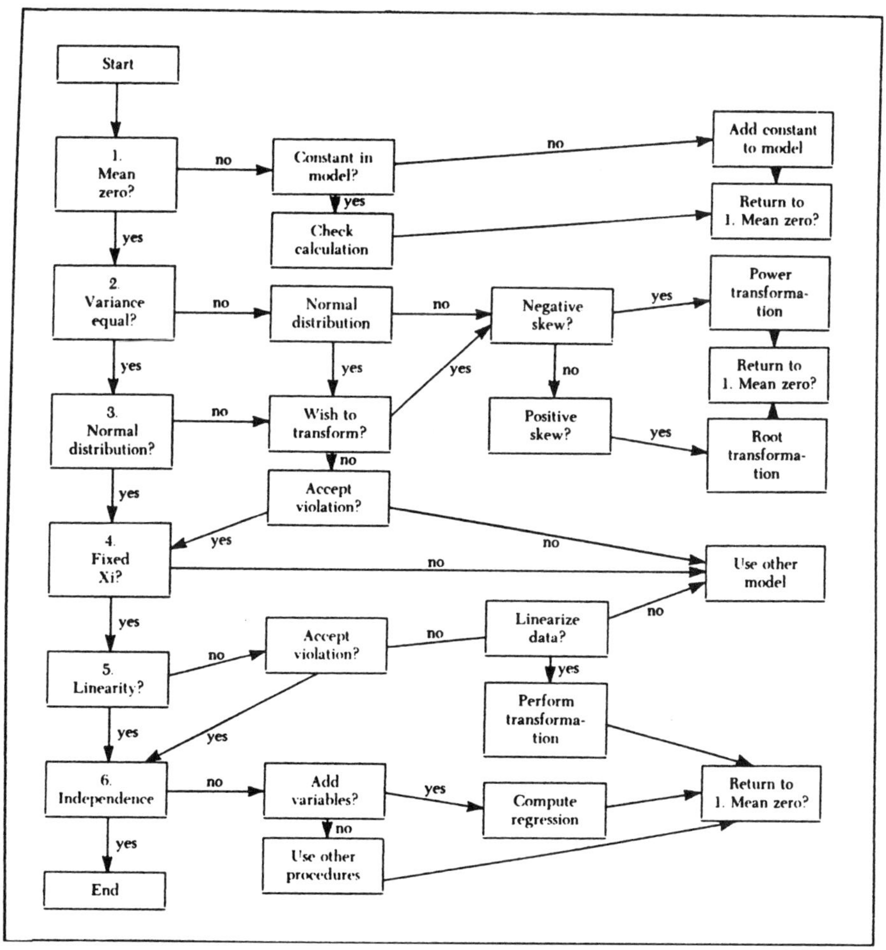

FIGURE 1 Flow Chart for Residual Analysis Procedure

TABLE 1 **Graphic and Statistical Means of Assessing Violations**

Violation	Graph	Statistical Test
1. Zero mean	Frequency distribution	95% confidence interval
2. Equal variance	Scatterplot	Split-half *F* test
3. Normality	Histogram	Shapiro–Wilk *W*
	Frequency polygon	Chi square
	Probability plots	
4. Fixed independent variables	Scatterplot	—
5. Linearity	Scatterplot	—
6. Independence	Scatterplot	Pearson correlation
		Durbin–Watson test
		Von Neuman ratio
		Runs test

reasonable confidence that the assumption of zero mean has not been violated. When an intercept or constant is fit as part of the linear estimation process, violation of this assumption is infrequent.

Normality

When investigating whether residuals fit a normal distribution, a variety of sources of information should be used. The manifestations of a nonnormal distribution can occur in a multitude of ways; therefore, data should be examined both graphically and statistically.

Graphic techniques for the test of the normality assumption include histograms, frequency polygons, and normal probability plots. For the researcher unfamiliar with the interpretation of probability plots, Daniel and Wood (1980) provide an excellent review of the variations that can occur within such plots.

Summary statistics include omnibus tests for deviation from a normal distribution. The Shapiro–Wilk *W* is considered a uniformly powerful test for deviations from normality (Huang & Bolch, 1974; Shapiro, Wilk & Chen, 1968). Although the *W* is an excellent test, its computation may be difficult and time-consuming if appropriate computer programs are not readily available. A chi-square goodness-of-fit test is hand computed easily and quickly provides a guide to normality that enhances the subjective information obtained from the graphic approach.

Variance Equality

Graphic analysis provides the best approach to the examination of residuals for the violation of equal variance. A scatterplot of standardized residuals; on the y axis, versus the predicted dependent variable, on the x axis, will demonstrate a random and equal scatter of points about the zero line of the residuals if there is no violation of this assumption. Alterations in scatter that indicate problems with variance are illustrated in Verran and Ferketich (1984).

A statistical test in support of the subjective interpretation of the scatterplot is a split-half *F* test (Younger, 1979). With this technique residuals may be split into two samples selected to best represent the observed unequal variance. An *F* test may then be performed on the variances of the residuals from the two samples.

Independence

Violation of the assumption of independence among the residuals may occur in a number of ways. Neter and Wasserman (1974) provide a helpful orientation to evaluating the data in regard to the independence assumption. They state that independence may be violated when one residual value depends on the value of another. This may occur when a variable is left out of the model, such as time, if the data were collected in a time sequence. Other variables, such as rater, care provider, or site, may cause relationships among the residuals that would not be discovered if only the more usual parameter of time were used for the residual plot. It is helpful to consider any other variable that may cause a correlation among the residuals and plot the standardized residuals against that particular variable or set of variables. If evidence of linear or nonlinear relationships is seen, follow-up statistical tests can be performed.

Summary statistical tests are selected on the basis of the evidence of the relationship observed in the graphic residual plot. For example, the statistical significance of a linear relationship can be supported by the use of a Pearson correlation coefficient. If residuals are sorted by the variable thought to cause dependency, the Durbin–

Watson test, the Von Neuman ratio, or the nonparametric Runs test may also be used (Zar, 1974).

A further technique to test the impact of an external variable on the model is, quite simply, to add the variable to the linear equation and examine its impact on the percent of explained variance. The decision to add a variable is both statistical and theoretical in nature. Theoretical considerations involve the logical assessment of fit between the new variable and other model concepts. For example, the investigator may find that the time the data were collected and the individual raters who obtained the data both evidence patterns with residuals. However, the differences in how raters collected the data may indicate measurement error rather than theoretical significance. A logical decision would then be to add time to the model but to correct the rater error in other ways such as dropping the cases attributable to the rater or raters evincing the most error. Statistical considerations include the relationship among the number of variables added to the model, the sample size, and the consequent number of *F* tests performed in the regression sequence.

Linearity and Fixed Independent Variables

The statistical procedure used to fit the model assumes a linear relationship among variables. Whether the linear function is appropriate for the data may be evaluated by the study of scatterplots of residuals. As noted earlier, when residuals are plotted versus the predicted dependent variable, a random scatter about the residual zero line is expected. A scatter that curves across this line indicates that the linear function is inappropriate for the data under analysis. Similar plots of residuals versus the independent variables in the equation are also helpful in determining the specific variable or set of variables that may result in the curved function. These latter plots are also used to indirectly estimate whether the distributions of the independent variables are fixed.

Conclusions

As nurse researchers develop or begin to use sophisticated methods of analyzing data, it is critical to fully evaluate the data for underlying relationships and for possible violation of model assumptions. The field of exploratory data analysis can provide valuable techniques to achieve full analysis of data. Hoaglin, Mosteller, and Tukey (1983) noted that a major theme of exploratory data analysis is use of residuals. This view asserts that the analysis of a set of data is not complete until an examination of the residuals is performed.

Residual analysis can assist in supporting theory across studies. Replication studies would be more comparable if there were evidence that estimated parameters were stable. Then, differences or similarities in results would be less likely due to an artifact of the statistical analysis and more likely due to population differences.

With the use of computers and packaged software programs, attention to examination of residuals becomes increasingly important. Researchers may tend to view the confirmation of relationships, evidenced by the computer printout, as the final step in analysis. But, further investigation, in an exploratory mode, may yield unexpected, yet theoretically valuable, information about relationships as well as provide evidence of the model's efficacy.

References

Anscombe, S. J., & Tukey, J. W. (1963). The examination and analysis of residuals. *Technometrics, 5,* 141–160.

Belsley, D. A., Kuh, E., & Welsch, R. E. (1980). *Regression diagnostics.* New York: John Wiley & Sons.

Daniel, C., & Wood, F. S. (1980). *Fitting equations to data.* New York: John Wiley & Sons.

Graybill, F. (1976). *Theory and application of the linear model.* North Scituate, MA: Duxbury Press.

Hartwig, F., & Dearing, B. E. (1979). *Exploatory data analysis.* Beverly Hills, CA: Sage Publications.

Hey, J. D. (1974). *Statistics in economics.* London: Martin Robertson & Company.

Hoaglin, D. C., Mosteller, F., & Tukey, J. W. (1983). *Understanding robust and exploratory data analysis.* New York: John Wiley & Sons.

Huang, C. J., & Bolch, B. W. (1974). On testing of regression disturbances for normality. *Journal of the American Statistical Association, 69,* 330–335.

Neter, J., & Wasserman, W. (1974). *Applied linear statistical models.* Homewood, IL: Richard D. Irwin.

Shapiro, S. S., Wilk, M. B., & Chen, H. J. (1968). A comparative study of various tests for normality. *Journal of the American Statistical Association, 64,* 1343–1372.

Verran, J. A., & Ferketich, S. L. (1984). Residual analysis for statistical model assumptions of regression. *Western Journal of Nursing Research, 6*(1), 27–40.

Younger, M. S. (1979). *A handbook for linear regression.* North Scituate, MA: Duxbury Press.

Zar, J. H. (1974). *Biostatistical analysis.* Englewood Cliffs, NJ: Prentice-Hall, Inc.

Log-Linear Contingency Table Analysis: An Illustration

Janet T. Ihlenfeld

Analysis of nominal-level data in nursing research is most often relegated to descriptive analysis. Frequency distributions, proportions, percentages, ratios, simple crosstabulations, and comparison of variables using row or column totals or cell means are used to describe and to show the relationship of various variables (Blalock, 1979). This may serve the needs of some research, but it does not give the complete story. Statistical methods exist to enable scholars to analyze nominal-level data so that the relationships of observed data can be compared to the models and equations based on theory.

Analyzing Nominal-Level Data

This article describes one such method of analyzing nominal-level data. Log-linear contingency table analysis tests whether observed frequencies of nominal-level variables approximate the expected frequencies for a particular model specified by theory (Knoke & Burke, 1980).

Log-linear contingency table analysis can be understood by first looking at the chi-square (χ^2) statistic. This is used to crosstabulate two or more nominal scale variables in a contingency situation. Here the observed frequencies are compared to the expected frequencies for each cell in the crosstabulation. The larger the χ^2, the greater the difference between the groups with confidence levels of statistical significance operating in full (Blalock, 1979). This statistical test gives approximate results in determining the independence of the variables.

The log-linear statistical method analyzes contingency table nominal-level data for goodness of fit of a model and tests whether the expected frequencies of given variables for a certain model specified by theory approximate the observed frequencies of the variables in the collected data (Knoke & Burke, 1980).

The general log-linear model does not assume whether one variable is dependent and affected by the independent variable(s). Simultaneous existence of variation within several nominal-level variables in a crosstabulation can be determined by using the likelihood ratio chi-square ($LR\chi^2$) to test a general log-linear model (Knoke & Burke, 1980).

Illustration

Nominal-level demographic data were collected from a sample of 103 baccalaureate- or higher-degree nursing faculty members in a larger study of friendship choice of women (Ihlenfeld, 1986).* Information on the demographic characteristics of the sample and of their three closest friends was compared for the simultaneous similarity or difference of the demographic variables of age (A), sex (S), marital status (M), educational level (E), and occupation (O). The variables of age, sex, marital status, educational level, and occupation are independent variables with the implied, and therefore not analyzed, dependent variable being whether the friend was chosen by the respondent. The simultaneous existence of the status characteristic variables as *same* or *different* is the basis of the equation to be tested.

Log-linear analysis uses nominal-level data which have been dichotomized into two mutually exclusive categories. Use of polytomous variables of three or more categories is discouraged because multiple beta coefficients would be produced for each variable, complicating explanation of results (Knoke & Burke, 1980). For example, variables should be divided as young/old, married/single, and so on. In the case of these data, to look at similarity between a respondent and the respondent's close friends, these data were dichotomized into same and different categories for the given variables. Specifically, if the faculty member was female and the friend also was female, sex was categorized as same. Age was dichotomized as same/different; same if the range was within plus or minus 5 years, different if the range was greater than plus or minus 5 years. All status characteristic variables were dichotomized similarly according to whether the self was same or different than the friend (i.e., single, married, separated, widowed, or divorced).

Janet T. Ihlenfeld, PhD, RN, is an associate professor in the Division of Nursing, D'Youville College, Buffalo, NY.

From *Nursing Research,* July/August 1988, *37,* 252–254.

* Data used in this illustration were gathered for the author's doctoral dissertation. All rights and privileges of the respondents were maintained.

The log-linear contingency table program must begin with completion of a crosstabulation of the observed frequencies of the data for the desired variables. A 2 × 2 × 2 × 2 × 2 table for Age by Sex by Marital Status by Educational Level by Occupation was generated. Prior to using the Everyman's Contingency Table Analyzer (ECTA) program, 0.5 cases were added to each cell to remove the zero cells while maintaining the relative percentages in each cell (Knoke & Burke, 1980). The observed frequencies from this table were then transferred to the data input section of the ECTA log-linear computer program.

From here a saturated model for the equation {ASMEO} was run. A saturated model is a fully identified model in which all variables in the equation are entered equally in the analysis. All possible effect parameters are present in this model: (a) the eta (η), which is the geometric mean of the cases in each crosstabulation cell and analogous to the intercept score in regression, and (b) tau (τ), which is the effect of the variables on the cell frequencies. In assessing the saturated model, the observed frequencies of the cells equal the expected frequencies for those same cells. This meaningless equation, the saturated model, though generated, is not in and of itself explanatory for log-linear analysis. The saturated model is a starting point for choosing the models that require fewer parameters and that test the goodness of fit of the model to the observed frequencies (Knoke & Burke, 1980). Fitted models are chosen, based on this goodness of fit.

Table 1 provides an examplc of parameters of the saturated model for the equation of age, sex, marital status, educational level, and occupational similarity {ASMEO}. The eta (grand mean) and the tau values for each parameter of the model are shown. The standardized lambda (which is the log of tau) is a standardized value wherein significance of $p = .05$ is reached at ±1.96. This is applicable only to saturated models (Knoke & Burke, 1980). Generally, in assessing the standardized lambda parameters, values less than approximately ±1.7 indicate that the variable combination is to be eliminated. Variable combinations with the best lambdas are indicated in Table 1. Values for singular variables are ignored.

Log-linear analysis is based on the hierarchical concept where the most complicated multivariate relationship also includes less complex relationships of those same variables (Knoke & Burke, 1980). For this reason, combinations of the {AS}, {SO}, {MO}, and {EO} variable relationships are fitted into the model because their standardized lambdas are greater than ±1.7. The different combinations of these variables are then run again in the ECTA program to determine the fitted models for each of these combinations resulting in determinations of LRχ^2, significance levels, and parameter effects.

TABLE 1 Saturated Model of Age, Sex, Marital Status, Educational Level, and Occupational Status {ASMEO}

	Lambda Effect	Standardized Lambda	Tau
Grand Mean Effect	**1.157**	—	**3.179**
Effect for Variables			
A	0.461	3.048	1.585
S	1.026	6.789	2.791
M	0.346	2.292	1.414
E	−0.206	−1.361	0.814
O	−0.410	−2.715	0.663
AS[a]	0.250	1.655	1.284
AM	0.071	0.472	1.074
AE	−0.050	−0.332	0.951
AO	−0.044	−0.291	0.957
SM	−0.139	−0.917	0.871
SE	0.142	0.939	1.153
SO[a]	0.276	1.825	1.318
ME	0.036	0.235	1.036
MO[a]	−0.255	−1.685	0.775
EO[a]	0.349	2.309	1.418
ASM	−0.075	−0.498	0.928
ASE	0.087	0.574	1.091
ASO	0.029	0.193	1.030
AME	−0.049	−0.323	0.952
AMO	−0.001	−0.004	0.999
AEO	−0.025	−0.163	0.976
SME	0.045	0.296	1.046
SMO	0.093	0.616	1.098
SEO	0.139	0.917	1.149
MEO	−0.033	−0.218	0.968
ASME	0.024	0.161	1.025
ASMO	0.009	0.058	1.009
ASEO	−0.024	−0.160	0.976
AMEO	0.031	0.202	1.031
SMEO	0.095	0.629	1.100
ASMEO	0.095	0.626	1.099

Standard error for all variables = .151

[a] Variables for fitted models

Table 2 reports the different fitted models chosen from the saturated model parameters above and their respective LRχ^2 values. The model with the smallest LRχ^2 and nonsignificant probability levels, $p \geq .05$, will turn out to be the best model for the equation, given that it contains the variables hypothesized in the theory. For Table 2, model

TABLE 2 Fitted Models for the Model, Age, Sex, Marital Status, Educational Level, and Occupational Status {ASMEO}

Fitted Model	$LR\chi^2$	*df*	*p*
{AS} {SO} {MO}	63.05	24	.000
{AS} {SO} {EO}	43.88	24	.008
{AS} {MO} {EO}[a]	22.85	23	.470
{SO} {MO} {EO}	102.39	24	.000
{AS} {SO} {MO} {EO}	12.07	22	>.5

[a] Best fitted model

TABLE 3 Parameters for Fitted Model {AS}{MO}{EO}

Term	Tau	Beta
Grand Mean	3.865	2.714
AS	1.159	0.294
MO	0.848	−0.330
EO	1.578	0.912

Log of odds of similarity versus differences

$$\phi \text{ ASMEO} = \eta + \beta + \beta \text{ MO} + \beta \text{ EO}$$
$$= 2.714 + .294 - .330 + .912$$
$$= 3.59$$

{AS}{SO}{MO}{EO} with a $LR\chi^2$ of 12.07, $p \geq .5$, looks to be the best fit; however, the high significance level indicates that this model fit is too good for the equation, meaning that it contains unnecessary variable parameters. Therefore, model {AS}{MO}{EO} is the best model because the relationships between all variables in the equations are identified and the $LR\chi^2$ of 22.85, though not the smallest, is not too significant to indicate that the observed frequencies are equal to the expected frequencies.

In general, log-linear analysis requires the best-fitted model to contain all of the variables in the theoretical equation, have a small $LR\chi^2$, and a probability level from .05 to roughly .35 (Knoke & Burke, 1980). The models {AS}{SO}{MO}, {AS}{SO}{EO}, and {SO}{MO}{EO} do not contain all variables and their probability levels are too small.

Following acceptance of the best-fitted model, the beta values (analogous to betas in multivariate regression analysis) can be formulated, as a beta is equivalent to two times lambda effects ($\beta = 2 \times \lambda$). These betas will indicate causal paths, if desired, or, as given here, may be added together to determine phi (Φ) which is the log of odds for the expected frequencies (Goodman, 1972). Table 3 gives the beta values for the model {AS}{MO}{EO} as well as for the grand mean of the equation (eta). The beta values may be interpreted as: (a) being similar with the friend in both age and sex results in a slight increase in overall similarity, (b) being similar in marital status and occupation causes a decrease in overall similarity, (c) being similar in educational level and occupation, however, causes a substantial increase in overall similarity with the friend. The log of the odds for similarity versus differences with the friend for age, sex, marital status, educational level, and occupation is 3.59.

Conclusions and Recommendations

Log-linear contingency table analysis can provide the detail of analysis of nominal-level data that other methods lack. Obtaining information from nominal-level data by converting them to dummy variables in multivariate regression is clumsy and results in difficulties when interpreting the dummy beta scores. Log-linear methods produce betas and can help the researcher describe and explain the patterns of phenomena.

Nurse scholars can use log-linear analysis in a variety of research studies. Any time path analysis is desired to show the effects of nominal-level variables in an equation, log-linear contingency table analysis can be used, as it can provide those beta statistics. This would be of more value than using simple correlation coefficients to see association when betas obtained here can predict the strength of parameter effects.

Nurse researchers are encouraged to obtain ECTA programs through university computer centers so that they can have access to another tool to analyze nursing research.

References

Blalock, H. M., Jr. (1979). *Social statistics* (rev. 2nd ed.). New York: McGraw-Hill Book Co.

Goodman, L. A. (1972). A modified multiple regression approach to the analysis of dichotomous variables. *American Sociological Review, 37,* 28–46.

Ihlenfeld, J. T. (1986). *Friendship, social support, and scholarly productivity in nursing faculty members: An exploratory test of the exchange hypothesis.* Unpublished doctoral dissertation, State University of New York at Buffalo.

Knoke, D., & Burke, P. J. (1980). *Log-linear models.* Sage University Paper Series on Quantitative Applications in the Social Sciences (Series No. 07-020). Beverly Hills, CA: Sage Publications.

Structural Equation Models and Nursing Research: Part I

Carol J. Boyd ■ Maureen A. Frey ■ Lauren S. Aaronson

Research using the analysis of linear structural equations (*LISREL*) is occurring with increasing frequency (Aaronson, 1984; Boyd, 1988; Chen & Land, 1986; Cox & Roghmann, 1984; Frey, 1988; Lavee, McCubbin & Patterson, 1985). Consequently, nurses need to know the appropriate uses of structural equation models and how to interpret research that uses the *LISREL* computer program. Part I of this article provides an introduction to structural equation models and a description of what one should expect to see in a report using *LISREL*, highlighting the utility of causal modeling for nursing research. Part II offers further information for researchers interested in actually using this approach.

Structural Equation Models

A structural equation model is an a priori causal model in which the sequence, sign, and direction of the paths in a graphic representation of the model are expressed as a series of algebraic equations. These specific relationships evolve from the investigator's substantive knowledge of the phenomenon of interest. Figure 1 is an example of a structural equation model.

Within a structural equation model, the dependent variables are referred to as *endogenous* variables. Endogenous variables are all those variables that are explained or presumed to be caused by other variables in the model—both exogenous and endogenous. On the other hand, *exogenous* variables are caused by factors outside the model and, therefore, are not explained within the specified model. Depending on its complexity, there can be multiple endogenous and exogenous variables in a specific model.

Variables within a structural equation model also are classified as *manifest* or *latent*. A manifest variable is the measured or observed indicator of the theoretical constructs in the model. An example of a manifest variable in Figure 1 is *family support,* where the observable event is a score on a self-report support scale. It is a manifest variable because it is the observable event, the measured score.

In contrast to a manifest variable, a latent variable is unobserved. It is a theoretical construct that is presumed to exist but for which no direct measurement is available (James, Mulaik & Brett, 1982). An example of a latent variable in Figure 1 is *stress.* Although a researcher is theoretically interested in the relationships among the latent variables, it is the manifest variables for which there are empirical data and through which relationships among latent variables are examined. In this example, stress is operationalized through two manifest variables: the Sarason, Johnson, and Siegel (1978) Life Experiences Survey and a subjective measure of perceived stress.

Until a few years ago, most path models and analyses were manifest variable designs; that is, each theoretical construct was represented by a single corresponding manifest variable. Although researchers paid lip service to the presence of measurement error when reporting reliabilities, statistically these models all assumed perfect measurement. That is, a measure or scale of social support was *social support,* the construct. This is not the case with structural equation models, which specify more than one manifest variable for each latent variable.

Hypothesized relationships among variables in structural equation models are depicted by arrows. A straight, single-headed arrow (→) represents a direct causal connection between variables. Two single-headed arrows (⇄) represent a reciprocal or bidirectional causal relationship between variables. Models that contain reciprocal causation or feedback among variables are referred to as nonrecursive. A straight, double-headed arrow (↔) represents a correlation between endogenous variables for which there is no clear theoretical or empirical evidence to posit a causal relationship. A double-headed,

Carol J. Boyd, PhD, RN, is an assistant professor of psychiatric–mental health nursing, School of Nursing, University of Michigan, Ann Arbor.

Maureen A. Frey, PhD, RN, is an assistant professor of parent–child nursing, School of Nursing, University of Michigan, Ann Arbor.

Lauren S. Aaronson, PhD, RN, is an assistant professor of psychiatric–mental health nursing, School of Nursing, University of Michigan, Ann Arbor.

From *Nursing Research,* July/August 1988, *37,* 249–252.

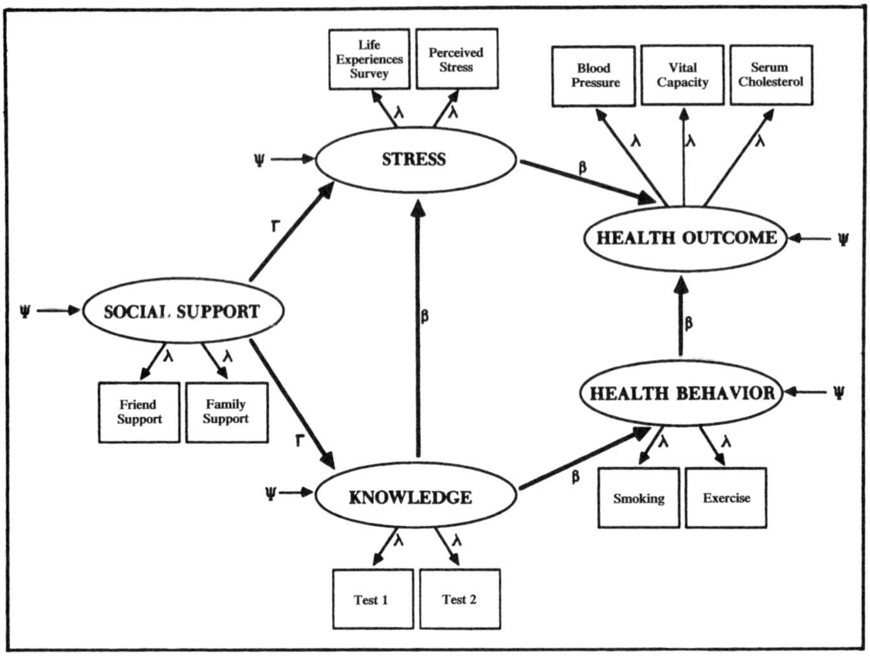

FIGURE 1 Hypothetical Structural Equation Model

curved arrow (⌒) represents a relationship between exogenous variables that is not specified in the particular model (e.g., one due to a common cause not in the model) and, as such, remains unanalyzed. If there is no arrow between two variables, the hypothesis of no direct relationship has been postulated. Models in which causation flows in only one direction are called *recursive* models. Figure 1 is a recursive model.

Each arrow between latent variables represents a theoretical hypothesis and has a structural parameter associated with it. The structural parameter reflects the amount of change in the caused variable that results from a unit of change in the causal variable, when all other causes are held constant. These structural relations are called *paths*. Although no arrow between two latent variables implies no direct relationship between these variables, the structural equation model may posit an indirect relationship. In Figure 1, no direct relationship is hypothesized between social support and health behavior, but an indirect path operating through knowledge is specified. This model proposes that if knowledge were held constant, there would be no relationship between social support and health behavior.

As exemplified in Figure 1, nurses frequently work with complex, theoretical constructs which demand multiple variables and hypotheses. Theoretical models used in nursing research (for example, social support theories) often are concerned with indirect and reciprocal relationships. Moreover, the complex phenomena (latent variables) nurses are concerned with often are better understood and measured by several indicators (manifest variables). Structural equation models allow researchers to use and test these complex constructs and their equally complex relationships. Thus, structural equation modeling is a valuable technique for nursing research.

LISREL

Although causal modeling has been in the general social science literature for some time, few nursing studies have taken advantage of this more powerful approach to data analysis. Computer programs for such analysis have been limited and most researchers have approached causal modeling with a series of regression analyses. In 1973, Karl Joreskog introduced a computer program that not only allows the simultaneous estimation of all statistical parameters in a single causal model, but also explicitly incorporates accounting for measurement issues. This program is known by the acronym, *LISREL,* which stands for the analysis of linear structural relations.

Since it was first proposed, *LISREL* has undergone several revisions. In addition to these revisions, two companion programs, *PRELIS* and *SIMPLIS*, have been developed. *PRELIS* is a preprocessor for *LISREL*. It provides a descriptive look at raw data and screens the data for potential problems (Joreskog & Sorbom, 1986). *SIMPLIS*, a limited and simplified version of *LISREL*, performs path analysis, confirmatory factor analysis, and structural equation modeling without requiring knowledge of Greek notation and matrix algebra. Although *LISREL* handles more models and uses more methods, *SIMPLIS* produces similar results. Further, inappropriate and poor-fitting models can be quickly identified with *SIMPLIS*, thereby eliminating the more costly *LISREL* analyses (Joreskog & Sorbom, 1987). Both *PRELIS* and *SIMPLIS* can be used with the more powerful current version of *LISREL*, *LISREL* VI.*

LISREL VI (Joreskog & Sorbom, 1984) is capable of providing a great deal of information regarding the proposed structural equation model. It can be used for estimating one model with a single sample, comparing multiple models with one sample, or assessing one model's fit to multiple, independent samples (Ladewig & McGee, 1986).

The *LISREL* program supplies several indicators of overall fit between a hypothesized model and the investigator's data, as well as statistics on the strength and direction of effects within the model. *LISREL* also provides estimates of the error variance for both the observed and the unobserved variables, and insight into possible misspecification within the model. This latter issue is discussed further in Part II.

Model/Data Fit

A prerequisite for assessing a model's fit to the data is that the model must be identified. This means having enough information to uniquely solve all of the equations implied by the model. Models may be overidentified, just-identified, or underidentified. Underidentified models cannot be estimated. (In Part II of this series, requirements for identification and how measures of model/data fit can be used with just-identified and overidentified models will be discussed further.)

There are several ways of determining whether the interrelationships designated within a model fit the data. First the *LISREL* program computes a maximum likelihood chi-square statistic. Unlike more familiar uses of the chi-square statistic, where one is looking for a large, statistically significant value to support a theoretically posited relationship, with structural equation models one is looking for a small, nonsignificant chi square. In this case, the small chi square provides evidence that the specified model and the investigator's data are congruent rather than different. A statistically significant chi square would mean that the model failed to adequately account for the covariances among the variables (Acock & Yang, 1982). As suggested by Joreskog and Sorbom (1984), the chi-square statistic should be used as an indicator of the goodness or badness of fit rather than as a test of significance. However, because chi square is sensitive to sample size and departures from normalcy, it is often difficult to achieve a nonsignificant chi square with samples large enough to support using *LISREL*.

A second measure of the model's fit is the relative likelihood ratio (RLR). This measure is the ratio of the chi-square value to its degrees of freedom (χ^2/df). The RLR offers a mental hueristic for assessing the significance of the chi-square value. It may be viewed as an indication of how well the hypothesized model compares to an alternative model containing all possible recursive paths. Ratios of approximately 2:1 or 3:1 are considered indicative of a good fit (Carmines & McIver, 1981).

Another measure of a model's fit is the Goodness-of-Fit Index (GFI) developed by Joreskog and Sorbom (1984). This index is a measure of the relative amount of variance and covariance jointly accounted for by the model. The GFI is believed to be relatively unaffected by sample size and departures from normalcy. However, because its statistical distribution is unknown, the GFI must be interpreted with caution (Joreskog & Sorbom, 1984; Liang, 1986). Further, the GFI, adjusted for degrees of freedom (AGFI), also should be reported. Generally, any GFI in the .90s is considered to indicate a good fit.

A structural equation model may demonstrate a good theoretical/empirical fit and yet be poorly determined (Joreskog & Sorbom, 1984). This means that the hypothesized model accounts well for the variances and covariances among the research variables (e.g., has a high GFI) but explains little of the variance in the endogenous variable(s).

LISREL provides information on the unexplained variance, reported as psi (Ψ) values, for each endogenous variable. This is important because some researchers report their high GFIs but fail either to include the psi values in their models or to discuss the explained variance within the model. For any model, a high GFI is notably less meaningful if the model fails to explain the variance in the dependent variable. After all, even if the theoretical sequencing of the variables is empirically supported, it means little if these variables fail to explain much of the dependent variable(s).

* At this time, *LISREL* VII is being tested but is not yet available for general use by the scientific community. *PRELIS* will be compatible with *LISREL* VII, but *SIMPLIS* will not. Whether *SIMPLIS* will be revised has not been decided. (L. Budd, Scientific Software, Inc., Mooresville, IN, personal communication, December 22, 1987.)

Structural and Measurement Parameters

The structural parameters are designated by the Greek letters, beta (β) and gamma (Γ). Betas are used for coefficients between endogenous variables and gammas are used for coefficients between exogenous and endogenous variables. They can be interpreted in the same manner as path coefficients, thus allowing the investigator to examine the strength and direction of the hypothesized relationships.

The structural parameters are tested with the *t* statistic. *T* values are determined by dividing the parameter estimates by their standard errors. Parameters with *t* values larger than 2.0 are generally considered significantly different from zero and, therefore, statistically significant (Joreskog & Sorbom, 1984).

The aspect of *LISREL* analysis that examines how well the constructs (latent, unobserved variables) are measured or modeled by the observed (manifest) indicators is called the *measurement model.* Lambdas (λ) are used to designate these links between latent and manifest variables. Lambdas may be viewed as factor loadings and are analogous to reliability coefficients. The measurement model is discussed in greater detail in Part II.

Perhaps because of the newness of *LISREL* analyses, there is little consensus on the optimal content or format for reporting the results of research findings using this technique. However, published reports should include enough data for the reader to be able to evaluate the fit of the model, the significance of the hypothesized relationships, the amount of variation explained by the structural model, and the adequacy of the selected measures as indicators of the theoretical constructs. Of course, a discussion of the findings in terms of the theoretical basis of the model is critical.

Conclusion

Because nurses describe health, illness, and people in complex, interactive, and holistic terms, the concept of causation is often problematic. Nonetheless, the analysis of structural equation models permits specifying conditions that are, at least partly, responsible for the phenomena of interest (Huston & Robins, 1982). Causal modeling is based on traditional multiple regression analysis. Although parameter coefficients estimated in structural equation models are not proof of causation (Pedhazur, 1982), these estimates do suggest functional relations.

As nurse researchers become more involved and sophisticated in developing nursing theory, they must begin to use data analysis strategies that enable them to test complex relationships among multiple variables. The use of structural equation models provides a means to parsimoniously develop and test theory, one of the most critical endeavors in nursing today.

References

Aaronson, L. S. (1984). Health behavior in pregnancy: Testing a general model (Doctoral dissertation, University of Washington, 1983). *Dissertation Abstracts International, 44,* 11A, 349S.

Acock, A., & Yang, W. (1982). Parental power and adolescents' parental identification. *Journal of Marriage and the Family, 44,* 487–494.

Boyd, C. J. (1988). Relationships among the correlates within the construct of mother-daughter identification: Mutual identification, attachment, conflict and identity in adult Polish-American women (Doctoral dissertation, Wayne State University, 1987). *Dissertation Abstracts International, 48,* 4A. (University Microfilms No. 87-14,530).

Carmines, E. G., & McIver, J. P. (1981). Analyzing models with unobserved variables: Analysis of covariance structures. In G. W. Bohrnstedt & E. F. Borgatta (eds.), *Social measurement: Current issues* (pp. 65–115). Beverly Hills, CA: Sage Publications, Inc.

Chen, M., & Land, K. (1986). Testing the Health Belief Model: *LISREL* analysis of alternative models of causal relationships between health beliefs and preventive dental behavior. *Social Psychology Quarterly, 49,* 45–60.

Cox, C., & Roghmann, K. (1984). Empirical test of the interaction model of client health behavior. *Research in Nursing and Health, 7,* 275–285.

Frey, M. (1988). Health and social support in families with children with diabetes mellitus (Doctoral dissertation, Wayne State University, 1987). *Dissertation Abstracts International, 48,* 4A.

Huston, T. L., & Robins, E. (1982). Conceptual and methodological issues in studying close relationships. *Journal of Marriage and the Family, 44,* 901–925.

James, L., Mulaik, S., & Brett, J. (1982). *Causal analysis: Assumptions, models, and data.* Beverly Hills, CA: Sage Publications, Inc.

Joreskog, K. G. (1973). A general method for estimating a linear structural equation system. In A. S. Goldberger & O. D. Duncan (eds.), *Structural equation models in the social sciences* (pp. 85–112). New York: Seminar Press.

Joreskog, K., & Sorbom, D. (1984). *LISREL VI* (4th ed). Uppsala, Sweden: University of Uppsala.

Joreskog, K., & Sorbom, D. (1986). *PRELIS.* Uppsala, Sweden: University of Uppsala.

Joreskog, K., & Sorbom, D. (1987). *SIMPLIS.* Uppsala, Sweden: University of Uppsala.

Ladewig, B., & McGee, G. (1986). Occupational commitment, a supportive family environment, and marital adjustment: Development and estimation of a model. *Journal of Marriage and the Family, 48,* 821–829.

Lavee, Y., McCubbin, H., & Patterson, J. (1985). The double ABCX model of family stress and adaptation: An empirical test by analysis of structural equations with latent variables. *Journal of Marriage and the Family, 47,* 811–825.

Liang, J. (1986). Self-reported physical health among aged adults. *Journal of Gerontology, 41,* 148–260.

Pedhazur, E. (1982). *Multiple regression in behavioral research* (2nd ed.). New York: Holt, Rinehart & Winston.

Sarason, I. G., Johnson, J. H., & Siegel, J. M. (1978). Assessing the impact of life change: Development of the life experiences survey. *Journal of Consulting and Clinical Psychology, 46,* 932–946.

Structural Equation Models and Nursing Research: Part II

Lauren S. Aaronson ■ Maureen A. Frey ■ Carol J. Boyd

Part I of this article (Boyd, Frey & Aaronson, 1988) introduced and defined the basic concepts of structural equation modeling with a focus on understanding and evaluating research that uses *LISREL*. Part II elaborates technical aspects and related issues about structural equation modeling for investigators who are considering this method for their own research.

Structural Models Using *LISREL*

Figure 1 is the graphic representation of a hypothetical structural equation model (temporarily omitting multiple indicators of the constructs). This model can be represented with the following set of algebraic equations:

$$X_1 = e_1$$
$$X_2 = \beta_{21}X_1 + e_2$$
$$X_3 = \beta_{31}X_1 + \beta_{32}X_2 + e_3$$
$$X_4 = \beta_{42}X_2 + e_4$$
$$X_5 = \beta_{53}X_3 + \beta_{54}X_4 + e_5$$

Both Figure 1 and the corresponding set of equations (shown above) identify *social support* (X_1) as the only exogenous variable in this model. As such, social support is completely determined by causes that lie outside the specified model. Thus, within this model, X_1 equals its disturbance or *error term,* e_1. On the other hand, the endogenous variable stress (X_3) is hypothesized in this model to be a linear, additive function of social support (X_1), knowledge (X_2), and all other causes of stress (e_3).

Taken alone, the equation for stress (X_3) should be familiar as the basic, multiple regression equation in its standardized form. For both practical and substantive reasons, structural equations are commonly presented in their standardized form. In this form, the intercept term, *a,* is equal to zero, and, therefore, omitted. Use of the standardized form facilitates demonstrating algebraic manipulations and allows comparisons among coefficients within a particular model. As with multiple regression, one cannot meaningfully compare unstandardized coefficients if they are based in different measurement units.

Although the principles of multiple regression and path analysis are applied with *LISREL,* the actual statistical operations are different. Unlike the least squares procedure used with multiple regression, the maximum likelihood procedure used in *LISREL* is an iterative approach for estimating population parameters (Joreskog & Sorbom, 1984). The iterative approach is a computational procedure that arrives at a final solution by repeating a series of operations through successive approximations. Another difference between multiple regression and *LISREL* is that the set of equations representing the proposed model is simultaneously, rather than serially, estimated. That is, all the equations implied by a model are solved as set in contrast to solving each equation with a separate regression analysis. Simultaneous estimation prevents a faulty and erroneous specification of an underidentified model.

The Identification Problem

Models may be underidentified, overidentified, or just-identified. Identification is a critical issue in all causal modeling because a model that is underidentified cannot be estimated. Identifying a model involves fixing, a priori, enough parameters so that the remaining free parameters can be uniquely estimated. If an insufficient number of parameters are fixed, the model will be underidentified. The technical as well as theoretical issues that arise from problems of identification are particularly evident with fully recursive and nonrecursive models.

As discussed in Part I, a *recursive* model is one in which causation flows in one direction. In a fully recursive model, all possible recursive paths are specified. A fully recursive model is just-identified as long as it meets the assumption, required of all recursive models, that

Lauren S. Aaronson, PhD, RN, is an assistant professor of psychiatric–mental health nursing, School of Nursing, University of Michigan, Ann Arbor.

Maureen A. Frey, PhD, RN, is an assistant professor of parent–child nursing, School of Nursing, University of Michigan, Ann Arbor.

Carol J. Boyd, PhD, RN, is an assistant professor of psychiatric–mental health nursing, School of Nursing, University of Michigan, Ann Arbor.

From *Nursing Research,* September/October 1988, *37,* 315–317.

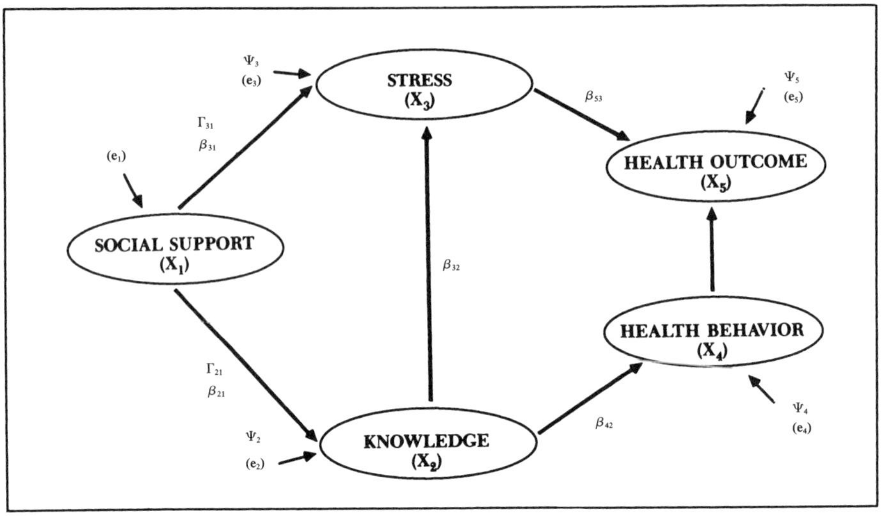

FIGURE 1 Hypothesized Structural Equation Model

the disturbance terms are mutually uncorrelated. Figure 1 would be a fully recursive model if arrows from social support to health behavior, social support to health outcome, knowledge to health outcome, and stress to health behavior were added. The resulting set of equations for this new, fully recursive, just-identified model would be:

$$X_1 = e_1$$
$$X_2 = \beta_{21}X_1 + e_2$$
$$X_3 = \beta_{31}X_1 + \beta_{32}X_2 + e_3$$
$$X_4 = \beta_{41}X_1 + \beta_{42}X_2 + \beta_{43}X_3 + e_4$$
$$X_5 = \beta_{51}X_1 + \beta_{52}X_2 + \beta_{53}X_3 + \beta_{54}X_4 + e_5.$$

With a just-identified model, only the fit of that model to the data can be assessed (see section on measures of goodness of fit, Part I) because there are no degrees of freedom left with which to test a competing model. On the other hand, overidentified models not only can be estimated, but hierarchically related versions of the model can be tested against each other for improvement in fit. Two models are hierarchically related if they include the same variables and if one model contains as a subset of its relationships, all of the relationships specified in the other model. For example, Figure 1 could be tested against the fully recursive model.

Identification is particularly troublesome for nonrecursive models and reciprocal causation. Empirical evidence and theoretical beliefs may lead one to put forth any number of relationships among the variables in a particular model. These may, and often do, include reciprocal causation. For example, in Figure 1, one might argue that stress affects knowledge as well as it is affected by knowledge. Adding an arrow from stress to knowledge changes the equation for knowledge to:

$$X_2 = \beta_{21}X_1 + \beta_{23}X_3 + e_2$$

This seems both simple and reasonable. However, doing so in this model would result in an underidentified model.

Thus, while reciprocal causation is theoretically possible in structural equation models, certain conditions for identification must be met. These are the *order* and *rank* conditions. The order condition is necessary but not sufficient. It requires that K-1 variables be omitted from each equation in a model with K endogenous variables. The rank condition, though sufficient for identification, is not as easily stated. To meet this condition, at least one nonzero determinant of K-1 rows and columns must be formed for each equation from a matrix of coefficients omitting the row of the targeted equation and all columns with nonzero entries in the omitted row (Namboodiri, Carter & Blalock, 1975).

Meeting these conditions is necessary to estimate unique solutions for the structural parameters β_{23} (representing the effect of stress on knowledge) and β_{32} (representing the effect of knowledge on stress). Generally speaking, if one identified an exogenous variable that is another cause of knowledge but not a cause of stress, and a separate exogenous variable that is a cause of stress but not of knowledge, this model, including the reciprocal causation between stress and knowledge, would again be identified. However, finding additional exogenous variables that meet these conditions is not easy, nor always possible. Thus, the *identification problem* (Namboodiri et al., 1975) is the point at which theoretical conceptualizations encounter the limits of presently known mathematical laws and properties.

Measurement Models in *LISREL*

Both complex relations and the reality of less-than-perfect measurement (measurement error) is accounted for when using *LISREL* (Boyd et al., 1988). Measurement error is handled through the measurement model. In a measurement model, all the latent variables are defined as exogenous and allowed to freely intercorrelate. This separates issues involved in fitting the measurement model from the issues involving the structural relations among the latent variables. Figure 2 is the measurement model for the hypothetical model used in these articles.

The measurement model is a factor analytic model. However, the difference between *LISREL* and the more common, exploratory factor analysis is that with *LISREL* the approach is one of *confirmatory* factor analysis. In exploratory factor analysis, the empirical measures may load on any factor and any number of factors may be extracted. In contrast, the confirmatory approach requires the investigator to determine, a priori, which measures (manifest variables) will load on which factors (latent variables).

The same principles of causal modeling that govern the structural equation model govern the measurement model. The relationship between the unobserved, latent variables and the observed, manifest variables is assumed to be causal. For example, in Figure 2, the construct social support is assumed to be something each individual has in varying amounts and this entity *causes* individual's responses to the items in the two empirical scales, family support and friend support. It is further assumed that the only reason the two manifest variables (family support and friend support) are empirically associated is due to their common cause, the latent variable (social support).

If one is not convinced the latent variable, as a common cause, is the only reason for the empirical association between two indicators, *LISREL* allows correlated measurement error to be specified. This means freeing the particular element in the relevant matrix and drawing a double-headed curved arrow between the two disturbance terms for the involved indicators. Like the *psis* associated with endogenous, latent variables (discussed in Part I), each manifest variable has a disturbance term associated with it—called *theta deltas* for exogenous indicators and *theta epsilons* for endogenous indicators.

Because the latent variables have no metric, the *lambda* for one arbitrary indicator of each latent variable is conventionally set or fixed to 1.0. This establishes an arbitrary metric for the latent variable. The arbitrary nature of this metric is another reason why standardized results of *LISREL* analyses are typically reported. Further, if one has only one indicator for a latent variable, this indicator must be assumed to perfectly measure the latent variable and the latent variable would take on the indicator's metric.

After the measurement model is established, the accepted indicators are added to the theoretical model (Figure 1) for testing the full structural equation model (see Figure 1, Part I). In the structural model, effects

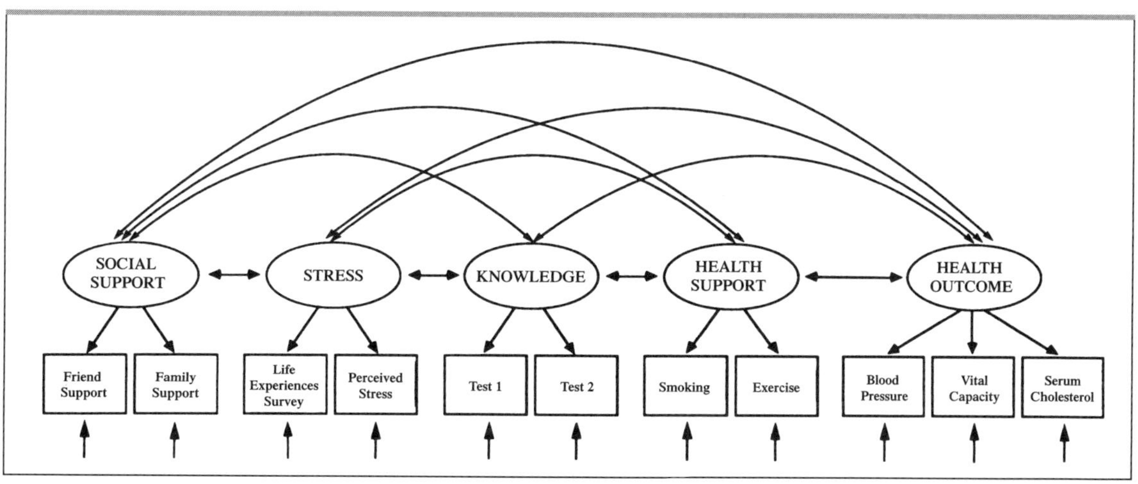

FIGURE 2 Hypothetical Measurement Model

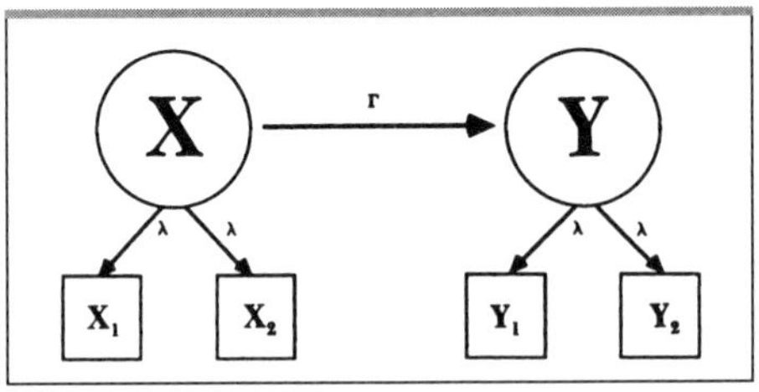

FIGURE 3 Two-Variable Model

among latent variables are estimated using data on these indicators. For example, in Figure 3, a simple two-variable model, the empirical correlation, $r_{x_1y_1}$, is viewed as a function of the relationship between x_1 and X, X and Y, and Y and y_1. Similarly, $r_{x_1y_2}$ is a function of the relationship between x_1 and X, X and Y, and Y and y_2. The remaining correlations, $r_{x_2y_1}$ and $r_{x_2y_2}$, also are viewed in this way. Consequently, *LISREL* has several pieces of information with which to determine a unique, best estimate of *gamma*, the structural coefficient for the effect of the exogenous latent variable, X, on the endogenous latent variable, Y.

Diagnosis of Sources of Poor Fit

In Part I a number of measures of goodness-of-fit were introduced. These measures assess the fit of the entire model but not the sources of poor fit. Specific sources of poor fit can be identified with the matrix of normalized residuals and with the modification indices provided by *LISREL*.

The matrix of normalized residuals shows the differences between the covariance matrix of the observed variables and the covariance matrix recreated from the parameter estimates. For example, using the two-variable model above, once *gamma* is estimated, the empirical correlations ($r_{x_1y_1}$, $r_{x_1y_2}$, $r_{x_2y_1}$, and $r_{x_2y_2}$) are each reproduced as products of *gamma* and their respective *lambdas*. In general, a normalized residual greater than 2.0 indicates that the model does not do a good job in accounting for that particular relationship, suggesting a specific specification error of the model (Joreskog & Sorbom, 1984).

Modification indices, on the other hand, are measures associated with the derivatives of the fitting function with respect to the structural parameters. The values of the modification indices each represent the relative decrease in the chi square that would occur if its associated parameter alone was freed and estimated with the rest of the model remaining unchanged. Generally, values greater than 5.0 suggest a need for modification of the model (Joreskog & Sorbom, 1984).

Summary/Conclusion

Structural equation modeling is a powerful approach with great potential for advancing nursing research and theory. It is no substitute, however, for sound thinking, careful conceptualization, and meticulous measurement. The old computing adage, "garbage in, garbage out," aptly applies to hasty and sloppy attempts at structural equation modeling by ill-prepared investigators.

In these two short papers the authors introduced structural equation modeling using *LISREL*. Part I was directed at those with no prior exposure to causal modeling. The purpose was to equip readers with enough knowledge to understand research reports using this technique. Part II provided more specific information about issues involved in using this technique. However, considering the complexity of *LISREL*, Part II is only a further introduction to structural equation modeling. Readers who want to use *LISREL* in their own research are encouraged to read the articles and books in the bibliography cited below.

References

Boyd, C. J., Frey, M. A., & Aaronson, L. S. (1988). Structural equation models and nursing research: Part I. *Nursing Research, 37*, 249–252.

Joreskog, K., & Sorbom, D. (1984). *LISREL VI* (4th ed). Uppsala, Sweden: University of Uppsala.

Namboodiri, K., Carter, L. F., & Blalock, H. M. (1975). *Applied multivariate analysis and experimental designs.* New York: McGraw-Hill Book Co.

PART FIVE

Measures and Measurement Issues

What Constitutes a Publishable Report of Instrument Development?

Jane S. Norbeck

In reviewing manuscripts about instrument development for nursing research journals, I have found that many investigators submit fragmented reports of this activity. Often my response is, "The instrument appears promising, but a more systematic report of its reliability and validity is needed before it is ready for publication." Why aren't these articles publishable at this stage? The answer lies in assuming the perspective of the reader.

The main consumers of articles on instrument development are other researchers who are interested in evaluating an instrument for possible use in their own research. The goal of communicating work in instrument development to other researchers is achieved if the reader can say, "I understand the conceptual basis for this instrument, how it is constructed, what types of subjects and research situations it is suitable for, and I am satisfied with the psychometric properties (reliability and validity) that have been established." Reports that fail to provide a complete picture in these areas are not ready for publication.

Partial reports on instrument development are of limited value because if every step of the instrument validation process were published in separate articles, the full picture of the reliability and validity of an instrument might be spread out across 8 to 10 articles. This method of reporting would lead to needless repetition of background information; and, researchers would have difficulty locating all the sources of information to evaluate the instrument.

This article outlines material that should be included in reports of instrument development to guide researchers in planning data collection efforts so that a report about the instrument is unified and complete.

Methodological texts can guide the actual conduct of instrument development and validation; however, little is written about reporting this work. Suggestions in this article are drawn from the APA (1974) *Standards for Educational and Psychological Tests*. In addition to the content suggested here, it is helpful to locate an example in the literature of a comprehensive report that may serve as a model for one's own data collection and reporting.

Jane S. Norbeck, DNSc, FAAN, is associate professor and chair of the Department of Mental Health and Community Nursing, University of California, San Francisco.

From *Nursing Research,* November/December 1985, *34,* 380–382.

Methodological Considerations

In selecting an instrument for use in a study, minimal levels of reliability and validity need to be established. A report describing a new instrument should provide a sufficient basis for evaluating these psychometric characteristics in a systematic way. In fact, there is a logical interconnection among the elements of instrument validation. For example, if an instrument lacks content validity, it is pointless to establish its reliability. Similarly, unreliable instruments are not worth further investigation of their validity because reliability is a prerequisite for validity. A basic core of reliability and validity is needed to evaluate any instrument.

What constitutes minimal reliability and validity for evaluating an instrument? Opinions vary, of course, but from the range of types of reliability and validity testing outlined in Table 1 a *minimal* standard for publishing the results of psychometric testing should include: at least one type of content validity, test–retest reliability, internal consistency reliability, and at least one type of criterion-related or construct validity. Ideally, most reports should include much more than this minimal amount of psychometric testing, but such a standard implies that reports with less should not be accepted for publication. Depending on the nature of the instrument or its intended use, more than this minimal standard might be needed to justify publication of a given report.

The psychometric testing should have been conducted according to the methodological guidelines of measurement theory (e.g., Allen & Yen, 1979; Nunnally, 1978). These guidelines, sampling adequacy, and other issues about the quality of the research are not addressed here but are considered by manuscript referees. Results that show unacceptable levels of reliability and validity should not be published; instead, the instrument should

TABLE 1 Outline of Types of Reliability and Validity Testing*

Reliability estimates
1. Test-retest reliability estimates
2. Parallel-forms or alternate-forms reliability estimates
3. Internal-consistency estimates of reliability

Validity estimates
1. Content validity
   a. Face validity
   b. Logical or sampling validity
2. Criterion-related validity
   a. Predictive-validity estimates
   b. Concurrent-validity estimates
3. Construct validity
   a. Testable predictions based on group differences, changes, correlations, or processes
   b. Multitrait/multimethod validity
   c. Factorial validity

* Described by Allen and Yen (1979).

be modified and retested until acceptable levels of the minimal types of reliability and validity are established.

Of course, there are exceptions to the reporting standard suggested here. Perhaps the item-generation technique used in the development of an instrument was sufficiently remarkable that readers would find this interesting and useful in itself. Other features of instrument development might warrant publication, independent of the goal of describing a new instrument to an audience of potential users.

The concept of a minimal list of types of reliability and validity does not imply that further work is not important. Establishment of validity is an ongoing process; additional validity testing and perhaps normative data will eventually warrant a second report.

However, unless extensive additional psychometric testing of the instrument is intended, all of the planned psychometric testing should be included in the initial report. A small follow-up report of testing the instrument is unlikely to reach publication because it probably will not be considered sufficiently substantive to compete for limited journal space.

In my experience, even when additional psychometric testing is planned, one complete report is the most desirable method of reporting, not only for the needs of users but also for the authors. For example, several authors have referred to the first article of the psychometric testing of the Norbeck Social Support Questionnaire (Norbeck, Lindsey & Carrieri, 1981) and raised questions about the exclusive use of students for respondents. Although normative data and validity testing from a general population sample were presented in a second article published 15 months later in the same journal (Norbeck, Lindsey & Carrieri, 1983), these readers apparently were not aware of the second phase of testing and based their evaluative judgments of the instrument only on the first published report.

Nonetheless, continuing work with the instrument will take place, and readers should communicate with the authors of the initial report to learn if additional data about the instrument are published or otherwise available. Over time, research articles will be published in which the instrument was used. These reports, although not methodological in intent, contribute valuable information about the reliability and validity of the instrument in the specific context in which it was used, as well as information about the appropriateness of the instrument for the study population.

Substantive Considerations

Descriptive information about the instrument is also needed to evaluate its suitability for inclusion in research. To make this evaluation, readers need to know the conceptual basis underlying the instrument, the methods and results of item generation and refinement, characteristics of the intended respondents (e.g., age, educational level), ease of use and method of administration, method of scoring, type of data obtained, and other features that are specific to the instrument. Descriptive statistics of variable means, standard deviations, and range of scores should be provided to give readers a picture of how the variables were distributed in the study sample. These values are useful as comparative data for other populations. The initial article should also include a representative selection of sample items with an illustration of the instrument format or a complete copy of the instrument included in an appendix.

If the early work on an instrument has uncovered questions about conceptual soundness or some of the subscales, the instrument is not ready for publication, despite the results of the reliability and validity testing. In these cases, revisions must be made. The revised version must again be tested for reliability and validity. Again, the point of view of the reader dictates this: Why should a reader be interested in an article that describes an instrument that must be changed and reevaluated before it can be used?

Methodological research differs from other research in that data gathered during the process of instrument revision are usually not publishable. This is because these results reflect inadequacies of the instrument itself rather than information about the phenomenon under study. In contrast, pilot data from other types of research studies might represent a substantive contribution that would be of interest to researchers in the field.

Because there are many steps in the validation of an instrument, it may seem discouraging that the preliminary steps do not warrant publication. However, the various data sets that make up the complete report of psychometric testing often are embedded in larger substantive studies that in themselves are publishable reports. For example, the item generation activity that was used to modify existing life events questionnaires for use with female respondents (Norbeck, 1984) was part of a larger study of the needs and resources of single parents (Norbeck & Sheiner, 1982). Additional psychometric testing was conducted in conjunction with other studies. The actual article of the modified life events questionnaire was developed from three separate data sets, each serving both methodological and substantive purposes.

Procedural Considerations

Because of the nature of the variables studied in nursing research, many nurse researchers are engaged in instrument development. This work is important and needs to be shared with scientific colleagues.

If beginning work on the development of an instrument is usually not sufficient for publication, how are other researchers to learn about this work in progress? There are several avenues for communicating with research colleagues. Presenting poster sessions or papers at scientific sessions, publishing abstracts of preliminary work, and communicating through professional newsletters are some ways that researchers share work on instrument development before it is ready for publication. Often these preliminary communications result in collaborative arrangements that contribute to the overall work of validating an instrument.

Once an article describing a reliable and valid instrument is published, authors can expect to receive a good deal of correspondence about the instrument and requests for permission to use it. Publishing the results of work on the development of an instrument carries an implied willingness to share the instrument with the scientific community. Thus, a mechanism should be developed to make the instrument and any associated material available to researchers upon request. Such sharing is mutually beneficial because other researchers are often willing to contribute to the larger effort of establishing normative data for the instrument or to other aspects of psychometric testing.

References

Allen, M. J., & Yen, W. M. (1979). *Introduction to measurement theory.* Monterey, CA: Brooks/Cole Publishing Company.

American Psychological Association (1974). *Standards for educational and psychological tests.* New York: The Association.

Norbeck, J. S. (1984). Modification of recent life event questionnaires for use with female respondents. *Research in Nursing and Health, 7,* 61–71.

Norbeck, J. S., Lindsey, A. M., & Carrieri, V. L. (1981). The development on an instrument to measure social support. *Nursing Research, 30,* 264–269.

Norbeck, J. S., Lindsey, A. M., & Carrieri, V. L (1983). Further development of the Norbeck Social Support Questionnaire: Normative data and validity testing. *Nursing Research, 32,* 4–9.

Norbeck, J. S., & Sheiner, M. (1982). Sources of social support related to single parent functioning. *Research in Nursing and Health, 5,* 3–12.

Nunnally, J. C. (1978). *Psychometric theory.* New York: McGraw-Hill Book Co., Inc.

Validity, Reliability, and Neither

Thomas R. Knapp

Over 30 years ago, Cureton (1950) wrote an article entitled "Validity, Reliability, and Baloney." In that article he took to task the then-common practice of determining the scoring weights for test items by correlating item responses with some external criterion and then using that same criterion to assess the validity of the test. It taught the educational and psychological measurement community an important lesson: that particular practice was indeed "baloney."

The purpose of this paper is to call attention to a number of misuses of the terms validity and reliability that have appeared in the pages of *Nursing Research,* other nursing journals and books, and psychometric reports in other disciplines. Certain studies that have been categorized as validity or reliability studies should not be subsumed under either term. They are interesting and important, and not baloney. Associating them with validity or reliability, however, reflects a much too liberal use of those technical terms.

The Context of This Critique*

Measurement is the process of translating reality into numbers. Three key concepts are involved in every attempt at such a translation: the construct, C; the true score on the variable, T; and the obtained score on that variable, X. Validity issues arise when the fit between the construct and the true score is studied. Reliability issues arise when the fit between the true score and the obtained score is studied. Figure 1 summarizes this idea.

Consider two examples. The first involves the construct "spelling ability." One operational definition of spelling ability is the percentage of words in an unabridged dictionary that examinees could spell correctly if all of the words were dictated aloud and if they were asked to spell them (their true scores). The percentage of, say, 200 words randomly drawn from the dictionary that an examinee does spell correctly when the words are dictated is an obtained score. Operationalizing spelling ability this way may or may not be valid, or may be valid to some degree. Similarly, the obtained scores may or may not be reliable, or may be reliable to some degree. It is incumbent upon someone (the developer of the instrument and/or the researcher who plans to use it in a substantive study) to carry out one or more of the usual investigations of the spelling test's validity and reliability. It might be argued, for instance, that content validity is built in, but that a parallel-forms reliability study is crucial. (Form A would consist of one sample of 200 words and Form B would consist of another sample of 200 words, both randomly drawn from the same dictionary.)

The second example involves the construct "height." Height is not a construct in the usual psychometric sense, but it is a construct. One measure of a person's true height as indicated by a particular tape measure is the mean of all possible obtained measurements (just as the true percentage of words spelled correctly is the mean across all possible parallel forms). Using a particular tape measure may or may not be a valid or reliable way to operationalize the construct of height. But unlike spelling ability, the options for validity and reliability studies are rather limited. Subjective judgments could be made regarding the content validity of such a procedure, and criterion-related correlations with measurements made using an expensive, carefully calibrated hospital measuring device could be calculated. As far as reliability is concerned, however, since this test has no items and no parallel forms, a test–retest investigation might be the only empirical option.

A number of other aspects of spelling ability or height (or any other construct of substantive interest) can be explored. But many of these other characteristics are beyond any considerations of validity or reliability.

* Although this formulation of the measurement problem in terms of constructs, true scores, and obtained scores has some original features (e.g., the focus on two different kinds of fit), it is consistent with classical test theory (Carmines & Zeller, 1979) and with professional recommendations (American Psychological Association, in press). Table 1 contains some brief definitions of the various kinds of validity and reliability.

Thomas R. Knapp, EdD, is a professor of education and nursing at the University of Rochester, Rochester, NY.

From *Nursing Research,* May/June 1985, *34,* 189–192.

CONSTRUCT (validity)	TRUE SCORE (reliability)	OBTAINED SCORE
C	T	X
Example 1: Spelling ability	Percentage of words in the population that examinees could spell correctly	Percentage of words in the sample that examinees do spell correctly
Example 2: Height	Mean of all possible tape measurements	A single tape measurement

FIGURE 1 A Conceptualization of Validity and Reliability

Stability of Test versus Stability of Construct

A test–retest reliability study is meant to provide some evidence regarding the short-term consistency of the measurements yielded by a particular instrument. It is not concerned with the long-term consistency of the construct that is being measured. Unfortunately, the word stability is associated with reliability studies carried out over a brief time interval and with investigations concerned with the consistency of the construct over extended periods of time.

The line between a test–retest reliability study and a study of the stability of a particular construct is a fine one, but it must be drawn. To carry out a test–retest reliability study over a particular time interval, the researcher must assume that the construct does not change during that interval. The whole point in doing such a study is to see if the obtained test scores do change. If they do, the instrument is unreliable (to some degree).

If one cannot assume that the construct stands still from Time 1 to Time 2, a test–retest study yields ambiguous information. Changes in obtained scores are a hopelessly confounded combination of changes in true scores and random measurement errors. Measures of states as opposed to traits pose especially difficult problems in this regard, since by definition states are transitory.

TABLE 1 **Types of Validity and Reliability**

	Type	Definition
Validity	Content validity	The degree to which the items in an instrument adequately represent the universe of content.
	Criterion-related validity (concurrent or predictive)	The degree to which scores on an instrument are correlated with some external criterion.
	Construct validity	The degree to which an instrument measures the construct under investigation.
Reliability	Coefficient alpha (Cronbach's alpha)	A reliability index that estimates the internal consistency or homogeneity of a measure composed of several items or subparts.
	Split-half technique	A method for estimating the internal consistency (reliability) of an instrument by correlating scores on half the measure with scores on the other half.
	Test–retest reliability	Assessment of the stability of an instrument by correlating the scores obtained on repeated administrations.
	Parallel forms (alternative forms)	The administration of two equivalent forms to a sample of individuals in immediate succession, obtaining the correlation between the two sets of scores.

Source: Polit, D. E., and Hungler, B.P. (1983) (p. 392 and Glossary). The definition for parallel forms is paraphrased from the text on p. 392 and the other definitions are taken verbatim from the Glossary. A fifth type of reliability is interrater reliability (sometimes called objectivity), but it raises a host of special problems.

In a substantive study of the stability of a construct, the argument is reversed. One must take the test–retest reliability as a given when investigating the differences between the Time 1 scores and the Time 2 scores.

Some alleged test–retest reliability studies have been carried out over such long periods of time that they are actually studies of the stability of the construct and not the stability of the test. A recent example is the investigation by Roberts and Feetham (1982). Differences in scores on the Feetham Family Functioning Survey (FFFS) were determined for 22 mothers who were initially tested on one day and retested two weeks later. Two weeks is not a long time compared to some test–retest intervals in the literature, but it might be argued that the family situations could have changed dramatically during that time. The authors offer no defense for their choice of two weeks. They also report a test–retest reliability coefficient of .82 over a *five-year* period for Pless and Satterwhite's (1973) Family Functioning Index (FFI).

A second example of the failure to distinguish between stability of a test and stability of a construct is the study reported by Calloway (1982) of the test–retest reliability of the Home Observation for Measurement of the Environment (HOME) inventory. Data for 91 families were obtained over 6-, 12-, and 24-month intervals for children up to 3 years of age, and data for 33 families were obtained over an 18-month interval for children 3 to 6 years of age. Such studies are concerned with the stability of the home situation itself and not with the psychometric properties of the instrument used to measure it.

Chang's (1978) methodological article regarding her Situational Control of Daily Activities (SCDA) instrument provides a third example. She reported a test–retest correlation of .96 for 20 subjects who were retested three months after their initial testing. This amazingly strong relationship may be explained partially by the fact that the subjects were patients in a skilled nursing facility in which activities could have been highly routinized. But the agreement between the two testings was based solely on whether the patients were categorized on both occasions as generally "self-determined" or generally "other-determined." It was not a reflection of the consistency of responses to each of the 22 items from one time to the next.

As a fourth and final example, Stevenson (1982) reported subscale correlations of .80 and above for 66 subjects tested twice over a four-month interval on her Margin in Life (MIL) scale. The purpose of that study was to "assess stability of responses over time" (p. 224). It is not clear whether her interest was in the stability of the construct or in the stability of the test.

An example of proper consideration of the distinction between the two is the discussion of a seven-month stability study by Norbeck, Lindsey, and Carrieri (1983). The authors explicitly argued that the level of functional support should not have changed over that time period. Any difference between Time 1 scores and Time 2 scores would be reflective of a faulty test.

For a technical discussion of reliability and stability, the interested reader is referred to the article by Heise (1969).

Between-Spouse "Reliability"

Roberts and Feetham (1982) cited as additional evidence for the reliability of the Family Functioning Index (FFI) a correlation of .72 between husbands' scores and their wives' scores. It is encouraging that spouses agree on how their families function. However, this is not an issue of reliability, since it does not address the possible discrepancy between true scores and obtained scores.

Between-Level "Reliability"

Many standardized tests have versions that are appropriate for different grade levels. The Stanford Achievement Test and the Iowa Tests of Basic Skills are perhaps the best known. There are also three levels of the Wechsler Intelligence Scales for subjects of different ages (WPPSI, WISC, and WAIS) and two levels of the new Kaufman Assessment Battery for Children (K-ABC). In the manual Kaufman and Kaufman (1983) reported results of studies in which they administered both levels of the test to the same borderline-age subjects (ages 4 and 5). Such studies may be useful, but they are not reliability studies. They deal with the operationalization of the construct at different age levels. Such operationalizations are not "parallel" forms in the usual psychometric meaning of that term.

The Criteria in Criterion-Related Validity Studies

In an investigation of the criterion-related validity of a particular measuring instrument, the criterion against which the obtained test scores are to be validated should be a higher-status operationalization of the same construct that the test is trying to tap and not an operationalization of some other construct. Again, the line between a criterion-related validity study and a substantive study of some interesting hypothesis regarding the relationship between two variables is often a fine one, but it too must be drawn.

To take an example from a recent *Nursing Research* article, consider the work by Norbeck et al. (1983).

Under the heading "Study 3: Concurrent and Predictive Validity" (p. 7), they reported an investigation of the relationships among the Norbeck Social Support Questionnaire (NSSQ), the Life Experiences Survey (LES), and the Profile of Mood States (POMS). The POMS was the principal dependent variable in that study of the stress-buffering role of social support. The study actually exceeded the usual bounds of concurrent and predictive validity. The POMS is an operationalization of mood and the NSSQ is an operationalization of social support. Mood and social support are different constructs; the former should not be regarded as an external criterion for the latter.

Calloway's (1982) discussion of the HOME inventory includes under the heading "Criterion-Related Validity" (p. 255) a summary of a study of the relationship between scores on that instrument and Stanford–Binet Intelligence Test scores. The impact of home environment on intelligence is important. However, that study was a step beyond the assessment of the criterion-related validity of the HOME itself.

In the predictive validity study reported by Miller et al. (1982), the Miller Attitude Scale (MAS) was correlated with the Health Behavior Scale (HBS) at a six-month follow-up of 34 myocardial infarction patients. The subscales of the MAS and the corresponding subscales of the HBS were found to be related to varying degrees. That is interesting, but behavior and attitude are not the same construct.

Aptitude testing is the only situation for which an operationalization of a somewhat different construct is an appropriate criterion. By definition, a test is a valid indicator of musical aptitude, for example, if it is predictive of subsequent musical achievement. Thus, a high correlation between aptitude test scores and achievement test scores is necessary and often sufficient evidence for the validity of the aptitude test.

Some Additional Confusions

In addition to miscategorizations of certain kinds of research as validity or reliability studies, there are a few inappropriate categorizations within validity and reliability. In no particular order, here are a few of them.

Correlations between Parallel Forms as Evidence for Validity

In the manual for the Woodcock Reading Mastery Tests (Woodcock, 1973), which is otherwise a paragon of psychometric virtue, the author claims that high correlations between scores on Form A at Time 1 and scores on Form B at Time 2 are indicative of the test's predictive validity. That is a matter of reliability, not validity (or neither, if the time interval is too long). Hayter (1983) committed the reverse error when referring to the correlation between two different indicators of sleep behavior (a questionnaire and a sleep chart) as an index of the reliability of the questionnaire.

Construct Validity Circularity

It has sometimes been said that one may simultaneously test the validity of a theory and the validity of a test (e.g., Selltiz, Wrightsman & Cook, 1976, p. 174). That argument is unacceptable, because in a construct validity study there should be two or more alleged operationalizations of Construct A and two or more alleged operationalizations of Construct B. If the A operationalizations correlate high with one another and low with the B operationalizations, validity for measuring Construct A is claimed. In a substantive study of the relationship between Construct A and Construct B, on the other hand, the validity of Operationalization A and the validity of Operationalization B must have already been determined. One cannot have it both ways; the validity argument becomes circular otherwise.

Confusions between Construct Validity and Criterion-Related Validity

All variables are on equal footing in a study of the construct validity of an instrument, whereas one (or more) of the variables has a superior status in a criterion-related validity study. In their abstract, Farrand, Holzemer, and Schleutermann (1982) stated that differences between nurse practitioners and other nurses supported the claim for construct validity of their patient management problems (PMPs). This is not defensible. It may be an important finding, but if it is a matter of validity at all, it is criterion-related, not construct, validity. The implied criterion is job status (nurse practitioners should score higher than other nurses on PMPs).

Incorrect Designations of Coefficients

For their double testing of 22 mothers over a two-week period, Roberts and Feetham (1982) called the correlation of .85 an alpha reliability coefficient. Alpha coefficients are measures of internal consistency among the test items at one point in time, not temporal consistency from time to time.

Separations of Sections That Should Go Together

Derdiarian and Forsythe (1983) have separate sections for internal consistency and reliability. Internal consistency is one aspect of reliability, not a different property.** Calloway (1982) has separate sections for criterion-related validity and concurrent validity. Concurrent validity and predictive validity are both subsumed under criterion-related validity.

Summary

Some studies of measuring instruments are validity studies. Others are reliability studies. Still others, such as the investigation of the stability of a construct and the correlation between the scores on two different levels of the same test, are neither. Authors of test manuals and of journal articles dealing with certain tests should label them accordingly as substantive studies, not methodological investigations.

References

American Psychological Association. (in press). *Joint technical standards for educational and psychological testing.* Washington, DC: The Association.

Calloway, S. J. (1982). Home observation for measurement of the environment. In S. S. Humenick (ed.), *Analysis of current assessment strategies in health care of young children and childbearing families* (pp. 252–258). Norwalk, CT: Appleton-Century-Crofts.

Carmines, E. G., & Zeller, R. A. (1979). *Reliability and validity assessment* (Number 17 in the series devoted to quantitative applications in the social sciences). Beverly Hills, CA: Sage Publications.

Chang, B. L. (1978). Perceived situational control of daily activities: A new tool. *Research in Nursing and Health, 1,* 181–188.

Cureton, E. E. (1950). Validity, reliability, and baloney. *Educational and Psychological Measurement, 15,* 94–96.

Derdiarian, A. K., & Forsythe, A. B. (1983). An instrument for theory and research development using the behavioral systems model for nursing: The cancer patient. Part 2. *Nursing Research, 32,* 260–266.

Farrand, L. L., Holzemer, W. L., & Schleutermann, J. A. (1982). A study of construct validity: Simulations as a measure of nurse practitioners' problem-solving skills. *Nursing Research, 31,* 37–42.

Hayter, J. (1983). Sleep behaviors of older persons. *Nursing Research, 32,* 242–246.

Heise, D. R. (1969). Separating reliability and stability in test–retest correlation. *American Sociological Review, 34,* 93–101.

Kaufman, A. S., & Kaufman, N. L. (1983). *Interpretive manual for the Kaufman assessment battery for children.* Circle Pines, MN: American Guidance Service.

Miller, P., Wikoff, R., McMahon, M., Garrett, M. K., & Johnson, N. (1982). Development of a health attitude scale. *Nursing Research, 31,* 132–136.

Norbeck, J. S., Lindsey, A. M., & Carrieri, V. L. (1983). Further development of the Norbeck social support questionnaire: Normative data and validity testing. *Nursing Research, 32,* 4–9.

Pless, I. B., & Satterwhite, B. (1973). A measure of family functioning and its application. *Social Science and Medicine, 7,* 613–621.

Polit, D. E., & Hungler, B. P. (1983). *Nursing research: Principles and methods* (2nd ed.). Philadelphia: J. B. Lippincott Co.

Roberts, C. S., & Feetham, S. L. (1982). Assessing family functioning across three areas of relationships. *Nursing Research, 31,* 231–235.

Selltiz, C., Wrightsman, L. S., & Cook, S. W. (1976). *Research methods in social relations.* New York: Holt, Rinehart & Winston.

Stevenson, J. S. (1982). Construction of a scale to measure load, power, and margin in life. *Nursing Research, 31,* 222–225.

Woodcock, R. W. (1973). *Manual for the Woodcock reading mastery tests.* Circle Pines, MN: American Guidance Service.

** Derdiarian and Forsythe also claimed that "the instrument's strong internal consistency and reliability on all three measures reflect discernible validity of the instrument as well as of its theoretical underpinnings" (p. 265). That does not necessarily follow. A test can be reliable without being valid; and, as pointed out, the validity of a test and the validity of a theory do not automatically follow from one another.

Determination and Quantification of Content Validity

Mary R. Lynn

Validity is a crucial factor in the selection or application of an instrument, for validity is the extent to which that instrument measures what it is intended to measure. Although over 35 terms may be used to connote kinds of validity (Brown, 1980), only three types are in common usage today—content, criterion-related, and construct. There has been little argument about the relative merits of criterion-related and construct validity, but the legitimacy of content validity as a *real* type of validity has been questioned by a number of psychometricians (Carmines & Zeller, 1979; Cronbach, 1970; Messick, 1981). These challenges to the value and merit of content validity have arisen from the confusion of content validity with face validity, the unstandardized approaches to the determination of content validity, and the previously unquantified nature of content validity.

The purpose of this article is to differentiate content and face validity, present the process by which content validity can and should be determined, and demonstrate some means by which aspects of the content validity determination can be quantified.

Face validity, rather than a true psychometric assessment technique, has been defined as validity conferred by the lay person's acceptance that a procedure, statement, or instrument appears to be sound or relevant (Guilford, 1954; Waltz & Bausell, 1981). In addition to this appearance of validity, face validity includes validity by assumption (a nonstatistical assessment of the logical tie between the elements or items of an instrument and its purpose) and validity by definition (the determination by one or more content experts that the elements/items of an instrument represent the content domain being assessed) (Mosier, 1947). Face validity is not quantifiable and long ago fell out of favor in psychometric usage (Mosier, 1947), but the continued confusion between content validity and face validity could also lead to content validity's eventual dismissal as a legitimate form of validity.

Mary R. Lynn, PhD, RN, is a National Research Service Award postdoctoral fellow and research associate at the College of Nursing, University of Arizona, Tucson.

From *Nursing Research,* November/December 1986, *35,* 382–385.

Assessment of Content Validity

Content validity is the determination of the content representativeness or content relevance of the elements/items of an instrument by the application of a two-stage (development or judgment) process. When content validity has been viewed as a one-stage process (either development or judgment), it has been challenged most as a form of validity (Jensen, 1980; Messick, 1981). Using a two-stage process to determine and quantify content validity is fundamental to the validation of virtually all instrumentation.

Developmental Stage

The assessment of content validity begins in the earliest development of an instrument. The development stage of content validity determination has three steps: domain identification, item generation, and instrument formation (Carmines & Zeller, 1979; Nunnally, 1978; Williamson, 1981). These steps vary in context, depending on the measurement objective of the instrument, i.e., whether the measure is being developed for a cognitive or affective/personality measure (see Table 1).

For cognitive measures, the full content domain must be identified in Step 1. If, for example, an instrument is being developed to measure clients' knowledge about self-care measures to prevent hypertension, all self-care measures need to be identified and categorized for the next step in this stage to be addressed. Domain identification is often facilitated by the use of a table of specification or a blueprint of the content domain.

The second step in the development stage of a cognitive measure is to sample from the content domain identified and generate the items from these sampled areas. Rarely is it necessary for a cognitive measure to address each and every aspect of the content area to fully represent the scope of the content. Ideally, this sampling should be random, but such is rarely practical. It is sufficient to ensure that all areas or cells of the table of specifications or blueprint have been represented appropriately (see Mehrens & Lehmann, 1984).

TABLE 1 **Stages of Content Validity (CV) Determination**

Step	Cognitive Instrument	Affective Instrument
	STAGE I—DEVELOPMENT STAGE	
1	Identification of full content domain	Identification of dimension(s) and/or subdimensions of affective variable
2	Sampling and item generation	Generation of items for all dimensions and/or subdimensions
3	Assimilation of items into useable form	Assimilation of items into useable form
	STAGE II—JUDGMENT–QUANTIFICATION STAGE	
4	Judgment/quantification of CV of items	Judgment/quantification of CV of items
5	Judgment/quantification of CV of instrument	Judgment/quantification of CV of instrument

In the development of an affective/personality measure the first two steps differ from those just described. In affective measures the domain identification (Step 1) is accomplished through a thorough review of the literature on the topic of the measure so that all dimensions and subdimensions can be identified. This incorporation of the ideas of a variety of experts (perhaps limited to those published) is in contrast to the domain identification in a cognitive instrument that can reasonably be done by a single expert or an arbitrary number of experts.

In the second step for an affective/personality measure, items are generated for all dimensions and subdimensions identified in Step 1. Rarely is a domain for an affective/personality variable so large as to justify or even make possible sampling for item generation, and it is always better to generate too many items than too few (Carmines & Zeller, 1979; Nunnally, 1978).

The third step of the development stage is the same for cognitive and affective/personality instruments. The items generated in Step 2 are now assembled in a usable form, that is, items generated in the second step are refined (reworded as necessary) and arranged in a suitable sequence. Once the items have been finalized and the instrument assembled, the development stage of content validity determination is completed.

Judgment–Quantification Stage

Stage II, the judgment–quantification stage of content validity, has two steps that are the same for both cognitive and affective/personality measures. These steps entail the assertion by a specific number of experts that the items are content valid (Step 4) and that the entire instrument is content valid (Step 5). The number of experts needed in this stage and the proportion of those experts that must agree for content validity to be established can be decided by application of the standard error of the proportion; content validity can be quantified with application of the index of content validity (CVI), as outlined in Waltz and Bausell (1981, p. 71).

Determining the number of experts needed has always been somewhat arbitrary in content validity determination. The number of experts often depends on how many accessible and agreeable persons the instrument developer or user can identify, not on a population estimation principle. Although this practice is widespread, specific guidelines can and should be applied to the selection of experts for content validity determination. A minimum of five experts would provide a sufficient level of control for chance agreement: however, in some content areas it may be difficult to locate this many content/domain experts and to obtain their cooperation. Therefore, in content/domain areas of sufficient restriction to preclude large numbers of experts, a minimum of three experts should be used. The use of only two judges is not only statistically unjustifiable, but also it places the instrument developer at great risk of an erroneous conclusion that content validity has not been achieved when it actually has. The maximum number of judges that might be used has not been established, but it is unlikely to exceed ten.

After (or perhaps as a part of) determining the number of experts, the minimum number of judges who must agree for the items and total instrument to be assessed as content valid must be established. This can be done by calculating the proportion of the number of experts who might agree out of the total number planned for use, and then setting the standard error of the proportion to identify the cut-off for chance versus real agreement. In Table 2 the proportions of experts agreeing on the content validity of an item and the entire instrument and the standard error of those proportions are presented (as a function of the total number of experts). If there are five or fewer experts, all must agree on the content validity for their rating to be considered a reasonable representation of the universe of possible ratings. When six or more experts are used, one or more can be in disagreement with the others and the instrument will be assessed content valid.

Regardless of the number of experts used, a structured procedure for the evaluation of the content validity of the instrument must be given to the experts (Kerlinger, 1973). Although the persons selected have already been determined to have expertise in the content/domain area(s) of the instrument, it is not sufficient to supply them with the instrument and simply ask if it is content valid. They must be given a set of specific instructions by which to determine the domain or content relevance of the items and also of the instrument as a whole (McCain, 1984). The experts should be provided with either a delineation of the full content domain for cognitive instruments or dimensions of the affective variable, with specific questions pertaining to the content relevance of each item.

The most widely used quantification of content validity is the index of content validity (CVI), which is derived from the rating of the content relevance of the items on an instrument using a 4-point ordinal rating scale, where 1 connotes an irrelevant item and 4 an extremely relevant item. The actual CVI is the proportion of items that received a rating of 3 or 4 by the experts (Waltz & Bausell, 1981).

Use of the CVI in both steps of the judgment stage of content validity determination necessitates extension of the CVI to item evaluation as well as entire instrument evaluation. The CVI for each item (Step 4) is determined by the proportion of experts who rate it as content valid (a rating of 3 or 4); the CVI for the entire instrument (Step 5) is the proportion of total items judged content valid.

Waltz and Bausell (1981) posed two limitations to the CVI procedure for the assessment of content validity: The possibility of chance inflation (agreement) of the CVI and the dependence of the CVI on the number of categories used in the rating, in that a four-option scale is not universally used in CVI determinations. These limitations can be controlled by using the methods discussed in this article. The first limitation is addressed in the selection of the number of experts and the minimum number that must agree by using a significant combination from Table 2. The second concern would be controlled by establishment of a 4-option rating scale (1 = not relevant; 2 = unable to assess relevance without item revision or item is in need of such revision that it would no longer be relevant; 3 = relevant but needs minor alteration; 4 = very relevant and succinct) for all content validity assessments. The scale should be both mathematically and conceptually meaningful. Although a 3- or 5-point rating scale might be considered, the 4-point scale is preferable because it does not include the ambivalent middle rating common in odd number rating scales. Using a 4-point rating scale should provide the instrument developer with sufficiently delineated information upon which to calculate a meaningful CVI.

TABLE 2 Proportion of Experts (Above the Line) Whose Endorsement Is Required to Establish Content Validity Beyond the .05 Level of Significance

Number of Experts	Number of Experts Endorsing Item or Instrument as Content Valid: 2	3	4	5	6	7	8	9	10
2	1.00								
3	.67	1.00							
4	.50	.75	1.00						
5	.40	.60	.80	1.00					
6	.33	.50	.67	.83	1.00				
7	.29	.43	.57	.71	.86	1.00			
8	.25	.38	.50	.63	.75	.88	1.00		
9	.22	.33	.44	.56	.67	.78	.89	1.00	
10	.20	.30	.40	.50	.60	.70	.80	.90	1.00

NOTE: The caution over using the standard error of the proportion when $n \leq 10$ (Downie & Heath, 1974) does not apply in this situation because only when $p > q$ is there significance, and any nonunique p [x] q solutions are irrelevant.

The experts, in addition to judging each item, should identify any area(s) that have been omitted from the instrument. If omissions are identified although the entire instrument is assessed as content valid, further clarification may be necessary. If no omissions are identified and the instrument is judged content valid by the experts, in conjunction with the knowledge of the magnitude of the CVI values, the content validity of the instrument may be asserted. Should an expert identify no areas of omission, evaluate the items positively, and, yet, not assess the instrument as content valid, doubt about the person's expertise should lead to considering replacing that person as an expert. Suggestions for item improvement may be requested from the experts, however, without interfering with the content validity judgment.

Items that do not achieve the required minimum agreement of the experts (Table 2) should be eliminated or further revised. It is certainly possible that several items, and, therefore, the entire instrument, need to be evaluated more than once in order to obtain sufficient content validity. In this case, the instrument developer should determine whether to use the same experts or obtain new, but equally qualified, replacement experts. Should the same experts be used in repeated assessments of an instrument, a 10- to 14-day period between assessments should be a sufficient time interval (McCain, 1984).

This process for content validity determination may also be applied to existing instruments, for the validity of many such instruments either has never been reported or has been simply untested. Given that the instrument has been already created, Steps 2 and 3 may not be applicable if, by completion of the content validity process, acceptable content validity is determined. In the event that content validity is not sufficiently achieved, with the instrument developer's permission, Steps 2 and 3 (item and instrument revision) may also be incorporated to eventually obtain content validity.

Summary

The arbitrary assertion of two or three experts does not establish content validity. Application of a two-stage process that incorporates rigorous instrument development practices and quantifies the aspects of content validity is required. In the first stage of this process, the content domain or dimensions are identified and items are generated to reflect the scope of the content domain of a cognitive variable or each of the dimensions of an affective variable. Once generated, the items are assembled in a usable, testable format. The instrument and domain or dimension specifications are then presented to a panel of experts, the size of which is an a priori decision, for their judgment of the items using a 4-point ordinal rating scale. Using the item evaluation, CVI calculations are applied to both the items and the entire instrument. The experts are asked, as a part of the content validity assessment, to identify areas of omission and to suggest areas of item improvement or modification.

Admittedly, there are times when adherence to such rigor may not be feasible. When less stringent methods of determining validity are applied, it should not be said that content validity has been determined. Opponents of the process described in this article might argue that these specifications and expectations exceed practical application and that this process is therefore too rigorous. Content validity, by its nature and definition, demands rigor in its assessment, and its assessment is, in fact, critical. Such a rigorous process for content validity determination is offered because content validity is an inexpendable form of validity that is rapidly losing credibility due to its less than standardized and rigorous assessments. Content validity, different from all other forms of validity, is crucial to the understanding of research findings and their practical or theoretical applications. It is worth the rigor.

References

Brown, F. (1980). Perspectives on validity. *NCME Measurement News, 23*(3), 3–4.

Carmines, E. G., & Zeller, R. A. (1979). *Reliability and validity assessment.* Beverly Hills, CA: Sage.

Cronbach, L. J. (1970). *Essentials of psychological testing* (3rd ed.). New York: Harper and Row.

Downie, N. M., & Heath, R. W. (1974). *Basic statistical methods* (4th ed.). New York: Harper and Row.

Guilford, J. P. (1954). *Psychometric methods.* New York: McGraw-Hill.

Jensen, A. R. (1980). *Bias in mental testing.* New York: The Free Press.

Kerlinger, F. (1973). *Foundations of behavioral research* (2nd ed.). New York: Holt, Rinehart & Winston.

McCain, N. L. (1984). *A test of Cohen's developmental model for professional socialization with baccalaureate nursing students.* Unpublished doctoral dissertation. The University of Alabama in Birmingham.

Mehrens, W. A., & Lehmann, I. J. (1984). *Measurement and evaluation in education and psychology* (3rd ed.). New York: Holt, Rinehart & Winston.

Messick, S. (1981). Evidence and ethics in the evaluation of tests. *Educational Researcher, 10*(9), 9–20.

Mosier, C. I. (1947). A critical examination of the concepts of face validity. *Education and Psychological Measurement, 7,* 191–205.

Nunnally, J. C. (1978). *Psychometric theory* (2nd ed.). New York: McGraw-Hill.

Waltz, C. W., & Bausell, R. B. (1981). *Nursing research: Design, statistics and computer analysis.* Philadelphia: F.A. Davis.

Williamson, Y. M. (1981). *Research methodology and its application to nursing.* New York: John Wiley and Sons.

Evaluating Validity of Screening Tests

Elaine Larson

There are epidemiologic methods that can predict whether a screening test is truly able to discriminate between individuals with and without a particular characteristic. The purpose of this discussion is to describe several quantitative methods that can be used to evaluate the validity of these tests and to discuss their applicability to issues in nursing.

Screening tests are useful under the following conditions: (a) when there is an important health problem, (b) when the problem can be detected during an early stage, (c) when there is a useful treatment or intervention for the problem (it is usually not helpful to make an early diagnosis of a disease or problem if nothing can be done about it), and (d) when the screening test is simple, convenient, reliable, and cost-effective. It is useful, for example, to screen health care personnel in high-risk areas for infectious diseases such as rubella and hepatitis because simple, safe, and valid tests are available, knowledge of the results of the tests will affect practice, and the costs of the effects of the disease far outweigh the costs of screening. Screening tests, then, are not designed to be diagnostic, but to detect persons with a high probability of having a characteristic.

Characteristics of the Tests

Sensitivity of a test is the extent to which a true characteristic is classified correctly; it refers to those who have a particular condition who also have a positive test, or the rate of "true positives." A highly sensitive test will identify the majority of individuals with a given disease or characteristic. A high degree of sensitivity, however, is not an adequate criterion for a useful test. A test, for example, may identify all patients with a characteristic, but might also misclassify many without the characteristic, identifying them as diseased or false positives. To minimize the risk of many false positives, a test must also be highly specific.

Elaine Larson, PhD, FAAN, holds the M. Adelaide Nutting Chair in Clinical Nursing at the School of Nursing, The Johns Hopkins University, Baltimore, MD.

From *Nursing Research,* May/June 1986, *35,* 186–188.

Specificity is the extent to which the absence of a characteristic is correctly classified, or the proportion of those without a condition who also have a negative test, or the rate of "true negatives." A highly specific test will correctly identify individuals who are free of a given characteristic. Sensitivity and specificity together are a measure of the validity of a test.

The *predictive value* of a positive test is the probability that when a test is positive, the characteristic is truly present. The predictive value of a negative test is the probability that when the test is negative, the characteristic is truly absent. As will be seen, predictive value as well as sensitivity and specificity must be considered when evaluating the clinical usefulness of a test.

Screening tests would not be necessary if there were definitive standard tests that were inexpensive, harmless, and easily applied to large populations. Often, however, the presence of a disease or characteristic cannot be readily confirmed without invasive or expensive tests, or sometimes even until the patient dies and an autopsy confirms the diagnosis. Therefore, noninvasive screening tests to identify a large proportion of individuals with certain characteristics are important. Some of the diseases for which screening tests are used can be found in Table 1.

Sensitivity and specificity can be calculated by forming 2×2 tables and then comparing results from the test with a reference criterion "gold standard"). All cases are classified by both the reference criterion and the screening test to identify the degree of agreement/disagreement between the two (Figure 1a). This, of course, assumes that there is indeed a valid and reliable reference standard against which other tests can be compared. If no acceptable standard exists, it is not possible to calculate the sensitivity and specificity of any other test.

Application

The concepts of sensitivity and specificity can be applied to the evaluation of many nursing research and practice problems. For example, a newly developed nursing assessment tool to categorize patients as depressed could be compared to a standardized tool. Or a patient classification scheme designed to categorize patients into high

TABLE 1 Examples of Screening Tests

Disease/Condition	Test	Reference Standard
Tuberculosis	Tine test	Chest X-ray or PPD
Breast cancer	Mammogram	Biopsy
Coronary artery disease	Electrocardiograph or myocardial imaging	Arteriogram
Sepsis	Clinical signs and symptoms	Blood culture
Cervical cancer	Pap smear	Biopsy
Syphilis	VDRL	Microscopic identification of the organism from clinical specimens

and low acuity groups for the purpose of nurse staffing could be compared to standardized tools such as diagnostic related groups or the Horn (1981) Severity of Illness tool. Keep in mind, of course, that the sensitivity and specificity of any tool are always in comparison to a defined standard.

In Figure 1b, sensitivity and specificity have been calculated to evaluate the validity of the nurse's clinical assessment of whether a patient has a urinary tract infection. The reference criterion used in this example is a urine culture. As shown, the sensitivity of the nursing assessment is rather low and, hence, patients with urinary

1a. Formula

Reference ("gold") standard	Test: Yes	Test: No
Yes	a	b
No	c	d

a = True positives (TP)
b = False negatives (FN)
c = False positives (FP)
d = True negatives (TN)

1b. Example: Does the patient have a urinary tract infection?

Urine culture	Nurse Assessment: Yes	Nurse Assessment: No	
Yes	17	9	26
No	1	20	21
	18	29	47

Term	Definition	Formula	Example
Sensitivity	Proportion of those with the condition who have a positive test	a/a+b (TP/TP+FN)	17/26 = 65.4%
Specificity	Proportion of those without the condition who have a negative test	d/c+d (TN/FP+TN)	20/21 = 95.2%
Predictive value of a positive test	Proportion of those with a positive test who have the condition	a/a+c (TP/TP +FP)	17/18 = 94.4%
Predictive value of a negative test	Proportion of those with a negative test who do not have the condition	d/b+d (TN/FN+TN)	20/29 = 69.0%
False positive rate (1-Specificity)	Proportion of those without condition who have a positive test	c/c+d (FP/FP+TN)	1/21 = 4.8%
False negative rate (1-Sensitivity)	Proportion of those with the condition who have a negative test	b/a+b (FN/TP+FN)	9/26 = 34.6%

FIGURE 1 Calculating Sensitivity and Specificity

tract infections may not be identified by the nurse's clinical screening, i.e., the false-negative rate is high. On the other hand, almost all patients who are identified by nursing assessment as being free of infection indeed are, i.e., the false-positive rate is low.

Ideally, one would hope for a test in which there is no overlap in test results between those with and without a characteristic. Such a test would be 100% sensitive and specific (Figure 2a). Unfortunately, there is usually some overlap and misclassification in test results (Figure 2b). In such a situation, one must choose a test that provides the best balance between sensitivity and specificity. Since sensitivity and specificity are inversely correlated, increasing the sensitivity of a test by lowering the point at which a test is considered positive (the cutoff point) decreases the specificity of the test, and vice versa. In the example in Figure 1b, if the cutoff point for defining a urinary tract infection was lowered from the standard of $\geq 10^5$ colonies/ml of urine to $\geq 10^4$ colonies/ml, more individuals would be categorized as infected. In that case, the sensitivity of the nurse assessments would decrease and the specificity would increase.

Combinations of tests are often used to enhance sensitivity or specificity. Tests administered in series may increase specificity. For example, if the VDRL screening test for syphilis is positive, other more specific tests are then performed. The individual is not diagnosed as having syphilis unless *all* tests are positive. In the example of the urinary tract infection, the nurse may suspect, based on clinical signs and symptoms, that a patient is infected. The next test may be a clean catch urine. Even if this test is positive, a catheterized specimen, the most specific test, may be required to confirm the diagnosis. Again, if all tests are positive, specificity is enhanced.

In contrast, tests done in parallel may be used to increase sensitivity. In such a case, the individual would be considered positive if *any* of the tests done were positive. For example, some cases of breast cancer are diagnosed by physical examination and some by mammography; neither test alone will identify all cases.

To help determine where to set a cutoff point for any screening test, one must consider the emotional and monetary costs of a false-positive result, the importance of missing a case, the likelihood that a population will be rescreened soon, and the prevalence of the condition.

The validity of a test is influenced not only by its sensitivity and specificity, but also by its predictive value. Figure 3 gives an example of how the prevalence of urinary tract infection can influence the predictive value of the nurse assessment of symptoms. Even though the sensitivity and specificity of the test are high, when the prevalence of a condition is low, such as the prevalence of urinary tract infection in the general population (Figure 3b), the predictive value of a positive test is poor. That is, only a small proportion of those clinically judged to have infection actually do. On the other hand, in a setting such as a nursing home where urinary tract infections are common, the nurse's positive prediction is very accurate. Low prevalence results in a high proportion of patients with a positive test who do not actually have the condition. When urinary tract infections, for example, are uncommon in a population, there will be a relatively greater proportion of individuals with a positive nurse assessment who, in fact, are not infected (a greater proportion of individuals in cell c of the 4 × 4 table). For this reason, the use of screening tests, even when they are highly specific and sensitive, is usually limited to high-risk groups. For example, mammography is recommended

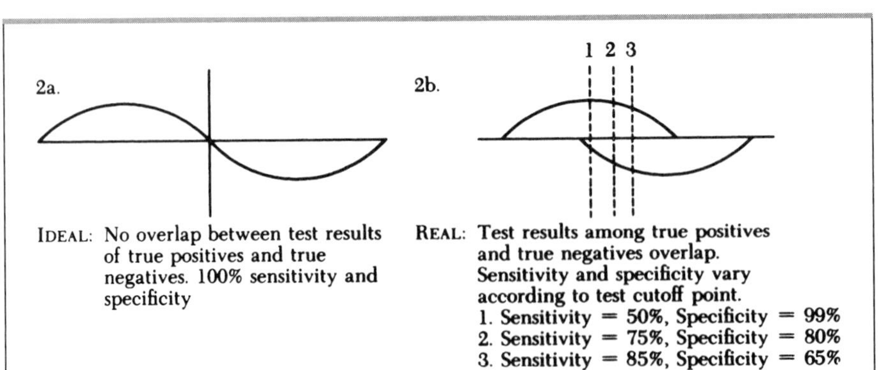

FIGURE 2 Ideal and Real Test Results

3a. Prevalence of urinary tract infection = 50%
(A sample of elderly in a nursing home)

		Nurse Assessment Yes	Nurse Assessment No	
Urine culture	Yes	450	50	500
	No	50	450	500
		500	500	1,000

Sensitivity = 90%
Specificity = 90%
False-negative rate = 10%
False-positive rate = 10%

Predictive value of positive test = 90%

3b. Prevalence of urinary tract infection = 1%
(A sample from the general population)

		Nurse Assessment Yes	Nurse Assessment No	
Urine culture	Yes	90	10	100
	No	990	8,910	9,900
		1,080	8,920	10,000

Sensitivity = 90%
Specificity = 90%
False-negative rate = 10%
False-positive rate = 10%

Predictive value of positive test = 8.3%

FIGURE 3 Effect of the Prevalence of a Characteristic on the Validity of the Test

only for women over the age of 45 and/or for those with a family history of breast cancer.

In summary, sensitivity and specificity are helpful in evaluating the validity of screening tests, but must be combined with a careful clinical assessment of the probability that a condition is present. Such quantitative techniques can be applied to the evaluation of a variety of nursing activities.

Reference

Horn, S. D. (1981). Validity, reliability, and implications of an index of inpatient severity of illness. *Medical Care, 19*(3), 354–362.

Reliability Estimates: Use and Disuse

Mary R. Lynn

Reliability has been defined as the ratio of true score variance to observed score variance (Lord & Novick, 1968; Magnusson, 1966), as the ratio of desired information (signal) to all obtained information (signal and noise) (Cronbach, 1970), and as the repeatability of a measure. Reliability is generally defined as the extent to which measurement error is minimized (Nunnally, 1978; Polit & Hungler, 1983); it is usually considered acceptable when the estimate is greater than or equal to .70 (Polit & Hungler, 1983). The empirical and unstable nature of reliability has not received sufficient attention from nurse researchers (Waltz & Strickland, 1982).

In 1981, Waltz and Strickland reviewed 191 articles published in *Nursing Research, Research in Nursing and Health,* and *Advances in Nursing Science* during the previous 21 months. They found that reliability estimates for the use of an instrument were cited in 42% of the non-instrument-development studies and in only 60% of the instrument-development studies. Although specific data for physiological measures were not given, reliability was not estimated in studies using this form of data collection.

This article reports a further analysis of the extent of reliability estimates in published nursing research. The focus of this study was to determine current emphasis on reliability estimation in nursing research by reviewing research published in two major nursing research publications. Two research questions were studied: To what extent are reliability estimates included in recently published nursing research? Did reporting of reliability estimates in published nursing research increase significantly over the study period?

Method

Traditionally, only pencil-and-paper tests or instruments have been considered in need of reliability estimates. Because any means of data collection has inherent potential for measurement error, a more comprehensive view of data collection devices than "instrument" was needed. Accordingly, the term *data collection strategy* (DCS) was developed to include all possible means of data collection. For this study, data collection methods were categorized as follows:

ESTABLISHED DATA COLLECTION STRATEGY (EDCS)—All methods of data collection that had been developed and used prior to the study.

NEW DATA COLLECTION STRATEGY (NDCS)—A method of data collection that had not been previously used.

COMBINATION DATA COLLECTION STRATEGY (CDCS)—EDCS and NDCS were used in combination in the study.

PHYSIOLOGICAL DATA COLLECTION STRATEGY (PDCS)—Exclusive use of physiological measures or instruments in the study.

OTHER DATA COLLECTION STRATEGY (ODCS)—Not classified as one of the other DCS (e.g., use of existing data).

Sample

All articles published in *Nursing Research* and *Research in Nursing and Health* between January 1978 and December 1982 were reviewed to identify research reports, after which the number of applicable articles for each year was determined for each journal. Inasmuch as the number of research articles per journal per year was relatively constant over the study period, a proportional allocation of articles from each journal was selected. This selection was accomplished through the use of a stratified random sampling approach, each year of publication being a strata. Of 70 articles selected, 50 were from *Nursing Research* and 20 from *Research in Nursing and Health.*

Procedure

An ex post facto survey design was used. To facilitate the data collection, a coding form was developed for recording the following data: article source and year of publi-

---

Mary R. Lynn, PhD, RN, is an associate professor in the School of Nursing, University of Mississippi, Jackson, MS.

From *Nursing Research,* July/August 1985, *34,* 254–256.

cation, intended application of the findings of the study (clinical, educational, administrative, or other), type of data collection strategy used, report of previous reliability estimates, if appropriate, and report of reliability estimates in the current study.

In a pilot test of the data collection form and process, ten articles were selected from the nonsampled articles. They were coded, using the developed form. One week later the same articles were again coded. Intrarater reliability of all coded data across the two codings was 98%.

Results

Of the 70 articles selected, 34 (48%) had clinical applications, 9 (13%) pertained to nursing education, and 2 (3%) were nursing administration studies. Twenty-five (36%) were instrument development studies or studies with combined applications and were classified as other.

When both the Lawshe-Baker nomograph for testing difference between percentages (Downie & Heath, 1974) and a chi-square test revealed no significant differences in the proportion (or frequency) of articles that contained reliability estimates across the two journals, data from the two journals were combined. This nonsignificant finding supported the selection of these two journals as a representation of the current state of published nursing research.

Simple frequencies were used to explore the extent of the reliability estimates in the selected articles. For the previous uses of EDCSs, reliability estimates were present in 15 of the 27 applicable articles, yet current reliability estimates were available in only 6 of the 27 articles. When NDCSs were employed in a study, reliability estimates were available for only 14 of the 27 studies. In studies in which EDCSs and NDCSs were used in combination (CDCSs), a different picture of reliability estimation emerged. For the EDCSs, no previous or current reliability estimates were offered but reliability estimates were given for 8 of the 9 NDCSs.

Physiological data collection strategies were used in only five studies with one study containing a previous report of reliability; none of the studies had a current reliability estimate. The ODCS studies were based on census data and product information data, for which the appropriateness of reliability estimates was not determined.

After the frequencies of reliability estimates were determined, the reliability estimates for the various DCSs for each year by journal were analyzed. The relationship between the proportion of articles with reliability estimates per year and the year of publication was determined, using Pearson product moment correlation. No significant correlations were obtained for the combined data set ($r = .13$, $p > .20$), or for each journal separately ($r = -.64$, $p = .16$ for *Nursing Research*; $r = .71$, $p = .14$ for *Research in Nursing and Health*). Using the Lawshe–Baker nomograph, all possible proportions of articles per year with reliability estimates were compared, yielding no significant differences. It was, therefore, concluded that there had been no significant change in the reporting of reliability estimates for all data collection strategies over the study period.

This study was limited by the fact that data were considered only if they appeared in the actual report of the studies; the data actually presented may not accurately represent the full study.

Discussion

Results of the Waltz and Strickland (1982) study and this study show that estimation of reliability is not receiving sufficient attention by nurse researchers nor is it being given significant emphasis in the decision to accept an article for publication in these nursing research journals. From this conclusion, it is suggested that there is a need for greater awareness by nurse researchers and prospective researchers of the critical role reliability plays in each data collection situation. In response to the apparent need, the following brief review of reliability (and its application) is offered.

Recommendations

Without sufficient and current estimates of the reliability of the measures used in a study, any and all results of that study must be viewed with caution. No study, no matter how sophisticated the design, analysis, theoretical background, or other component, can rise above the threat of nonreliability of the measures used in the study. There is no single or perpetual reliability coefficient for a test, instrument, or other data collection device. Reliability estimates are not a stable property of a data collection method but are specific to the use of that data collection method with any particular population (or sample) under any particular measurement condition (Cronbach, 1970; Nunnally, 1978). In other words, reliability is affected by the range of the variable being measured as well as by the conditions under which the measurement was conducted. Since reliability varies with population or sample and with the measurement conditions, the reliability of a data collection strategy must be reestimated with each subsequent use of the strategy. Presumably, researchers using EDCSs in this study who did not estimate the reliability of the current use of the EDCS assumed (incorrectly) that the "old" reliability would apply in the current use of the strategy.

When an EDCS is used, both previous reliability estimates and current estimates should be reported. Current estimates can be derived at the time of data analysis. In the development and use of a NDCS, a pilot test must be conducted for an initial reliability estimation before the DCS is used in the actual data collection. That the development of the instrument be the focus of a single study is often recommended; the data would be collected for the purpose of reliability estimation and would not be used to test the hypothesis of the "real" study that should follow the pilot study.

In terms of the various forms of data collection, different types of reliability estimation can be used. The type of reliability estimation is, in fact, paired with the specific forms of data collection. When a traditional pencil-and-paper instrument for measurement of a cognitive or affective variable is employed, the first type of reliability estimation should be internal consistency using the KR20 (cognitive) or Cronbach's coefficient alpha (affective or cognitive). Initial reliability estimation with these measures of internal consistency is advantageous because they are mathematically simple, offer an estimation of the lower bound of all other reliability estimates (Novick & Lewis, 1967), and address the major source of measurement error-content sampling (Nunnally, 1978).

Other means for reliability estimation for traditional DCSs include test–retest reliability. In spite of the limitations of test–retest reliability (necessity of two instrument administrations, potential memory effects, lack of statistical specificity of the correlation coefficient), it can be a useful addition to the internal consistency information already obtained.

Another form of reliability estimation, parallel or equivalent forms, is often of lesser value in nursing research. Since this reliability procedure requires the creation of two separate instruments, a worsening of the current state of instrumentation in nursing may occur. Use of this form of reliability estimation is valuable, and recommended, when a current instrument, with sound psychometric properties, is divided into two instruments (usually because the original instrument is too long). Although the reliability of an instrument whose length is altered in any fashion can be estimated using the Spearman–Brown prophecy formula, parallel forms reliability estimation gives more exact reliability information on the combined and separate uses of the instrument(s).

Interviews and observation strategies are also amenable to reliability estimation. When a single data collector is used, intrarater reliability is the only appropriate estimate. When multiple data collectors are used, interrater reliability is necessary, but intrarater reliability may also be appropriate, depending on whether the data collected by a single data collector are analyzed separately. If the data of a single data collector are to be analyzed independently of the data of other collectors, intrarater reliability estimates for that collector are required.

In studies that employ PDCSs, reliability estimates for the equipment should be provided by the manufacturer, as appropriate. When humans make judgments using physiological monitoring equipment (e.g., sphygmomanometers), inter- and/or intrarater reliabilities should be estimated as appropriate. No matter what type of PDCS is employed, there is always a possibility of measurement error and, therefore, a need for reliability estimation.

With the lack of reliability in published nursing research, much of the data with which nursing is currently attempting to build a "nursing science" cannot be considered as building blocks. Nursing's efforts toward scientific credibility will be seriously affected unless the reliability, and thereby the quality, of the measures used in research is addressed.

References

Cronbach, L. J. (1970). *Essentials of psychological testing* (3rd ed.). New York: Harper and Row, Inc.

Downie, N. M., & Heath, R. W. (1974). *Basic statistical methods* (4th ed.). New York: Harper and Row, Inc.

Lord, F. L., & Novick, M. R. (1968). *Statistical theories of mental test scores.* Reading, MA: Addison-Wesley Publishing Co.

Magnusson, D. (1966). *Test theory.* Reading, MA: Addison-Wesley Publishing Co.

Novick, M. R., & Lewis, C. (1967). Coefficient alpha and the reliability of composite measures. *Psychometrika, 32,* 1–13.

Nunnally, J. C. (1978). *Psychometric theory* (2nd ed.). New York: McGraw-Hill Book Co.

Polit, D., & Hungler, B. (1983). *Nursing research: Principles and methods* (2nd ed.). Philadelphia: J.B. Lippincott Co.

Waltz, C. F., & Strickland, O. L. (1982). Measurement of nursing outcomes: State of the art as we enter the eighties. In W. E. Field (ed.), *Proceedings of the First Annual SCCEN Research Conference.* (pp. 47–62). Atlanta: Southern Council on Collegiate Education for Nursing and the University of Texas at Austin School of Nursing.

Managing Measurement Error

Bonnie Mowinski Jennings ■ **Sandra Rogers**

Multiple regression is a valuable statistical technique that can be used not only with experimental research but also to reduce the tentativeness of conclusions derived from nonexperimental designs (Asher, 1983; Blalock, 1985; Cohen & Cohen, 1983). Confidence in the findings from regression procedures is derived from (a) trust in the reliability and validity of the instruments used and (b) assurance that mathematical assumptions undergirding the statistical tests are not violated.

From a quantitative research perspective, concept measurement is inseparable from the process of theory development. The purpose of this paper is to consider how measurement error affects building and testing theoretical models based on regression statistics, as faulty instrumentation can result in an inadequate test of the theoretical model.

Measurement—A Review

"Measurement can be the Achilles' heel of behavioral research," Kerlinger wrote (1979, p. 141). This vulnerability is particularly salient to nursing, because investigator-devised and first-generation measures are prevalent. The frequency of measurement error weakens the links between empirical indicants and their theoretical constructs. This, in turn, reduces the confidence with which the overall theoretical model can be regarded (Blalock, 1968; Cohen & Cohen, 1983; Pedhazur, 1982). Because many nursing concepts are often exceedingly abstract, the task of linking concepts to empirical indicants poses a special challenge to nurse researchers. The question is not whether error is operating, but to what degree (Carmines & Zeller, 1979; Nunnally, 1978), as there is an inverse relationship between error and instrument reliability and validity.

Bonnie Mowinski Jennings, DNSc, RN, a lieutenant colonel in the U.S. Army Nurse Corps, is a nurse researcher in the Health Care Studies Division, U.S. Army Health Services Command, Fort Sam Houston, TX.

Sandra Rogers, MS, RN, is a doctoral candidate in nursing, School of Nursing, University of California, San Francisco.

From *Nursing Research,* May/June 1989, *38,* 186–187.

Because reliability and validity are population-specific rather than inherent properties of an instrument, it is important for the researcher to select instruments that are not only psychometrically sound but also relevant to the population of interest so that the link between construct and empirical referent will be enhanced. However, because the state of instrument development in nursing is still in its infancy, it is highly probable that nurse researchers may have to decide whether to select an instrument with less than desirable psychometric properties or to use an investigator-developed measure with unknown psychometrics to tap the constructs depicted in the theoretical model.

The Consequences of Variable Position*

The multiple regression equation epitomizes the dynamics of error in theory testing and theory building. The following parameters of the regression equation are estimated from the sample data:

$$Y = A + BX_1 + BX_2 + BX_3 + E$$

where Y = dependent, criterion, or outcome variable; A = constant; B = regression coefficient; X = exogenous, independent, or predictor variables; E = error or residual.

Less reliable and valid referents have different ramifications depending on whether they represent dependent or independent variables.

Effects on the Dependent Variable

There are actually two lines of thinking in regard to the effects of instrument reliability on the dependent variable; one is theoretical, the other mathematical. The theoretical argument is perhaps most obvious.

The substance of a theoretical model predicated on an unreliable dependent variable must be questioned. Reliability, in a sense, is a precursor to validity. Without validity, theory is powerless because it does not explain

* The basis of these thoughts can be found in the pages cited in the Pedhazur reference. However, the authors were able to advance their thinking about these issues through discussion with David C. Heilbron, PhD, and Sandra Ferketich, PhD, RN, faculty at the University of California, San Francisco.

the phenomenon it purports to explain. A study that uses an unreliable outcome variable is meaningless because it is impossible to know what the independent variables are predicting.

From a mathematical perspective, the effect of error in the dependent variable is to reduce beta coefficients. Directionality in beta weights for the predictor variables remains unchanged, but the magnitude of those beta weights is altered. Therefore, the actual strength that may exist in depicted relationships cannot be detected (Pedhazur, 1982). The statistical tests thus fail to expose an actual association, and consequently the theoretical model has not been truly tested. The effect is not one of spuriousness, but failure to detect.

It is probable that the theoretical model test will remain sensitive if reliability in the dependent measure is .80 or above. However, as reliability coefficients diminish below .80, beta weights are more likely to be reduced (Nunnally, 1978). This reduction circumvents a reasonable test of the accuracy of the theoretical relationships depicted in the model. Despite the importance of attending to this reliability standard, it is necessary for researchers and consumers of research alike to appreciate the stringency of this criterion.

Effects on the Independent Variables

The Variable Order Unrealiability in the measures of the independent variables creates a different set of issues. The effects of the variables that enter the multiple regression equation first form the basis for the model; the effects of the remaining variables are essentially partialled on those variables. Therefore, if the least reliable indicants are the first to enter the equation, a cascade-like effect of unreliability is set into motion for all remaining independent variables, despite their individual reliability coefficients. The mathematical effect is not only one of magnitude; the direction of the relationships indicated by the beta coefficients can also be spurious. Mathematical chaos leads to theoretical confusion.

When the more psychometrically sound measures precede the weaker indicants in the equation, the effect is less profound. Rather than a shaky foundation for all the predictors, only those entering later are somewhat suspect. The pervasive effects of the unreliable predictors are not sustained throughout the model.

The best option is to avoid measures with less than desirable reliability, although they may have to be used, given the state-of-the-art in nursing instrument development. Although order of entry can diminish the adverse effects of unreliable instruments, it may conflict with the theory under scrutiny and preclude a test of the theoretical model. The onus is on the researcher, therefore, to analyze and balance the effects of inexact tests of theory and the use of unreliable measures.

The Type of Regression In simultaneous and stepwise regression, the computer, in a sense, selects the order of variable entry based on any number of predesignated criteria such as p values or F ratios. In hierarchical regression, the investigator forces the order of entry. In this case, selection of variable order cannot be arbitrary. It is not sufficient to merely enter the most reliable measure first. Rules of theoretical priority govern the entry of variables in a hierarchical regression.

If previous research can substantiate the order of entry, a hierarchical model is defensible. If there is no previous research and no sense of temporal ordering, the only tenable option afforded the investigator is to allow the correlations between the predictor and outcome variables to motivate the order of entry. In other words, preestablished computer criteria must objectively govern the order of variable entry. Therefore, it behooves all researchers who cannot designate the sequence of variable entry based on temporal ordering or previous research to seriously consider the effects of unreliability in all items. If an unreliable regressor enters early, all subsequent F-to-enters will be biased; variable selection itself may be biased.

Reliability Revisited

As an initial step in all research, instrument reliability must be examined for the population on which the study was conducted. Furthermore, as Hartshorn (1987) emphasized, the responsible researcher will also report the study-specific reliabilities. In that way, the researcher can consider possible effects of error introduced by the instruments and the research consumers can evaluate the adequacy of the model coefficients with full knowledge of how the instruments operated in that particular sample.

A dangerous misconception is that use of large sample sizes is a foolproof method to assure that empirical evidence is credible. Large samples are needed to meet basic mathematical assumptions inherent in statistical procedures and to have sufficient power to detect relationships among the variables. Equally important, but totally separate, is the issue of reliability. Increasing sample size will not correct for error. Reliability, not sample size, is the key indicant of error. Only through assuring that this psychometric property is as sound as possible can the effects of error be modified.

Conclusion

Kerlinger (1979) suggested that planning impeccable research is not possible without attending to measurement issues. Therefore, researchers must consider a priori how instrument selection will compound or reduce both error and judgments about the theoretical models being developed. Although the steady testing and revision of instruments to improve their psychometrics must be considered a priority, measurement error will always exist.

Consequently, the researcher must weigh the use of an unreliable measure against the effects of testing an incomplete theoretical model. When the unreliable measure is on the independent variable side of the equation, the risks of partialling on unreliable indicants must be considered. When the unreliable measure is on the dependent variable side of the equation, the contribution of the entire study must be questioned.

In either case, the judgment must be made thoughtfully if scientific inquiry is to provide a sturdy foundation for nursing knowledge.

References

Asher, H. B. (1983). *Causal modeling* (2nd ed.). Beverly Hills, CA: Sage Publications., Inc.

Blalock, H. M. (1968). The measurement problem. In H. M. Blalock and A. Blalock. (eds.), *Methodology in social research* (pp. 5–27). New York: McGraw-Hill Book Co., Inc.

Blalock, H. M. (1985). Simple recursive models and path analysis. In H. M. Blalock (ed.), *Causal models in the social sciences* (pp. 3–6). New York: Aldine de Grayter.

Carmines, E. G., & Zeller, R. A. (1979). *Reliability and validity assessment.* Beverly Hills, CA: Sage Publications, Inc.

Cohen, J., & Cohen, P. (1983). *Applied multiple regression/correlation analysis for the behavioral sciences* (2nd ed., pp. 79–132). Hillsdale, NJ: Lawrence Erlbaum Associates, Inc.

Hartshorn, J. C. (1987). Research-based practice: The need for, use, and reporting of instrument reliability and validity. *Heart & Lung, 16,* 100–101.

Kerlinger, F. N. (1979). *Behavioral research. A conceptual approach* (pp. 107–127, 141–143). New York: Holt, Rinehart & Winston.

Nunnally, J. C. (1978). *Psychometric theory* (2nd ed., pp. 190–255). New York: McGraw-Hill Book Co., Inc.

Pedhazur, E. J. (1982). *Multiple regression in behavioral research. Explanation and prediction* (2nd ed., pp. 34, 230–232, 251–254). New York: Holt, Rinehart & Winston.

Treating Ordinal Scales as Ordinal Scales

Thomas R. Knapp

In a recent article in this journal, Knapp (1990) summarized and tried to resolve the controversy regarding the treatment of ordinal scales as interval scales. He cited Agresti's (1984) book on the analysis of ordinal data as a source of a variety of techniques that have been developed explicitly to handle those bothersome scales that permeate so much of nursing research. The purpose of the present paper is to bring to the attention of nursing researchers a variation of one of the strategies for analyzing ordinal/ordinal relationships that is explained in Agresti's 1984 text and in his later (1990) expansion of that book. Two examples based on hypothetical data in McLaughlin and Marascuilo's (1990) nursing research text will be used for illustrative purposes.

The Examples

In one of the appendices to their book, McLaughlin and Marascuilo (1990) provide an interesting set of data for a hypothetical study of the effect of preoperative teaching on postoperative recovery for a sample of 246 subjects. Included among their variables are three classic ordinal scales: (a) cigarette smoking behavior (never smoked, less than one pack per week, less than one pack per day but more than one pack per week, one or more packs per day); (b) alcohol consumption (never used alcohol, less than one drink per day, more than one drink per day); and (c) severity of illness (mild, moderate, severe). These data provide a basis for a secondary analysis of two research questions: "What is the relationship between cigarette smoking behavior and severity of illness?"; and "What is the relationship between alcohol consumption and severity of illness?" (The relationship between the two independent variables, cigarette smoking behavior and alcohol consumption, is of lesser interest.)

In order to answer the first of those questions, most "liberal" researchers would code the levels of the smoking variable 1, 2, 3, and 4 and the levels of the illness variable 1, 2, and 3; calculate Pearson *r*, and test it for statistical significance ($r = .462$; $p < .001$). They would do the same sort of thing for the second research question ($r = .073$; *NS*).

Most "conservative" researchers would display the data for the first question in a 4×3 contingency table and carry out a chi-square test of the difference between the corresponding obtained and expected frequencies, perhaps accompanied by a calculation of the associated contingency coefficient ($\chi^2 = 71.80$; $df = 6$; $p < .001$; $C = .475$). They would do likewise for the second question ($\chi^2 = 5.33$; $df = 4$; *NS*).

Both approaches are technically incorrect, for opposite reasons. The "liberal" approach endows the two ordinal scales with interval properties that they do not in fact possess. The "conservative" approach deflates the ordinal scales to nominal scales, since neither chi-square nor the contingency coefficient takes into account the inherent order of the row and column categories. (Moses, Emerson, and Hosseini [1984] take clinical investigators to task for their similarly inappropriate analyses of the differences between two groups.)

A more defensible analysis treats both variables as no more than, and no less than, what they are—ordinal. The following discussion is concerned with one such technique based on the work of Williams (1952), Marascuilo and Levin (1983), Goodman (1984), and Agresti (1984, 1990).

The Analysis

This technique involves a (no more than) four-step process:

1. Set up the i x j cross-classification frequency table (contingency table) for the two ordinal variables, where i is the number of categories for the variable that has the larger number of categories and j is the number of categories for the variable that has the smaller number of categories. (If both variables have the same number of categories, it doesn't matter which is chosen as the row variable and which is chosen as the column variable.)

2. Test that table for independence by either the traditional Pearson chi-square statistic or the likelihood-

Thomas R. Knapp, EdD, is professor of nursing and education, The Ohio State University, Columbus, OH.

From *Nursing Research,* May/June 1993, *42,* 184–186.

ratio chi-square statistic, G^2 (the two approaches usually yield very similar results). If chi-square is not significant for some prespecified alpha level, for (i – 1)(j – 1) degrees of freedom, you may be all done. The hypothesis that the variables are unrelated in the population cannot be rejected, and any measure of the degree of relationship between the variables in the sample is of little interest. (If chi-square "just misses" statistical significance and/or if some of the discrepancies between the obtained and expected frequencies are fairly large, especially in the corners of the table, you may want to go on to the next step. (See the example in Agresti [1990], pp. 267–269.)

3. If chi-square *is* significant, use Goodman's (1984) log-linear approach to test the hypothesis that in the population the uniform association model holds, for "scores" of 1 to i for the row variable and "scores" of 1 to j for the column variable. If the associated chi-square for that test is not significant, for (i – 1)(j – 1)–1 degrees of freedom, the equally spaced scores are reasonable choices. Various functions of the local odds ratio (including a Pearson *r* approximation), and their corresponding confidence intervals, can be used to estimate the degree of relationship between the variables in the population from which the sample has been drawn (see Agresti, 1990).

4. If *that* (second) chi-square *is* significant, the uniform association model (equally spaced scores) does not fit the data very well, and the scores to be assigned to the categories of the two ordinal variables need to be estimated from the data, using a procedure that is similar to general-linear-model canonical correlation analysis. Williams (1952) provided the necessary formulas for doing so, and they have been incorporated in Goodman's work. (See also Marascuilo and Levin [1983], pp. 451–460.)

Applications to the Two Hypothetical Examples

The data in McLaughlin and Marascuilo (1990) for testing the relationship between cigarette smoking behavior and severity of illness are:

	Illness		
Smoking	*Mild*	*Moderate*	*Severe*
Never	67	34	7
< Pack/week	33	6	11
< Pack/day	20	19	13
> Pack/day	2	10	24

For these data the Pearson chi-square is 71.80, for $df = 6$. The likelihood-ratio chi-square is 74.96, also for $df = 6$. Both are well beyond the tabled values for the .05, .01, and .001 traditional significance levels (12.59, 16.81, and 22.46, respectively). The independence model therefore does not fit the data very well and the null hypothesis of no relationship in the population is rejected.

But what is the form of the relationship? A test of the goodness-of-fit of Goodman's (1984) uniform association model (see Appendix A for an SPSSX program that can be used to carry out that test) yields a Pearson chi-square of 18.07, for $df = 5$, which is significant at .05 and .01 (but not at .001). Therefore, that model does not fit the data well either, so assigning scores of 1 to 4 for Smoking and 1 to 3 for Illness is not a very good idea.

Williams' (1952) approach involves the calculation of the eigenvalues and eigenvectors of a matrix whose elements are functions of the frequencies in the 4 × 3 cross-tab (see Appendix B). The scores for the Smoking variable that best fit the data are –.74, –.27, .27, and 2.23 (or any nonzero multiplicative transformation thereof). The scores for the Illness variable are –.80, .01, and 1.75 (or, again, any nonzero multiplicative transformation thereof).

The data in McLaughlin and Marascuilo (1990) for testing the relationship between alcohol consumption and severity of illness are:

	Illness		
Alcohol	*Mild*	*Moderate*	*Severe*
Never used	66	30	31
< Drink/day	31	16	14
> Drink/day	25	23	10

For these data the test of independence yields a Pearson chi-square of 5.33, for $df = 4$, which is not statistically significant for any of the usual levels (the tabled value for the .05 level is 9.49), and none of the discrepancies between obtained and expected frequencies are very large. This is sufficient evidence to conclude that the independence model fits the data reasonably well and the null hypothesis of no relationship between Alcohol and Illness cannot be rejected. There is, therefore, little reason to pursue the data any further.

Summary

To investigate the relationship between two ordinal variables, one first tests their independence. If the independence model fits well (nonsignificant chi-square), the variables are said to be unrelated. If the independence model does not fit well (significant chi-square), one then tests for uniform association. If that model fits well (nonsignificant chi-square), the relationship is said to be approximately linear, scores of 1 to i and 1 to j are assigned to the categories of the row and column variables, respectively, and various measures of the direction and the strength of the relationship can be pursued. If that model does *not* fit well (significant chi-square), one uses Williams' method to estimate the scores that should be assigned to the categories of the two variables so that the correlation between them is as high as possible.

APPENDIX A

Goodman's test of uniform association can be carried out by using the log-linear routines in SPSSX or any of the major statistical packages. (You can use BMDP to get a graphical representation of the data through correspondence analysis [Greenacre, 1984].) For SPSSX the following commands are required (the variable names, data, etc. are those of the smoking/illness example in the McLaughlin and Marascuilo text):

```
BEGIN    DATA
1 1       67
1 2       34
1 3        7
2 1       33
2 2        6
2 3       11
3 1       20
3 2       19
3 3       13
4 1        2
4 2       10
4 3       24
END      DATA
DATA LIST LIST/SMOKING ILLNESS COUNT*
VALUE LABELS SMOKING 1 'NEVER'
    2 '<PACK/WEEK'
    3 '<PACK/DAY' 4 '>PACK/DAY'/
    ILLNESS 1 'MILD' 2 'MODERATE' 3 'SEVERE'
WEIGHT BY COUNT
COMPUTE UV = SMOKING* ILLNESS
COMPUTE U = SMOKING
LOG-LINEAR SMOKING(1.4)
    ILLNESS (1,3) WITH UV/
    DESIGN = SMOKING ILLNESS UV/
    PRINT = ESTIM/
FINISH
```

The expected counts on the first full page of output are the expected frequencies, *given that the uniform association model holds.* They are compared to the observed counts, and both the likelihood ratio chi-square and the Pearson chi-square are calculated and provided at the bottom of that same page. There is a "loss" of one additional degree of freedom for estimating those expected counts from the sample data.

APPENDIX B

To apply Williams' procedure for estimating the "scores" that should be assigned to the row and column categories, you must first create a matrix M of the same size as the contingency table, whose elements are the table entries divided by the square root of the product of the corresponding row and column totals. For example, the element in the first row, first column of the M matrix for the Smoking and Illness data is equal to 67 divided by the square root of 122 times 108, i.e., .5837.

Next, a vector V of i elements is created by taking the square root of the quotient of each row total and the sample size. For the Smoking and Illness data, the first element is equal to the square root of 122/246, i.e., .7042. The remaining elements are determined in like manner.

Next, the matrix M is multiplied by its transpose and the eigenvalues and eigenvectors of that matrix product are determined. The *second largest* eigenvalue is the square of the maximum correlation between the two variables. (The largest eigenvalue will always be equal, within rounding error, to 1.) For the Smoking and Illness data, that correlation, *R,* is .5058.

Finally, the scores for the row categories are determined by dividing the elements of the eigenvector associated with the second largest eigenvalue by the corresponding elements of the vector V defined above (they are –.7449, –.2741, .2686, and 2.2275 for the Smoking and Illness data); and the scores for the column categories are determined by dividing each row score by *R,* multiplying those quotients by the corresponding cell frequencies in a given column, summing, and dividing by the column total. For example, the score for the first column category for the Smoking and Illness data is obtained by dividing the –.7749, the –.2741, the .2686, and the 2.2275 by .5058, multiplying *those* by 67, 33, 20, and 2, respectively, summing the four products and dividing that sum by 122. The result is –.7961. The other two column scores are obtained in like manner.

As far as computer packages for Williams' method are concerned, MINITAB can be easily programmed to do all of the calculations, since it has built-in matrix operations. Some of the other packages could be "fooled" into getting the necessary eigenvalues and eigenvectors the same way they get eigenvalues and eigenvectors for factor analyses, discriminant analyses, or canonical correlation analyses.

References

Agresti, A. (1984). *Analysis of ordinal categorical data.* New York: Wiley.

Agresti, A. (1990). *Categorical data analysis.* New York: Wiley.

Goodman, L. (1984). *The analysis of cross-classified data having ordered categories.* Cambridge: Harvard University Press.

Greenacre, M. J. (1984). *Theory and applications of correspondence analysis.* New York: Academic Press.

Knapp, T. R. (1990). Treating ordinal scales as interval scales: An attempt to resolve the controversy. *Nursing Research, 39,* 121–123.

Marascuilo, L. A., & Levin, J. R. (1983). *Multivariate statistics in the social sciences: a researcher's guide.* Monterey, CA: Brooks/Cole.

McLaughlin, F. E., & Marascuilo, L. A. (1990). *Advanced nursing and health care research: Quantification approaches.* Philadelphia: Saunders.

Moses, L. E., Emerson, J. D., & Hosseini, H. (1984). Analyzing data from ordered categories. *New England Journal of Medicine, 311,* 442–448.

Williams, E. J. (1952). Use of scores for the analysis of association in contingency tables. *Biometrika, 39,* 274–289.

Instrumentation in Cross-Cultural Research

Elaine G. Jones ■ **Margarita Kay**

Cross-cultural studies are designed to uncover cultural universals and cultural specifics in human experience. This requires reconciling *emic* concepts with overall *etic* labels. Emic concepts are derived from the culture under study, while etic concepts are derived from the researcher's standard. Goodenough (1963) described the concept of culture as "standards for deciding what is, standards for deciding what can be, standards for deciding how one feels about it, standards for deciding what to do about it, and standards for deciding how to go about doing it" (pp. 258–259). Cultural standards of people are learned by attending to how they talk about the standards (Agar, 1980). Instruments are then devised to reflect those concepts as they are uniquely described by the culture. Group culture may be defined by common ethnicity, language, socioeconomic status, or participation in a particular cultural scene such as jogging, which has its own lingo. The purpose of this article is to propose a systematic approach to preparing quantitative instruments for use in cross-cultural research.

Preliminary Qualitative Studies

The first step in developing instruments for cross-cultural research is to conduct a preliminary qualitative study. To study bereavement in Mexican American widows, it was necessary to develop instruments for use by both Spanish-speaking and English-speaking Mexican Americans. It was necessary to learn the words that the widows themselves used. In a previous study, widows were interviewed in English or Spanish, according to the women's stated language preference. The interviews were audiotaped and transcribed verbatim. The words that described emotional and somatic symptoms associated with bereavement and their emic concepts were drawn from the transcripts and used to design symptom scales (Kay & Portillo, 1989). The words were reviewed by an expert panel, and by 12 widows who were bilingual in English and Spanish.

Elaine G. Jones, PhD, is an assistant professor of family and community health nursing, College of Nursing, the University of Arizona, Tucson, AZ.

Margarita Kay, PhD, RN, is professor emerita, College of Nursing, University of Arizona, Tucson, AZ.

From *Nursing Research*, May/June 1992, *41*, 186–188.

Cross-Cultural Research Goals

An important step in designing a cross-cultural study is identifying the goal of the study as operational or comparative. The goal of the study will guide the translation procedures and interpretation of research findings. The validity of cross-cultural research findings has been compromised in the past when there was a mismatch between the implicit goal of a particular cross-cultural study and the translation strategy used to develop a new language version of the instruments. The underlying error seems to have been in the researchers' assumption that a particular concept was universal and could be indexed with the same test items across cultures simply by translating the original test into a second language. Irvine and Caroll (1980) noted that such practices disregard the distinction between operational use (criterion-referenced meaning) and comparative use (construct-referenced meaning) of the test scores generated.

A classic example of the consequences of failing to distinguish between construct-referenced meaning versus operational use of test scores can be found in the early use of intelligence tests in which scores were considered indexes of inherent intelligence, that is, construct-referenced. Later, the same tests were redefined operationally as correlates of academic abilities or school performance rather than basic intelligence (Anastasi, 1982). The usefulness of distinguishing between construct-referenced and criterion-referenced tests is illustrated by Mindel and Vernon's (1981) comment about early misinterpretation of deaf subjects' test scores: "deaf and hard of hearing people have essentially the same distribution of intelligence as the general population. . . .[however] Educational achievement [of deaf people] stands in sharp contrast with the facts on equal intellectual ability" (p. 87). Explicit identification of the cross-cultural research goal as operational or comparative will guide translation of the quantitative instrument and interpretation of scores.

Developing Instruments in a Target Language

Matching Translation Strategy to the Study Goals

Werner and Campbell (1970) defined two categories of translation: symmetrical (or decentered) and asymmetrical (or unicentered). The goal of symmetrical translation is loyalty of meaning and equal familiarity and colloquiality in each language. A symmetrical translation includes test items common to both (or all) the cultures under study. Symmetrical translation involves supralinguistic translation of cultural symbols and is essential when the study goal is comparative. If a test is specific to one of the cultures, it must be replaced with an item that references the construct in both cultures. Judgments about the cultural relevance of test items must be based on thorough familiarity with both cultures and results of preliminary qualitative work.

A potential problem with symmetrical translation arises when the original instrument has a history of use in the original language and has sound psychometric properties, and the researcher is unwilling to tamper with the content of the original items as they are translated (Chapman & Carter, 1979). The researcher must be aware that enhancing the validity of a comparative study through symmetrical translation may compromise reliabilities because some items on the original instrument may require changes to achieve conceptual equivalence across cultures.

Asymmetrical translation emphasizes loyalty to one language, usually the source (original) language (Werner & Campbell, 1970). Asymmetrical translation is most appropriate for cross-cultural studies with operational goals. Asymmetrical translation often results in a translated version that seems exotic and unnatural in the new language, though the target language version is faithful to the original text. If the goal of testing is to measure responses of one culture against responses of another culture in a situation specific to one of the cultures, then asymmetrical translation is the appropriate method.

Translation Procedures

Researchers often hire a single bilingual person to perform a translation or, if the researcher is bilingual, the researcher may personally develop the translated instrument. These approaches always call into question the quality of the translation and, therefore, the validity of the study findings. Back translation is appropriate, whether the research goals are comparative or operational, once the content of the items has been established. In addition, the back translation procedures should be applied to the test instructions as well as the items themselves.

The preferred translation procedures involve use of panels of experts and multiple interpreters who engage in multistage back translation procedures (Werner & Campbell 1970). The panel of experts and the interpreters should include (a) professional interpreters, (b) lay people who are monolingual and representative of the populations under study, (c) people who are bilingual with the source language as their first language, and (d) people who are bilingual with the target language as their first language.

The most common and highly recommended procedure for translating an instrument from the source language to the target language is back translation (Brislin, 1970; Chapman & Carter, 1979). In back translation, two interpreters are used. One translates the first half into the target language, the other the second half. The interpreters then switch positions and translate the words of one another back into English. The investigator ends with two versions in English, and through them a triangulation onto the target language version (Werner & Campbell, 1970).

For example, in a study of deaf parents (Jones, 1986; Jones, Strom & Daniels, 1989) two sign language interpreters were each assigned to translate half the items from written English into American Sign Language. One interpreter was bilingual, with American Sign Language as her first language (her parents were deaf), and American Sign Language was a second language for the second professional interpreter. After the investigator and interpreters discussed the items that did not seem equivalent on either the English or the sign language versions, changes were made and the back translation process repeated until the investigator and the interpreters were satisfied that the English and signed versions were equivalent. In addition, deaf parents critiqued the translations at each stage of the translation process.

Translation of rating scales can present another kind of challenge. Subjects in the widows' study responded to questionnaires with several Likert scales (Kay & Portillo, 1989). Because the use of five degrees of difference was difficult for the subjects, who always chose the middle, neutral point, the scale was reduced to four degrees. The anchoring points were not translated literally. Rather, everyday Spanish was used to roughly represent the semantic distance of the original English rating scale. For example, the meaning of *bastante* (enough) corresponded more closely to the English word "moderately" than did *moderamente* (moderately), the literal translation (Fernandez Esquer, 1990).

Test-Related Factors

The last step in developing a target language version of the original instrument is pilot testing. Pilot testing the translated instrument with members of the target culture serves as a check not only for the quality of the translation, but also for practical aspects of test administration. Cultural differences may extend to the subject's test-related skills and methods of test administration, as well as to the actual test content.

Failure to consider test-related factors in cross-cultural research can lead to significant errors in interpreting test results, even if the researcher has been meticulous in developing a sound target language version of the instrument.

Determining Psychometric Properties

Although the emphasis in this article is on preparation of quantitative instruments for use in cross-cultural study, the assumption is that the study design includes qualitative as well as quantitative data (Mitchell, 1986). Whether the qualitative data is used in triangulation or for assessing validity, the concern is with correspondence of findings across methods.

Comparison of psychometric properties of the quantitative source and target language instruments provides additional data for assessing equivalence of both versions of the instrument. Most commonly, claims for adequacy of translation are based on finding similarity in reliability, validity, and factor structure for the forms in both languages (Werner & Campbell, 1970). The ideal means of comparing the psychometric properties of the source and target language versions of the instrument is to administer both versions to persons fluent in both languages (Chapman & Carter, 1979) during pilot testing. Total scores of the bilingual subjects on the two versions of the measure should demonstrate a high correlation across forms. Correlation of total scores on two forms of the questionnaire should be followed with item analysis. Simple correlation of total scores may hide inconsistencies within individual item translations (Jones, 1987). In addition, item analysis may indicate that specific items perform differently on the two forms. Additional comparisons should be made in terms of reliability coefficients. According to Nunnally (1978), the target language version can be treated like a new instrument. Therefore, an alpha of .70 may be considered adequate.

Evaluation of the conceptual equivalency of the two versions of the instrument can be assessed through comparison of factor structure if there are sufficient numbers of subjects. As an alternate, cluster analysis can be performed when there are insufficient numbers for factor analysis (Jones, 1987; Romesburg, 1984).

Ensuring Validity

Validity issues are at the heart of any discussion about interpreting the findings of cross-cultural research. The most common cause of inaccurate representation of subjects in cross-cultural research is failure to recognize the difference in interpreting results of cross-cultural studies with operational versus comparative goals. Clarification of research goals, preliminary qualitative work, appropriate translation strategies, and interpreting results consistent with the study goal can contribute to a stronger research foundation for improved understanding of people from various cultures.

References

Agar, M. H. (1980). *The professional stranger.* New York: Academic Press.

Anastasi, I. (1982). *Psychological testing,* (5th ed.). New York: Macmillan.

Brislin, R. W. (1970). Back-translation for cross-cultural research. *Journal of Cross-cultural Psychology, 1,* 185–216.

Chapman, D. W., & Carter, J. F. (1979). Translation procedures for the cross-cultural use of measurement. *Educational Evaluation and Policy Analysis, 1*(3), 71–76.

Fernandez Esquer, M. E. (1990). Cultural issues relevant to instrument development and administration for Mexican American Widows. In *The efficacy of support groups for Mexican American widows* (SIROW Working Paper No. 25, p. 40). Tucson, AZ: Women's Studies, University of Arizona.

Goodenough, W. H. (1963). *Cooperation in change.* New York: Russell Sage Foundation.

Irvine, S. H., & Caroll, W. K. (1980). Testing and assessment across cultures: Issues in methodology and theory. In H. C. Triandis & J. W. Berry (eds.), *Handbook of cross-culture psychology: Methodology* (vol. 2, pp. 181–244). Boston: Allyn and Bacon.

Jones, E. (1986). *Deaf adults as parents.* Unpublished doctoral dissertation, University of Arizona, College of Nursing, Tucson.

Jones, E. (1987). Translation of quantitative measures for use in cross-cultural research. *Nursing Research, 36,* 324–327.

Jones, E., Strom, R., & Daniels, S. (1989). Evaluating the success of deaf parents. *American Annals of the Deaf,* 332–336.

Kay, M., & Portillo, C. (1989). Depression and grief in Mexican American widows. *Health Care for Women International, 11,* 273–293.

Mindel, E., & Vernon, M. (1981). *They grow in silence.* Silver Spring, MD: National Association for the Deaf.

Mitchell, E. S. (1986). Multiple triangulation: A methodology for nursing science. *Advances in Nursing Science,* 18–26.

Nunnally, J. (1978). Psychometric Theory. New York: McGraw-Hill.

Romesburg, H. C. (1984). *Cluster analysis for researchers.* Belmont, CA: Lifetime Learning Publications.

Werner, L., & Campbell, D. T. (1970). Translating, working through interpreters and the problem of decentering. In R. Naroll & R. Cohen (eds.), *American Handbook of methods in Cultural Anthropology* (pp. 398–420). Garden City, NY: Natural History Press.

Standardization of the Visual Analogue Scale

Margaret E. Cline ■ **JoAnne Herman** ■ **Elizabeth R. Shaw** ■ **R. Donald Morton**

Much current nursing research is focused on the measurement of subjective feelings, perceptions, sensations, and symptoms. The visual analogue scale (VAS) has become a commonly used instrument for the measurement of these subjective feelings because it is easy to administer, simple for the subject to understand, and can be a valid method for measuring subjective feelings that yield interval level data (Edwards, Herman, Wallace, Pavy & Pavy, 1991; Gift, 1989; Lee & Kieckhefer, 1989). Operationally, the VAS is a vertical or horizontal line, 100 mm in length, anchored by terms that represent the extremes of the subjective phenomenon the researcher wishes to measure. Subjects are asked to indicate the intensity of a sensation by placing a line across the VAS at a point that represents the intensity of the sensation at that moment in time. Responses are scored by measuring the distance from the lowest anchor point to the subject's mark across the line.

The VAS has been used both in descriptive and experimental research to measure phenomena such as pain, anxiety, nausea, fatigue, dyspnea, and hunger (Carrieri, Janson-Bjerklie & Jacobs, 1984; Edwards et al., 1991; Gift, 1991; Gift, Plaut & Jacox, 1986). While literature about the general psychometric properties of the VAS is available, there is little literature that describes the technical construction of the VAS. In addition, the VAS has been used most frequently with chronically ill populations, not critically ill patients. The purposes of this article are to describe the construction of a VAS, describe the technical aspects of duplicating the VAS, and outline the procedure for producing a scoring template.

Margaret E. Cline, MS, RN, is a colonel in the U.S. Army Nurse Corps. She is currently a doctoral candidate, College of Nursing, University of South Carolina, Columbia, SC.

JoAnne Herman, PhD, RN, is the associate dean, research and evaluation, College of Nursing, University of South Carolina, Columbia, SC.

Elizabeth R. Shaw, MSN, RNC, is a doctoral candidate, College of Nursing, University of South Carolina, Columbia, SC.

R. Donald Morton, MA, is the media arts specialist, College of Nursing, University of South Carolina, Columbia, SC.

From *Nursing Research,* November/December 1992, *41,* 378–380.

Construction of the VAS

The need for a VAS that could be used with critically ill subjects grew out of a project to measure anxiety in patients maintained on ventilators. These subjects had short attention spans, were under stress, had restricted movement, and generally had poor vision. Because of these characteristics, a number of decisions needed to be made about the construction of the VAS.

First, the VAS line was oriented vertically. Research findings have indicated that the vertical line is more sensitive and easier for patients to use, especially for those under stress with a narrowed visual field (Gift, 1989; Gift et al., 1986). Second, a 1/2 inch perpendicular line was placed at each end of the VAS, since Edwards and Herman (1988) found that subjects marked off the scale, unless perpendicular lines were present. Third, no intermediate marks, gradations, or terms were placed on the VAS line since Gift (1989) argued that using gradations decreased sensitivity, imposed another's language on the subject, and required a higher reading level. The short attention span of the critically ill subjects was another reason to avoid a complex VAS. The words selected to anchor the VAS in this particular study were "not nervous at all" and "the most nervous I have ever been."

The Macintosh IIci computer, a high-resolution color monitor (M0401), and the Claris-MacDraw II (Version 1.1) software were used to construct the 100 mm vertical line. The software has a selection of rulers that appear as grids on the monitor and allow exact measurement on several scales, including millimeter. Accuracy of the 100 mm was obtained using the software's zoom feature that allows magnification of 3,600%. Claris-MacDraw II (Version 1.1) has the capability to measure the length of a line and provide that measure to the user to an accuracy of .001 mm.

The program is very versatile, allowing the user to lock parts together and visualize the entire page and quickly move or change items on that page. Several possible alternatives for line width, shadings, fonts, size of anchor words, position of the line on the page, placement of additional markings, and other ways to make the VAS easy to see were previewed using these program options. Changes in line widths did produce some distortion in line length, which could be easily managed once identified. Figure 1 displays the final VAS.

The VAS line and verbal anchors were enclosed in a lightly shaded box to contrast with the rest of the page and help the subjects focus on the VAS. The size of the letters in the anchor words were varied to highlight the term of interest. The verbal anchors were set in bold type and capitalized to stand out. The box and VAS were positioned in the top half of the 8 1/2″ × 11″ paper. The VAS could then be placed on a clipboard and angled for appropriate viewing by a subject in bed with limited movement. Once the VAS was completed, all the parts were locked and saved as a unit.

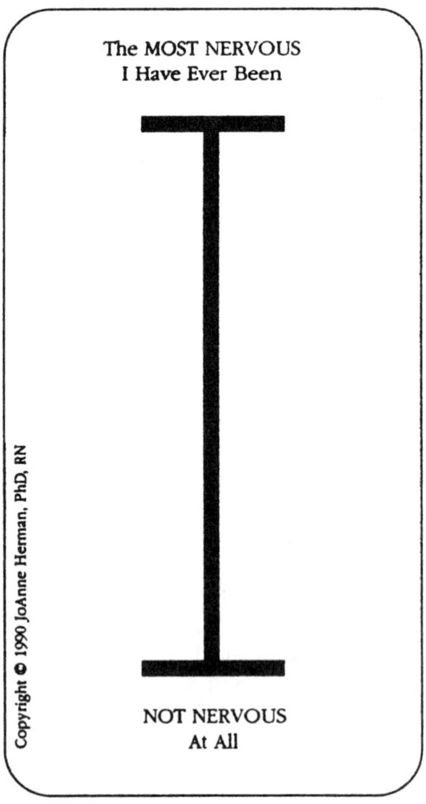

FIGURE 1 The Visual Analogue Scale

Construction of the Scoring Template

The original VAS image was copied onto a new file to create a scoring template. The MacDraw features allowed duplication of two exact copies of the 100 mm VAS and perpendicular anchor lines. These two lines were placed parallel, and the anchor lines were connected. The resulting rectangle was centered in the shaded box. Therefore, the original VAS fell between the two parallel images of the template when the overlay was positioned for scoring.

Using high magnification and the millimeter grid, a series of thin horizontal lines were added to the template at 2 mm intervals from 2 to 98 mm (Figure 2). These horizontal lines resembled rungs on a ladder and extended slightly beyond the bolder vertical lines. The numerical values were placed on alternate lines for easy reading. Once all portions of the lines were even and exact, shading of the surrounding box was reversed, making the box on the template clear rather than shaded. Finally, the parts of the template were locked, saved as a unit, and printed using the laser printer. Reproduction of the template to a transparency was done using the Xerox Model 5090 copier.

To score the VAS, the template is positioned over the subject's VAS and aligned using the three structural and visual references: the box that frames the VAS line, the perpendicular anchor lines, and the reverse shading effect. The multiple reference points make alignment easy and accurate. The subject's mark can be seen through the template and the score can be read using the horizontal rungs and the template scale.

Reproduction of the VAS

Once completed, the VAS was printed using a high-quality, clay-surfaced white paper in the Apple LaserWriter II. The contrast of white and black with the lightly shaded area was sharp and clear.

The VAS was also reproduced using the Xerox Model 5090 copier. The copier specifications state that reproduction of images is 100%. Numerous copies were measured with both a millimeter ruler and the template and found to be true reproductions. Both Gift (1989) and Lee and Kieckhefer (1989) stated that photocopying the VAS resulted in a distortion of the line. However, the current availability of photocopiers with 100% reproduction capability, instead of the former 101%, makes photocopying a cost-effective alternative. Using this option, the VAS consistently measured 100 mm from the outside edge of the lower anchor line to the outside edge of the upper anchor line.

While the image size is reproduced at 100%, it is impossible to prevent some movement of the total image on

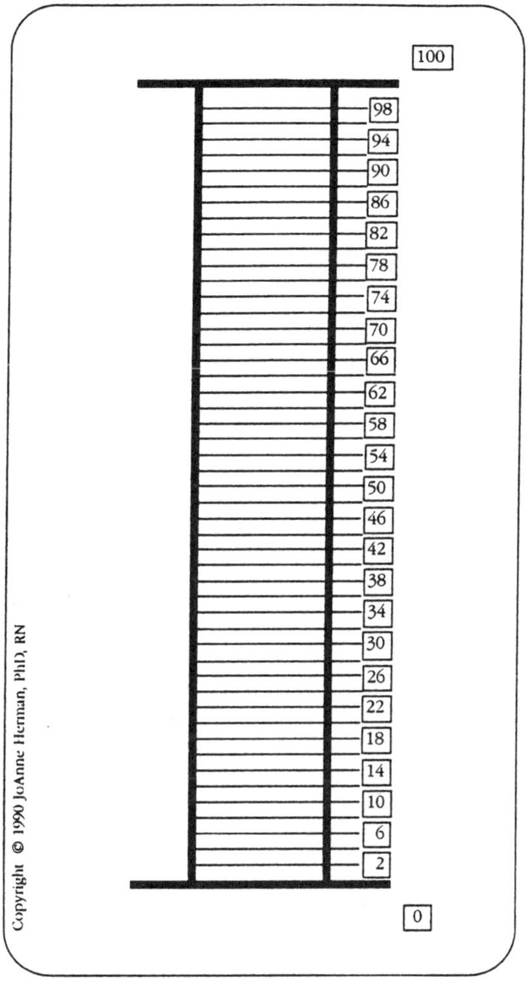

FIGURE 2 Scoring Template of the Visual Analogue Scale

the page during photocopying. Therefore, reference points such as the box around the VAS line and the perpendicular anchor lines should always be included on the VAS, because page edges will not be reliable reference points.

This particular VAS is visually appealing, easy to read, and structured to focus attention on the salient content. The scoring template constructed from the same file as the VAS ensures that the VAS line and the scoring template are exact duplicates. The structural and visual cues on the VAS allow for exact placement of the template and reliable measurement.

References

Carrieri, V. K., Janson-Bjerklie, S., & Jacobs, S. (1984). The sensation of dyspnea. *Heart Lung, 13,* 436–446.

Edwards, J. N., & Herman, J. A. (1988). The effectiveness of patient controlled antiemetic therapy in patients receiving chemotherapy. *South Carolina Nurse, 3*(1), 22.

Edwards, J. N., Herman, J. A., Wallace, B. K., Pavy, M.D., & Pavy, J. (1991). Comparison of patient controlled and nurse controlled anti-emetic therapy in patients receiving chemotherapy. *Research in Nursing and Health, 14,* 249–257.

Gift, A. (1989). Visual analogue scales: Measurement of subjective phenomena. *Nursing Research, 38,* 286–288.

Gift, A. (1991). Psychologic and physiologic aspects of acute dyspnea in asthmatics. *Nursing Research, 40,* 196–199.

Gift, A. G., Plaut, D. M., & Jacox, A. K. (1986). Psychologic and physiologic factors related to dyspnea in subjects with chronic obstructive pulmonary disease. *Heart and Lung, 15,* 595–601.

Lee, K. A., & Kieckhefer, G. M. (1989). Measuring human responses using visual analogue scales. *Western Journal of Nursing Research, 11,* 128–132.

PART SIX

Special Analytic Techniques

Meta-Analysis

Alice I. O'Flynn

Glass (1976) outlined three levels of analysis: primary analysis, secondary analysis, and meta-analysis. *Primary analysis* is the original analysis of data. This level is commonly found in research journals, reported by the primary investigators. *Secondary analysis* is a re-analysis of data aimed at (1) answering the original research question, often bringing to bear more sophisticated or better statistical techniques or (2) using old data to answer new questions. *Meta-analysis* is the integration of findings, the analysis of analyses using statistical approaches.

There are a variety of techniques available that fall under the rubric of meta-analysis; all generate different solutions. We will consider the following: (1) the overall significance/ probability of pooled data from combined studies, (2) the average effect size across studies, and (3) the interactions or relationships between variables. One or more techniques may be applied to a particular set of data. Rosenthal (1978) suggests that more than one of these meta-analytic approaches be applied to the data.

Overall Probability of Pooled Data

Finding a single grand conclusion may be the primary goal. The question is do all the studies in concert support or reject the hypothesis? To quantitatively make this judgment, the reviewer adds the level of significance for each statistic and derives an overall z score, which is the normal standard deviate. To derive this overall probability, ts, Fs, or χ^2 may be used. Rosenthal (1978) described how to convert one statistic to another in order to combine them. Pillemer and Light (1980, p. 184) write that "the z's are added across studies, and their sum is divided by the square root of the number of studies that are combined. The probability value associated with the resulting overall score provides the level of significance for the combined statistical test."

Alice I. O'Flynn, PhD, RN, is an assistant professor at the Medical College of Georgia, School of Nursing, Augusta, GA.

From *Nursing Research,* September/October 1982, *31,* 314–316.

The advantage to this form of meta-analysis is its computational ease and low informational requirement. The "how to's" are demonstrated in detail by Glass (1976, 1978), McGaw and Glass (1980), and Rosenthal (1978). It is important for the reviewer to ascertain that the support for the hypothesis goes in the same direction in each case. If the hypothesis is consistent with most of the other hypotheses, the value will be given a (+) positive value. However, if the results are not consistent, for example, if the control group outperforms the experimental group a (–) negative value is assigned. This is easily understood as a principle of reverse scoring.

If a reviewer is examining the hypothesis that husband-coached labor results in a shorter duration of labor, all the studies that reported findings consistent with this statement would be assigned a (+) plus and study findings that indicated a longer labor time would be assigned a (–) minus. The important principle is consistence in the assignment of positive versus negative support of the hypothesis.

In a hypothetical example, five studies were performed to assess the effectiveness of cognitive strategies used to improve dietary intake in low nutritional status populations. All the studies derived a t statistic and in all except Study Five the cognitive strategy group scored higher than the control. Note the negative value assigned to the t statistic for the fifth study (Table 1).

The resulting z using the z table is compared at the degrees of freedom for the combined studies, in this case $df = 300$ and the probability of this value of z occurring by chance is $p < .004$.

In the preceding example, the studies were weighted equally. However, there may be a rationale for differentially weighting studies according to some criterion, such as sample size, power, judgment of validity, research design, and so forth. When weighting is desired, this is accomplished by first computing a z statistic for each study and multiplying the z by the assigned weight (w). The w may be a function of the N of the study or some other logical system devised by the reviewer.

TABLE 1 **Five Hypothetical Studies of Strategies to Improve Dietary Intake in Low Nutritional Populations**

Study	t	df	$df/(df-2)$
1	3.08	40	1.0526
2	1.40	20	1.1111
3	.82	30	1.0714
4	1.46	190	1.0106
5	−.65	20	1.1111
Sum	6.11	300	5.3568

The Formula for z:

$$z = \frac{\Sigma t}{\sqrt{\Sigma(df/df-2)}} = \frac{6.11}{\sqrt{5.3568}} = \frac{6.11}{2.3144} = 2.6399$$

NOTE: z = a standard normal deviate
t = the sum of the tx
$\Sigma\,(df/df\!-\!2)$ = the sum of each study's degrees of freedom divided by the degrees of freedom minus 2.

The sum of the weighted z scores is divided by the square root of the sum of the squared weights.

$$\text{Weighted } z = \frac{W_i z}{\sqrt{W^2 i}}$$

Where W_i are the weights for each study.

An overall probability or overall significance is important and paramount in deciding if something is significant or not. Yet statistical significance does not answer all the questions raised in a review. To understand if a treatment, intervention, or program really makes a difference, the researcher may be more interested in the effect size (ES). Average effect size is an estimate of the practical significance or average size of treatment effect. "An average effect size provides a single summary value for an entire area of study" (Pillemer and Light, 1980, p. 185).

A study may indicate a statistically significant difference due to a large N in the study, but if this only means a change of a few raw score points—dollars, hospital days, or whatever the outcome measure is—what difference does this make? As a summary statistic, ES is commonly thought of as a measure, in standard deviation units, of degree of departure from the null hypothesis and is defined as the difference between the means of the two groups in the outcome divided by the pooled within-group standard deviation (Hall, 1978). This statistic is valid and valuable, especially when the outcomes (dependent measures) are normally distributed. Calculation is simple when means and standard deviations are reported. The formula for ES is:

$$ES = \frac{\overline{X}_e - \overline{X}_c}{S}$$

ES is the effect size; $\overline{X}_e$ is the means for experimental group; $\overline{X}_c$ means for control group; S is the within-group SD.

There may be more than one outcome measure per study and each one may be used to derive an effect size. For instance, a study may have more than one dependent (outcome) measure or it may have a single dependent variable measured repeated. Each can be used as an estimate of effect size. In the 375 psychotherapy studies examined by Smith and Glass (1977), 833 effect sizes were estimated for a variety of outcome measures ranging from behavior change to scores on rating scales. Effect size can be thought of as a common metric because it is based upon standard deviations from the mean. Effect size scores are related directly to the changes resulting from treatment, interpretable and reliable (McGaw and Glass, 1980). For instance, an effect size of 1 would indicate that the experimental group's average score was one standard deviation better than the control group's average score in terms of an outcome. In other words, the experimental group's mean score was 34% higher than the control group's mean score.

The effect size is akin to the standard deviation unit. Therefore, it is important to conceptualize the normal curve (Figure 1). Smith and Glass (1977) and Smith, Glass, and Miller (1980) found that psychotherapy resulted in .68 superiority (.68 SD) in terms of average effect size for the experimental group, that is, the treatment group moved on the average to the 75 percentile on the outcome measure. This improvement as a result of psychotherapy is impressive, considering that some circles believe that therapy is a waste of time and being on a waiting list has the same effect as being in treatment. The merit of using ES in evaluating programs and procedures seems to have potential for aiding policy makers in decision-making. Average ES may be used to study

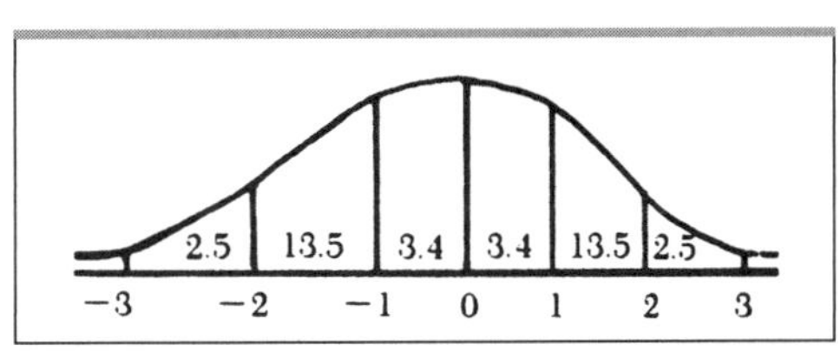

FIGURE 1 The Normal Curve

relationships between variables in the same way as a correlation analysis. (ES as dependent variable and another variable as the independent variable.)

Averaging Effect Sizes

The formula when means and standard deviations are given is:

$$ES = \frac{\overline{X}_e - \overline{X}_c}{S}$$

with ES equaling the effect size; $\overline{X}_e$ the means for experimental group; $\overline{X}_c$ the means for control group; and S is the within-group *SD*.

After ES is calculated for each study, the ESs are averaged across the studies. The effect of birth education classes on attitude toward spouse's coping ability was investigated in six studies (Table 2).

An average effect size of .61 indicates that the average spouse's attitude (coping ability) improved from, on average, the 50th percentile in the control group to the 72 percentile. In this example the studies were weighted equally.

The Form of the Relationship

The two procedures outlined above aggregate sets of data into a cohesive whole. In some situations, it is beneficial to search for variation or discrepancies in results in order to explain them.

Smith and Glass (1977) used ES as the dependent variable and developed 16 independent variables coded from various features of the psychotherapy studies. Their independent variables included duration of therapy, group vs. individual therapy, therapist's experience, age of client, and many others. They performed numerous regression analyses on these features. From the results they predicted outcomes of therapy and/ or which variables accounted for most of the variance in outcome.

Regression technique provided the vehicle for the investigation of similarities and differences. The discovery and explanation of differences is a valuable part of the synthesis process. Knowing why, for instance, a weight program works in one situation and fails in another aids in developing theories and hypotheses worthy of testing. Investigating atypical responses to treatment is fertile ground. Perhaps the treatments were dissimilar or the interaction with other variables caused the difference. Single studies may not provide sufficient data to examine relationships. However, synthesizing multiple studies can pave the way for these investigations.

TABLE 2 A Hypothetical Averaging Effect Size from Six Studies

Study	*df*	ES
1	38	.68
2	21	.38
3	18	.57
4	54	.74
5	84	.52
6	10	.81
	225	3.70

$$\text{ES (Average Effect Size)} = \frac{\Sigma \text{ES}}{\text{N}}$$

$$\text{ES} = \frac{3.70}{6}$$

$$= .6166$$

NOTE: ΣES = Sum of Es_s; *N* = Number of studies.

Limitations

It is unwise to apply any technique without being aware of its limitations. Harrop (1980) cautioned us not to abuse these techniques and assume they answer all review or synthesis types of questions. Some tend to overuse meta-analysis and develop "metamegaly." A continued critical appraisal of all studies, including those performed within the framework of meta-analysis, is warranted.

In meta-analysis, the spirit is to engender graphs, tables, and figures. With this method much of the contextual richness of the qualitative approach is lost. Meta-analysts lack the firsthand experience of the primary research team. Therefore, researchers may not have an adequate grasp of the actual treatment or program under investigation. Rosenthal (1978, 1979) commented on another problem referred to as the "file drawer." Some journals have a predilection for publishing studies with significant findings. This is compounded by the fact that novice researchers often fail to submit manuscripts to editors when the analysis reveals nonsignificant results. Findings that are nonsignificant and unpublished often end up in the file drawers. Rosenthal states that, "the fundamental idea in coping with the file drawer problem is simply to calculate the number of studies averaging null results that must be in the file drawer before the overall probability of Type I error is brought to any desired level of significance, say, $p = .05$" (Rosenthal, 1979, p. 639). As the number of meta-analysis studies increases, the file drawer hypothesis can be safely ruled out. Rosenthal's example is that if 300 studies have an average z of + 1, it would take 32,960 studies hidden, filed, or thrown out to bring the probability level below significance.

Recommendations and Implications

In terms of meta-analysis and practical significance, journals should report the means and standard deviations or the effect sizes of studies. This information, so basic to research reporting, is often lacking. Glass (1977). Rosenthal (1978), and Judd and Kenny (1983) provide examples of how to transform data into effect sizes and other common metrics. Editors need to become more open to publishing secondary and meta-analyses.

Meta-analysis should be viewed as exploratory and explanatory research, depending upon the questions asked. Findings can be placed on computer disks. Then the meta-analyst can simply acquire the disks and use the appropriate studies. As researchers become more familiar with sharing results, the body of nursing knowledge will increase proportionately.

Before undertaking a meta-analysis, the researcher needs to be very familiar with the topic under study. The decision as to whether meta-analysis is appropriate within a certain area must be made. For instance, are there sufficient studies to warrant a meta-analysis? Perhaps the primary needs are for replications, new instruments or procedures, or for secondary analyses. Even if a meta-analysis is performed, that does not necessarily indicate that every issue has been effectively handled in a particular area. Meta-analysis is an extremely efficient approach to the integration of studies and when appropriately used will expedite nursing's future endeavors.

References

Glass, G. V. Primary, secondary, and meta-analysis of research. *Educ Res* 10:3–8, 1976.

Glass, G. V. Integrating findings. The meta-analysis of research. *Rev Res Educ* 5:351–379, 1977.

Hall, J. A. Gender effects in decoding nonverbal cues? *Psychol Bull* 85:845–857, 1978.

Harrop, J. W. *A Meta-Review of Meta-Analysis of Psychotherapy Outcome Research.* Kingston, University of Rhode Island, 1980. (Unpublished paper)

Judd, C. M., and Kenny, D. A. *Design and Analysis of Social Research in Applied Settings.* New York, Cambridge University Press, Chap. 10, 1983.

McGaw, B., and Glass, G. V. Choice of metric for effect size in meta-analysis. *Am Educ Res J* 17(3):325–337, 1980.

Pillemer, D. B., and Light, R. J. Synthesizing outcomes: How to use research evidence from many studies. *Harvard Edu Rev* 50, 1980.

Rosenthal, R. Combining results of independent studies. *Psychol Bull* 85(1): 185–193, 1978.

Rosenthal, R. The file drawer problem and tolerance for null results. *Psychol Bull* 86(3):638–641, 1979.

Smith, M., and Glass, G. V. Meta-analysis of psychotherapy outcome studies. *Am Psychol* 32:752–757, Sept. 1977.

Smith, M. L., Glass, G. V., and Miller. *Benefits of Psychotherapy.* Baltimore, Johns Hopkins University Press, 1980.

Measurement of Quality of Primary Studies for Meta-Analysis

Sharon A. Brown

As a method for making sense out of conflicting research data, meta-analysis can be a critical step between individual studies and application of findings to practice (Massey & Loomis, 1988). In the future, meta-analysis will be used more extensively to build a body of knowledge, particularly knowledge that is applicable to clinical practice. Consequently, it is imperative that meta-analytic procedures and issues be clarified, so that nurse researchers use the method accurately and appropriately.

Meta-analysis has been somewhat controversial since it became popular in the early 1980s. While the rigor of meta-analyses has improved, one important question that has consistently emerged is what to do about the variability in quality of the original studies (Cooper, 1984). Conflicting results from a group of studies of the same phenomenon may be artifactual, and variability in the quality of the primary studies may contribute to inconclusive and conflicting findings (Hunter & Schmidt, 1990; Hunter, Schmidt & Jackson, 1982). The purposes of this article are to review briefly the issue of research quality and its effects on research outcomes and to propose a method for measuring research quality specifically for meta-analysis.

Effects of Research Quality on Study Outcomes

Some meta-analysts have suggested that only superior studies should be included in research synthesis; however, how does one decide what criteria to use as indicators of a "superior" study? And, if superior studies are identified, what does one do with the poorer studies? Omission of all but superior studies could reduce considerably the available database for meta-analytic efforts. Glass, McGraw, and Smith (1981) stated that "many weak studies can add up to a strong conclusion" (p. 221). Perhaps by pooling a group of studies and thus increasing sample size, increased power could overwhelm some of the methodological flaws.

Sharon A. Brown, PhD, RN, is associate professor and associate dean for research, School of Nursing, The University of Texas Health Science Center-Houston, Houston, TX.

From *Nursing Research,* November/December 1991, *40,* 352–355.

Quality has not been shown to alter significantly effect size estimates, at least not in a linear fashion (Rosenthal, 1984; Brown, 1990b). Rosenthal cites a study of differences in effect-size estimates based on quality of primary studies in which well-designed studies produced larger effect sizes than both poor and intermediate studies. McCain and Lynn (1990) reported moderate mean effect sizes for studies of excellent quality, while studies of lower quality produced effects not significantly different from zero.

Brown (1990b) also found no linear relationship between quality and weighted effect sizes in a meta-analysis of studies conducted on effectiveness of diabetes patient education. In this study, attrition as a threat to internal validity of studies was the only quality indicator found to be significantly and negatively correlated with outcome effect sizes ($r = -.52$, $p = .002$). In a recent secondary analysis of these data, collapsed into two categories of low and high quality, no consistent pattern was found across outcome variables based on quality; however, higher quality studies produced larger effects for weight loss and lower effects for metabolic control. An interesting result was that low quality studies produced the only 95% confidence intervals containing zero, specifically for weight loss and psychological outcomes (Brown, 1990a). While there may be few consistent differences in magnitude of effect sizes based on quality, more variability in effect sizes may occur in poorly designed studies as compared to those that are well designed (Wolf, 1986).

The current approach to addressing the research quality issue appears to be to measure quality whenever conducting a meta-analysis and to determine if differences exist between poor and good studies. Further, an attempt should be made to demonstrate whether quality of primary studies affects relationships between variables of interest, such as treatment type, diagnosis, and effect sizes (Mintz, 1983). In other words, threats to the internal and external validity of the studies as well as characteristics that might produce inadequacy should be coded and characteristics should be tested as moderator variables (Hunter et al., 1982).

Measuring Research Quality of Primary Studies for Meta-Analysis

Most researchers agree that meta-analyses should include some type of quality measure or results cannot be "meaningfully utilized" (Lynn, 1989; Mullen & Ramirez, 1987; Wolf, 1986; Cooper, 1984). Sacks et al. (1987) found in reviewing meta-analyses (a meta-meta-analysis) that only 19% fully addressed the quality issue, and 53% did not mention quality of primary studies at all. To increase assessment of research quality in meta-analyses, a rigorous yet realistic method of measuring quality must be developed.

A number of instruments to measure research quality are described in the literature, some of which were designed specifically for measuring research quality of primary studies included in meta-analyses (McCain & Lynn, 1990; Smith, 1988). Many instruments are quite lengthy and measure long lists of study characteristics thought to be potential threats to the adequacy and validity of studies. Reported interclass correlations for quality rating schema ranged from $r = .19$ (Cicchetti & Eron, 1979) to $r = .54$ (Scarr & Weber, 1978); intercoder agreement for a 68-item instrument ranged from $r = .75$ to $r = .83$ (Smith, 1988). A shorter quality rating scale reported by McCain and Lynn (1990) was found to have a reliability of .66, using Pearson's correlation coefficient calculated on two raters' scores.

Some authors suggest using Campbell and Stanley's (1963) list of threats to internal and external validity and coding studies for presence or absence of these threats (Cooper, 1984). Many lists have been generated for this purpose; however, the threats have not been weighted with regard to the seriousness of the influence of individual threats on study outcomes. And, in many cases, the "elegance of rating schema often exceeds the availability of information reported in the primary studies" (Mullen & Ramirez, 1987, p. 217). Therefore, while it may be that measuring research quality of primary studies in meta-analyses is necessary, it is not clear how to accomplish the task reliably and realistically.

A Meta-Analytic Example

Two meta-analyses have been conducted by this author to evaluate studies of effectiveness of diabetes patient education. The first study (Brown, 1988), incorporated Duffy's (1985) Research Appraisal Checklist (RAC) accompanied by operational definitions of Campbell and Stanley's (1963) threats to validity. The RAC was selected because it was similar to other research quality instruments recommended for use in meta-analyses and more importantly, reliability and validity had been established. The RAC contained 51 criteria listed under eight categories. Each criterion was evaluated on a six-point Likert-type scale, from 1 (*not met*) to 6 (*fully met*), for a total of 306 possible points.

The process of evaluating the quality of the 47 studies included in the first meta-analysis was difficult, particularly in evaluating threats to validity. An interrater reliability level of $r = .89$ was achieved; however, this level of reliability required four months of training and practice. Furthermore, results of quality ratings did not agree with raters' intuitive perceptions of study quality, which were generally considerably lower than total scores indicated. The correlation between total RAC scores and total number of threats to validity was near zero ($r = .03$, $p = .85$), indicating that each method, RAC and number of threats, was measuring a different construct.

Two major validity concerns arose during quality assessment. First, each criterion was equally weighted on the RAC and the list of threats to validity. Consequently, on the RAC clarity of a title contributed as much to the total quality score as did an adequate sample size. Certainly, sample size poses more of a threat to study quality than does the title.

A second major concern was whether the RAC measured the quality of the research or the quality of the writing. For example, if the study did not have an explicit conceptual framework, was it because of space limitations imposed by journals or a deficiency in the study? Should the study be penalized by deducting quality points? Other quality criteria also might be compromised by editorial decisions and preferences rather than by methodological omissions of authors/researchers. In a review of nursing research literature, Jacobsen and Meininger (1985) reported that only 5% of the sample of studies reported prior sample size calculation, 14% reported their method of randomization, 74% reported complete data on equivalence of randomized groups, and only 50% mentioned attrition rates. Certainly, quality of the reporting affects the meta-analyst's ability to evaluate quality of the study in terms of validity.

The second meta-analysis (Brown, 1990c) was a replication of the first and was conducted because the database had almost doubled ($n = 82$) in the period since completion of the first study. Because the quality instrument used in the first study had posed such problems, a different quality coding scheme was developed according to Sackett and Haynes' (1976) model for measuring quality of studies on compliance. A detailed code book was developed to define and describe the coding process for the meta-analysis, part of which guided coding of research quality. Table 1 depicts coding criteria for research quality assessment used in the second meta-analysis.

A number of critical quality indicators are not readily apparent in the quality scoring method shown in Table 1. For example, adequacy of sample size and instrument quality were not measured directly. These criteria are embedded in Selection and Specification of Study Sample and Outcome Measure, respectively. Two major considerations formed the basis for development and selection of the quality rating criteria shown in Table 1. First, data

TABLE 1 Research Quality Scoring Method*

Variable	Coding Guidelines for Allocation of Points
Study Design	3=randomized trial 2=nonrandomized control group 1=pretest/posttest
Selection and Specification of Study Sample	3=random population sample or 3 or more hospitals/clinics in a geographic area or regional program/referral center (includes description of 4–5 of: age, sex, race, SES, or other demographic variables) 2=as for 3, but inadequate demographic description or not randomized population sample but randomized to groups only with adequate demographic description 1=grab sample or single clinic, including adequate description of demographic features of sample 0=grab sample or single clinic not otherwise specified 1 bonus point for all categories if any of the following are met: • description of patient access to clinic (referral) • ndication of proportion of patients excluded • indication of consecutive admissions or all patients during stated time period or a random sample of a single clinic population with at least 80% follow-up
Specification of Illness or Condition	3=replicable diagnostic criteria stated with inclusion/ exclusion criteria 2=diagnostic criteria stated 1=diagnosis only 0=no diagnosis or where diagnosis can only be inferred 1 bonus point for all categories if co-morbidity is described
Description of Educational Condition	2=complete description that would permit the reader to replicate the intervention 1=incomplete description (no description of two or more of the features of the intervention) 0=no description or when intervention can only be inferred 1 bonus point for all categories if co-intervention with a second regimen is precluded by study design or is noted when it occurs
Construct Definition of Outcome	2=replicable by reader in own setting 1=vague definition 0=no definition
Outcome Measure (Most Direct Measure Only)	4=objective direct measures taken longitudinally For example, glycosylated hemoglobin is most direct measure, but must be measured on more than one occasion 3=immediate direct For example, blood levels, direct observation of behavior change 2=objective indirect measures For example, test of knowledge or performance accuracy, keeping appointments, etc. 1=subjective measures For example, interview of patient, i.e., self-reporting or review of records 0=not stated 1 point bonus for codes 1, 2, and 3 when random as opposed to scheduled determination or when patient is unaware of purpose of determination
Total Quality Points	Sum of variables above—a total of 21 points possible

*Adapted from Sackett, D. L., & Haynes, R. B. (eds.) (1976). *Compliance with Therapeutic Regimens.* Baltimore: The Johns Hopkins University Press.

for each criterion needed to be readily available in most research reports in order for the criterion to be useful. Second, minimal subjectivity was desired in applying the criteria. Otherwise, measurement of research quality would be a cumbersome and lengthy process and adequate interrater reliability difficult, if not impossible, to achieve.

Using the critical quality scoring method, interrater agreement between two raters was 89%, and this level was achieved with very little practice. Instead of determining interrater reliability for a randomly selected subsample of studies, as was done in the first meta-analysis, interrater agreement was determined for the entire set of studies in which diabetes patient education was evaluated. This was possible since the task of coding was much simpler. The intuitive perception of quality for each study was more in concert with its final quality score. Consistent with previous research, no relationship was found between quality scoring and weighted effect-size estimates for patient outcomes. Threats to validity were also coded in the second meta-analysis, and the relationship between total number of threats and total quality score was statistically significant, $r = .58$, $p = .001$, indicating an association but not redundancy. Higher quality studies were associated with fewer threats.

Discussion

In measuring research quality for meta-analysis, a compromise should be made between application of exhaustive lists of quality indicators and use of an approach that assesses critical aspects of a study without sacrificing scientific rigor. That is, what are the aspects of a study that, if seriously flawed, bias outcomes and/or generalizability as a result of variation in quality? Each meta-analysis is unique in that the variables and study characteristics that are coded, including quality criteria, differ somewhat according to the specific content domain. Therefore, meta-analysis may differ in the degree to which effect sizes are influenced by research quality. In other words, finding that quality influences effect-size estimates in one meta-analysis does not necessarily indicate that quality would influence effect sizes to the same degree or in the same manner in other meta-analyses. The inability to generalize regarding study quality supports the notion that measurement of research quality should be a required standard of each meta-analysis so that conclusions drawn from such integrative studies are based on sound evidence.

The lack of generalizability of research quality and its effects on study outcomes has been demonstrated by previous investigators. In general, few study characteristics, including those criteria used to measure study quality, have been found to correlate with effect sizes (Hunter et al., 1982, p. 138; Hunter & Schmidt, 1990). The only significant relationships between quality criteria and outcome effects found in meta-analytic studies conducted by this author have involved attrition and research design (control group versus one group pretest-posttest designs). In a meta-analysis of studies on psychoeducational interventions with surgical patients, Devine and Cook (1986) found inconsistency between the size of patient outcome effects and quality criteria. For some outcomes, studies assessed as having higher validity yielded higher mean effect sizes than did studies with lower validity. For other outcomes, the reverse was true (McCain & Lynn, 1990).

Clearly, there are no perfect studies, particularly when studying the complexities of human behavior in natural environments; therefore, quality remains an important issue in meta-analytic studies. Critical aspects of the study, some of which may be individualized for the particular area of research, should be assessed and related to findings. Selected criteria should be used, and validity and reliability issues pertaining to the measurement of quality should be addressed. The example of a quality measure in Table 1 was found to be very useful and measured important research design variables that could be modified and incorporated into any meta-analysis. Using operational definitions for validity threats and obtaining acceptable levels of interrater reliability was difficult. Improved definitions for these threats are still needed, and this author is attempting to refine the list.

The rigor of meta-analyses must parallel that of other types of research, particularly since meta-analytic methods are useful for promoting application of research in clinical practice and for guiding difficult health care policy decisions. Given the present state of nursing research and the dearth of research topics that have been studied extensively enough or conducted in a manner to warrant a meta-analysis, it may have limited current value (Lynn, 1989). In the future, meta-analysis should prove to be a useful tool for making sense out of large numbers of nursing intervention studies and clinical research data.

The call for improved rigor in meta-analysis must be accompanied by improved reporting of research in primary studies. For meta-analysis to be useful, accurate and complete data must be available. In some instances, basic research information is missing from research reports, perhaps due to author oversight or editorial changes imposed by space constraints of journals. For example, to calculate effect sizes, means and standard deviation units must be reported for both experimental and control groups. Further, clarity about sample size is necessary if effect-size estimates are to be weighted according to sample sizes of individual studies (Hedges & Olkin, 1985). In many studies, sample size is a confusing issue; authors do not distinguish or clearly report beginning sample size and subsequent sample size (after attrition) at the time of postintervention outcome measurement. Another problematic omission in reported research is inadequate description of the intervention, which precludes meta-analytic determination of the most effective strategies.

More work needs to be done to determine the answer to the critical question of what aspects of a study, if compromised, bias outcomes. It is apparent that quantitative procedures for synthesizing a body of research are useful. To do an adequate synthesis, research must be available in a form conducive to extracting necessary information. And, assessment of quality of primary studies must be part of every meta-analytic study.

References

Brown, S. A. (1988). Effects of educational interventions in diabetes care: A meta-analysis of findings. *Nursing Research, 37,* 223–230.

Brown, S. A. (1990a). Characteristic of diabetes patient education programs: A meta-analysis of factors influencing effectiveness. Manuscript submitted for publication.

Brown, S. A. (1990b). Quality of reporting in diabetes patient education research: 1954–1986. *Research in Nursing & Health, 13,* 53–62.

Brown, S. A. (1990c). Studies of educational interventions and outcomes in diabetic adults: A meta-analysis revisited. *Patient Education and Counseling, 16,* 189–215.

Campbell, D. T., & Stanley, J. C. (1963). *Experimental and quasi-experimental designs for research.* Boston: Houghton Mifflin Company.

Cicchetti, D., & Eron, L. (1979). The reliability of manuscript reviewing. *Journal of Abnormal Psychology, 22,* 596–600.

Cooper, H. M. (1984). *The integrative research review.* Sage University Paper series on Quantitative Applications in the Social Sciences, volume 2. Beverly Hills, CA: Sage Publications.

Devine, E. C., & Cook, T. D. (1986). Clinical and cost-saving effects of psychoeducational interventions with surgical patients: A meta-analysis. *Research in Nursing & Health, 9,* 89–105.

Duffy, M. E. (1985). A research appraisal checklist for evaluating nursing research reports. *Nursing & Health Care, 6,* 539–547.

Glass, G. V., McGraw, B., & Smith, M. L. (1981). *Meta-analysis in social research.* Beverly Hills, CA: Sage.

Hedges, L. V., & Olkin, I. (1985). *Statistical methods for meta-analysis.* New York: Academic Press.

Hunter, J. E., & Schmidt, F. L. (1990). *Methods of meta-analysis: Correcting error and bias in research findings.* Newbury Park, CA: Sage.

Hunter, J. E., Schmidt, F. L., & Jackson, G. B. (1982). *Meta-analysis: Cumulating research findings across studies.* Sage University Paper series on Quantitative Applications in the Social Sciences, volume 4. Beverly Hills, CA: Sage.

Jacobsen, B. S., & Meininger, J. C. (1985). The designs and methods of published nursing research: 1956–1983. *Nursing Research, 34,* 306–312.

Lynn, M. R. (1989). Meta-analysis: Appropriate tool for the integration of nursing research? *Nursing Research, 38,* 302–305.

Massey, J., & Loomis, M. (1988). When should nurses use research findings? *Applied Nursing Research, 1,* 32–40.

McCain, N. L., & Lynn, M. R. (1990). Meta-analysis of a narrative review: Studies evaluating patient teaching. *Western Journal of Nursing Research, 12,* 347–358.

Mintz, J. (1983). Integrating research evidence: A commentary on meta-analysis. Journal of *Consulting and Clinical Psychology,* 51, 71–75.

Mullen, P. D., & Ramirez, G. (1987). Information synthesis and meta-analysis. *Advances in Health Education and Promotion, 2,* 201–239.

Rosenthal, R. (1984). *Meta-analytic procedures for social research.* Sage University Paper series on Quantitative Applications in the Social Sciences, volume 6. Beverly Hills, CA: Sage.

Sackett, D. L., & Haynes, R. B. (eds.) (1976). *Compliance with therapeutic regimens.* Baltimore: The Johns Hopkins University Press.

Sacks, H. S., Berrier, J., Reitman, D., Ancona-Berk, V. A., & Chalmers, T. C. (1987). Meta-analysis of randomized controlled trials. *New England Journal of Medicine, 316,* 450–455.

Scarr, S., & Weber, B. (1978). The reliability of reviews for the American Psychologist. American Psychologist, 33,935.

Smith, M. C. (1988). *Meta-analysis of nursing intervention research.* Birmingham, AL: Author.

Wolf, F. M. (1986). *Meta-analysis: Quantitative methods for research synthesis.* Sage University Paper series on Quantitative Applications in the Social Sciences, 07-059. Beverly Hills, CA: Sage.

An Application of Hierarchical Linear Models to Meta-Analysis in Nursing Research

Yow-Wu B. Wu

Researchers conduct meta-analyses that heavily rely on quantitative methods for research synthesis. Typically, these methods have involved estimating treatment effect magnitude from each of a series of studies and then averaging the estimates to obtain a single index of effect magnitude. Because meta-analysis relies on data in the form of summary statistics (derived from primary analysis of studies), it is an analysis of the results of statistical analyses. One of the criticisms of using meta-analysis is that logical conclusions may not be drawn by comparing and aggregating studies that include different measuring techniques and definitions of variables and subjects.

One solution is to use the standardized mean differences (d_j), also known as effect size, to demonstrate the treatment effect:

$$d_j = (\overline{Y}e_j - \overline{Y}c_j)/S_j \qquad (1)$$

where d_j is the effect size for Study j, $\overline{Y}e_j$ is the mean of experimental group in Study j, $\overline{Y}c_j$ is the mean of control group in Study j, and S_j is the pooled within-group standard deviation for Study j.

Researchers are most interested in attempting to obtain the true effect size (δ_j). Figure 1 illustrates that the effect size for any given study (d_j) is one of many estimates of δ_j. Sampling error and reliability of d_j are important to researchers. The purpose of this report is to demonstrate the use of hierarchical linear models (HLM) to improve the estimation of true effect size δ_j, by weighing reliability. This article will demonstrate how to use the empirical Bayes estimate to achieve this goal.

Hierarchical Linear Models

HLM are multilevel data analysis techniques. Traditional regression analysis is usually used to analyze data at either the individual or the aggregated level (such as organizations or experiments). In meta-analysis, researchers only have the summarized data, such as the effect size of the individual study (d_j). The variation within each study usually is not considered in estimating the overall effect size across studies. The strength of HLM is that this analytical approach examines both within- and between-study variations.

HLM can be used in meta-analysis to (a) estimate the average effect size across a set of studies, (b) estimate the variance of the effect-size parameters, (c) derive empirical Bayes estimates of each study's effect, (d) test a series of linear models to explain variation in effect size, and (e) estimate residual variance of the effect size parameters for each linear model.

An Application of HLM to Meta-Analysis

Smith, Holcombe, and Stullenbarger (1994) surveyed 428 studies and selected 28 experimental intervention studies to investigate the intervention effectiveness for symptom management in oncology nursing. Smith et al. used binomial effect size to display the percentage of improvement in each of the 28 studies.

Is it possible for researchers to average these 28 effect sizes and obtain an overall effect size to best represent the effect of the experimental intervention? HLM can be used to estimate the overall effect size by applying empirical Bayes to estimate each study's effect size.

The level 1 (within-study) model in HLM can be described as a model in which individual observed effect size from Study j consists of the true effect size and the error. The equation can be written as:

$$d_j = \delta_j + e_j \qquad (2)$$

This model explains that each individual effect size (d_j) from separate studies consists of two parts: One is the population true effect size, δ_j; the other is the error, e_j. Each individual study, j, has its own within-study (or error) variance, V_j, and it is assumed that meta-analysis presents the analyst with a series of independent effect estimates, each normally distributed with known variance at level 1.

Bryk and Raudenbush (1992) stated that within-study variance can be calculated by the number of subjects in experimental and control groups and the square of true effect size. This error variance can be obtained by summing up two ratios: One is the total number of sub-

Yow-Wu B. Wu, PhD, is an associate professor, School of Nursing, State University of New York at Buffalo, Buffalo, NY.

From *Nursing Research,* September/October 1997, *46,* 295–298.

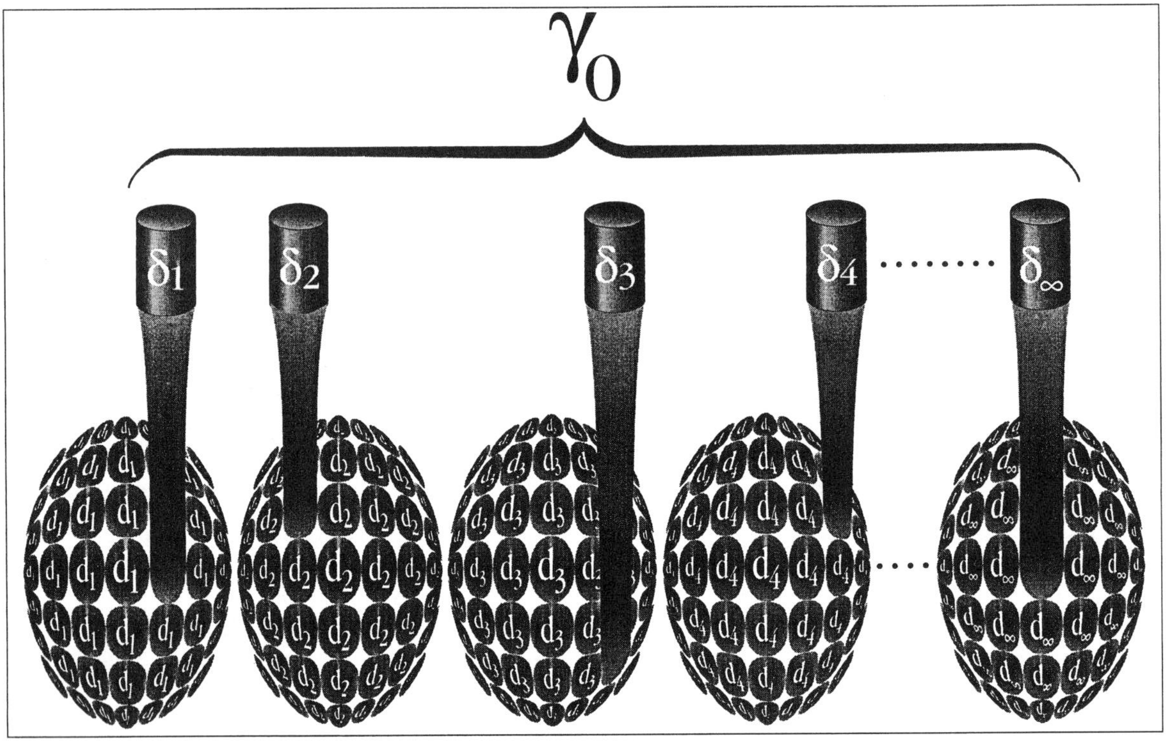

FIGURE 1 Conceptual Framework

jects over the product of the number of subjects of experimental and control group; the other is the ratio of the square of the true effect size to twice of total sample size. This equation can be written as:

$$V_j = (n_{ej} + n_{cj})/(n_{ej}n_{cj}) + \delta_j^2/[2(n_{ej} + n_{cj} \qquad (3)$$

where V_j is the within-study or error variance, n_{ej} is the sample size for experimental group in Study j, n_{cj} is the sample size for control group in Study j, and δ_j^2 is the square of the true effect size. Sample size has a negative relationship with error variance; that is, the larger the sample size, the smaller the error variance.

Level 2 (between-studies) was modeled as the true effect size of Study j equals the grand mean of all true effect sizes plus error. This equation can be expressed as follows:

$$\delta_j = \gamma_0 + u_j \qquad (4)$$

where γ_0 is the grand mean of all true effect sizes across infinite studies and u_j is the difference between each study's true effect size δ_j and the grand mean γ_0 of all true effect sizes. The variance of u_j, also known as parameter variance, is τ.

This model is referred to as an unconditional model because it estimates the true effect sizes and parameter variance across infinite studies without modeling any predictors in the model. Owing to the lack of information on the second level and simplifying the second level model, an unconditioned model is selected. Researchers can add in-between study predictors, such as quality of each individual study, and test the conditional model.

For the unconditional model, researchers need three pieces of information: identification number for each study, observed effect size (d_j) of each study, and error variance (V_j) within each study. The required information for this demonstration was prepared in columns 1, 3, and 7 in Table 1. HLM software will generate estimates of true population mean effect size γ_0 and parameter variance τ, which will be used to calculate the reliability and the empirical Bayes estimate for each individual study.

Reliability and Empirical Bayes Estimate

Reliability is a function of parameter variance and error variance. Reliability equals the ratio of parameter variance to observed variance, which is parameter variance plus error variance (Bryk & Raudenbush, 1992). Relia-

TABLE 1 **Reliability, Effect Size, Empirical Bayes Effect Size, Sample Size, and Error Variance**

Study j	Reliability λ_j	Effect Size d_j	Empirical Bayes Effect Size δ_j^*	Sample Size		Error Variance V_j
				Experimental n_{ej}	Control n_{cj}	
1	.147	.87	.548	10	10	.2180
2	.177	.69	.527	12	12	.1766
3	.217	.45	.483	15	15	.1367
4	.309	.36	.451	25	23	.0848
5	.273	.23	.420	20	20	.1007
6	.360	.27	.412	30	30	.0673
7	.121	.45	.487	7	8	.2746
8	.279	.17	.402	20	21	.0980
9	.018	−7.93	.342	10	7	2.0924
10	.160	1.78	.697	14	14	.1994
11	.211	.71	.538	15	15	.1417
12	.265	.63	.529	20	20	.1050
13	.441	.23	.377	40	44	.0480
14	.093	.13	.458	6	5	.3674
15	.167	1.83	.715	15	15	.1891
16	.273	.70	.549	21	21	.1011
17	.254	.14	.403	18	18	.1114
18	.342	.07	.348	27	28	.0728
19	.238	.66	.532	19	16	.1214
20	.082	1.47	.572	6	6	.4234
21	.210	.73	.542	16	14	.1428
22	.131	.23	.458	8	8	.2517
23	.180	.54	.501	12	12	.1727
24	.308	.42	.470	24	24	.0852
25	.148	.83	.542	10	10	.2172
26	.117	1.07	.560	8	8	.2858
27	.187	.31	.458	11	14	.1643
28	.145	.23	.454	9	9	.2237

bility will be higher if parameter variance is large and error variance is small.

Reliability of Study j = parameter variance/(parameter variance + error variance of Study j)

or:

$$\lambda_j = \tau/(\tau + V_j) \tag{5}$$

The empirical Bayes estimate, δ_j^* is a weighted d_j based on the reliability of each individual study. If the individual study is reliable, more weight will be placed on d_j; otherwise more weight will be placed on the population effect size γ_0. The following equation represents the empirical Bayes estimate of an individual effect size:

$$\delta_j^* = \lambda_j d_j + (1 - \lambda_j)\lambda \tag{6}$$

where the weight λ_j equals the reliability of d_j as an estimation of δ_j and γ_0 is the grand mean of all true effect sizes across infinite studies.

Results

Table 2 presents the estimates of the population true effect size, $\hat{\gamma}_0$, and the level 2 between studies variance or parameter variance, $\hat{\tau}$. The estimated population true effect size $\hat{\gamma}_0$ is .49, which is larger than the mean of the 28 samples observed effect size ($\bar{d}$) The estimated variance of population effect size is $\hat{\tau} = .038$. The χ^2 test indicates that the variability among δ_j is significantly different from 0 ($p < .001$), which means there is a variation among true effect sizes.

Table 1 illustrates the relationship between sample size, effect size, and the error variance; the larger the sample size, the smaller the error variance. Study 9 best exemplifies this relationship. The error variance of Study 9 is:

$$V_9 = (10 + 7)/(10 \times 7) + (-7.93)^2/[2(10 + 7)] = 2.0924$$

TABLE 2 **Unconditional Model for the Meta-Analysis of the Smith et al. (1994) Study**

Fixed Effect	**Coefficient**	***SE***		***t* Ratio**
Grand mean, γ_0	0.491	0.080		6.111
Random effect	Variance component, τ	*df*	χ^2	*p* value
True effect sizes, δ_j	0.038	27	66.983	< 0.001

NOTE: SE = standard error.

where 10 and 7 are numbers of subjects in experimental and control groups, respectively, and −7.93 is the observed effect size that was used to substitute the true effect size δ_9. (See Equation 3.)

The reliability of Study 9 was calculated by Equation 5:

$$\lambda_9 = 0.038/(0.038 + 2.0924) = 0.018$$

where .038 is the parameter variance ($\hat{\tau}$) and 2.0924 is the error variance (V_9).

With the reliability, we can calculate the empirical Bayes estimate of the effect size of Study 9 using Equation 6:

$$\delta_9^* = 0.018 \times (-7.93) + (1 - 0.018) \times 0.491 = 0.34$$

where 0.018 is the reliability (λ_9) of Study 9, −7.93 is the observed effect size (d_9), and 0.491 is the estimate of the true effect size ($\hat{\gamma}_0$).

This example reflects that larger error variance is associated with lower reliability; therefore, effect size d_j may mislead the interpretation of the true effect size. However, the empirical Bayes estimate will place less weight on the sample effect size and place more weight on the grand mean effect size if the reliability is low for a specific study. Table 2 also shows that the variance of the empirical Bayes effect size is smaller than the variance by observed sample effect size.

Conclusion

Based on this unconditional model, there are three major findings. First, the empirical Bayes estimate of effect size is more precise after taking the reliability of d_j as an estimate of δ_j into consideration in estimating the true effect size of each study. Second, the variance of empirical Bayes estimates of individual studies is smaller compared with the unadjusted effect size. Third, different factors that influence the variation of the second level effect size δ_j can be further modeled by HLM. For example, if a quality index for each study is available, a researcher will be able to study the variation of these effect sizes in relation to the quality of each study.

References

Bryk, A. S., & Raudenbush, S. W. (1992). *Hierarchical linear models.* Newbury Park, CA: Sage.

Smith, M. C., Holcombe, J. K., & Stullenbarger, E. (1994). A meta-analysis of intervention effectiveness for symptom management in oncology nursing research. *Oncology Nursing Forum, 21,* 1201–1209.

Use of a Meta-Analytic Database Management System

Cheryl Tatano Beck

Reynolds, Timmerman, Anderson, and Stevenson (1992) noted that nurse investigators have used meta-analysis almost exclusively for experimental research, but that it has yet to be used to its fullest extent. These authors call for making maximum use of meta-analysis by synthesizing descriptive as well as experimental research.

While most of the steps of a meta-analysis are intellectually stimulating and rewarding, the numerical computations are tedious. The purpose of this article is to describe the use of a meta-analytical software system designed to perform these statistical computations. It is hoped that if computations are less laborious, nurse researchers will conduct meta-analyses more frequently.

The Advanced BASIC Meta-Analysis is a software system designed to perform a full range of meta-analytic statistical computations (Mullen, 1989). It is a revised version of an earlier interactive software system (Mullen & Rosenthal, 1985), which allows the researcher to create meta-analytic data files containing all the statistical information needed for the hypothesis tests. The software system contains options to save data files to disk for editing and revision. After a data file has been entered into the system, any one of the multiple statistical computations needed for a meta-analysis can be performed. In addition, the package allows the user to generate various meta-analytic graphic displays, including scatterplots, funnel plots, and frequency distributions.

The integrated database management system consists of five different modules: (a) *The Database Management System Proper*. This is the module the user enters when calling up the system. It includes the basic functions of creating and handling data files. (b) *Editing Existing Data Files*. This module permits the researcher to add or delete hypothesis tests or predictors and to change a specific hypothesis test. (c) *General Combinations and Comparisons*. Using this module, the user can perform the basic combinations and diffuse comparisons, disjoint cluster analysis, and blocking. (d) *Effects of Predictors and Model Testing*. The basic focused comparisons for testing both simple and complex effects of predictors are performed in this module. (e) *Meta-Analytic Graphics Displays*. Meta-analytic graphic displays of scatterplots, frequency distributions, and funnel plots are performed in this module.

The database management system is designed to generate statistics to answer three general analytic questions of a meta-analysis: central tendency, variability, and prediction. The research questions involved in central tendency are, "What is the combined significance level?" and "What is the mean magnitude of effect?" To achieve an in-depth understanding of a phenomenon under meta-analytic review, variability around the average effect needs to be determined. The research question related to variability is, "How much variability is there around the average effect size?" Mullen (1989) refers to this type of comparison as the diffuse comparison of effect sizes and their significance levels. In the Advanced BASIC Meta-Analysis, both research questions of central tendency and variability can be answered by selecting the option Combination and Diffuse Comparisons of Significance and Effect Size in the General Combinations and Comparisons module.

Focused comparisons are used to answer the third general analytic question of prediction and explanation: "To what extent do the significance levels and effect sizes vary in meaningful, predictable ways as a function of practically important or theoretically illuminating variables?" (Mullen, 1989, p. 87). Both simple and complex comparisons can be generated. Complex effects can involve looking at the combined effects of two or more predictors on the effect size and level of significance.

This article uses data from the author's meta-analysis on the relationship between postpartum depression and infant temperament to discuss and illustrate selected tasks from these modules (Beck, 1996).

Create Data File

When creating a data file, the meta-analyst is prompted to name the data file using no more than eight characters.

Cheryl Tatano Beck, DNSc, CNM, FAAN, is a professor, College of Nursing, University of Rhode Island, Kingston, RI.

From *Nursing Research,* May/June 1996, *45,* 181–184.

For the author's example, the data file name PPDTEMP was entered. The next prompt is to enter the exact number of hypothesis tests to be included and the number of predictors. The default value of 200 hypothesis tests will operate on a machine with 256 kilobytes (K) of random access memory (RAM). The maximum number of predictors is 10. Next, the meta-analyst is prompted to enter a name for each predictor. Up to eight characters can be used. The 10 predictors used in the meta-analytic example were year the study was published, type of publication, country where the research was conducted, sample size, research design, postpartum depression measures, quality score, socioeconomic status, type of postpartum depression, and infant temperament measurement. The quality score of each study was computed by a scoring scheme of 10 criteria, specifically tailored for postpartum depression research.

The next step involves entering the following data for each hypothesis test in the meta-analysis: (a) type of statistic (chi-square, *t* test, *F* test, correlation coefficient, *Z* score, or one-tailed *p* value); (b) value of the test statistic; (c) sample size; (d) degrees of freedom; (e) direction of effect; and (f) values of all of the predictors. When entering data in the database management system, some restrictions apply. Only chi-squares with 1 *df* and only *F* tests with 1 *df* in the numerator can be entered. Mullen (1989) warns that an *F* with more than 1 *df* in the numerator can represent an unfocused general comparison between several means. Also, chi-squares with more than 1 *df* can represent varying patterns of findings for different analyses. Only the absolute values of the statistics are entered, with the direction of effect identified later in the program by a plus (+) or minus (−).

Display Data File in Memory

When this task is selected from the menu, all the statistical information and predictors for each hypothesis test in the database are displayed on the screen, one hypothesis test at a time. In addition, the common metrics of *Z* and one-tailed *p* for significance, Fisher's *Z*, *r*, r^2, and *d* for effect size are displayed. Figure 1 illustrates the printout of one hypothesis test of the relationship between postpartum depression and infant temperament included in the meta-analysis.

General Combinations and Comparisons is the third module. If the option Combinations and Diffuse Comparisons of Significance and Effect Size is selected, the system will compute the following statistics:

1. Combination of significance: *Z* for combined significance, associated one-tailed *p*, and fail-safe number for the $p = .05$ level of significance.

2. Combination of effect size: mean Fisher's *Z*, mean *r*, mean r^2, and mean *d*.

3. Diffuse comparison of significance: chi-square and associated one-tailed *p*.

4. Diffuse comparison of effect size: chi-square and associated one-tailed *p*.

The database management system can generate the statistics for the combinations and diffuse comparisons of significance and effect sizes three different ways: unweighted, weighted by sample size, and weighted by a predictor chosen by the meta-analyst. Figure 2 illus-

ADVANCED BASIC META-ANALYSIS **DATA FILE IN MEMORY: PPDTEMP**

META-ANALYTIC DATABASE MANAGEMENT SYSTEM

DISPLAY DATA FILE	
HYPOTHESIS TEST #15	PREDICTORS:
R = .37	YEAR = 1993
SAMPLE SIZE = 88	PUB = 1
DEGREES OF FREEDOM = 86	COUNTRY = 4
DIRECTION OF EFFECT = +	SAMPLE = 88
SIGNIFICANCE LEVEL:	DESIGN = 2
Z = 3.547917	PPDMEAS = 1
P = 1.942512E-04	QUALITY = 21
EFFECT SIZE:	SES = 2
FISHER'S Z = .3884231	PPD = 2
R = .37	DVMEAS = 2
R2 = .1369	
COHEN'S D = .7965282	

FIGURE 1 Display Data File: Hypothesis Test #15

ADVANCED BASIC META-ANALYSIS
DATA FILE IN MEMORY: PPDTEMP
GENERAL COMBINATIONS AND COMPARISONS

17 HYPOTHESIS TESTS (WEIGHT BY QUALITY)

COMBINATION OF SIGNIFICANCE LEVELS
Z FOR COMBINATION = 11.29346
ASSOCIATED ONE-TAILED P = 1.328782E-24
FAIL-SAFE NUMBER (P = 0.5) = 809.3819

COMBINATION OF EFFECT SIZES
MEAN FISHER'S Z = .3648982
MEAN R = .3495212
MEAN R2 = .1221651
MEAN COHEN'S D = .7461001

DIFFUSE COMPARISON OF SIGNIFICANCE LEVELS
CHI-SQUARE (16) = 6.490507
ASSOCIATED ONE-TAILED P = .9818785

DIFFUSE COMPARISON OF EFFECT SIZES
CHI-SQUARE (16) = 18.1331
ASSOCIATED ONE -TAILED P = .316161

FIGURE 2 General Combinations and Comparisons (Weighted by Quality)

trates the printout of combinations and diffuse comparisons of significance and effect size for the author's meta-analysis. The predictor used to weight hypothesis tests in this example was named Quality.

As indicated in Figure 2, the combined level of significance for the relationship between postpartum depression and infant temperament in the 17 studies included in the meta-analysis is highly significant at p = 1.32E-24. The mean magnitude of effect is in Cohen's (1988) moderate range: mean r = .35. The fail-safe number of 809 indicates that 809 unretrieved studies averaging null results would be needed to overturn the conclusion of this meta-analysis. Both the diffuse comparisons of significance levels (p = .98) and effect sizes (p = .31) are nonsignificant, which indicates that the significance levels and effect sizes of the 17 hypothesis tests included in this meta-analysis are not significantly different from one another.

Another option available in the General Combinations and Comparisons module is blocking. The meta-analyst enters the name of the predictor that will be used to block hypothesis tests into subsets. If this task is chosen, the database management system will compute the statistics for combination and diffuse comparison within levels of the blocking predictor.

In the fourth module, Effects of Predictors and Model Testing, the following options are available: (a) Effects of a Single Predictor, (b) Comparisons Between Two Levels of a Blocking Predictor, (c) Combined Effects of Two Predictors, and (d) Effects of One Predictor Within Levels of a Blocking Predictor. The first option is used to illustrate this module using a printout from the author's meta-analysis. When it is selected, a prompt is given to enter the name of the predictor to be used. The database management system then generates correlations between the predictor and each of the effect-size indicators: Fisher's *Z, r,* and *d.* The formula for the best-fitting regression line for each of these three indicators of effect size is presented. Mullen (1989) warns that these primary level inferential statistics are not completely appropriate to apply to a meta-analysis, but they do serve as helpful illustrations of patterns in the meta-analysis. Lastly, focused comparisons for effect sizes and levels of significance are computed.

The extent to which the mean effect size of the relationship between postpartum depression and infant temperament can be accounted for by the predictor of sample size of the individual studies included in the meta-analysis can be examined by the correlations computed in Figure 3. The correlation between r and sample size is −.81, indicating a strong negative relationship. The larger the sample size of the study included in the meta-analysis, the smaller was the effect size. The focused comparison of effect sizes was significant at the p = .0009 level, thus indicating that hypothesis tests in the meta-analysis yielded smaller effects if the sample size was larger. The probability associated with the focused comparison of significance levels for sample size was p = .46, indicating that hypothesis tests did not yield more significant results due to sample size. In his work, Mullen (1989) does stress that the correlation between study outcomes and predictors be used as a preliminary gauge of the predictive power of the specific predictors since the assumptions required for primary-level inferential statistical tests are not likely to be met by the meta-analytic data points.

Options in the fifth module, Meta-Analytic Graphics Displays, include Scatterplot of Effect Size and Predictor, Frequency Distribution of Effect Size, and Funnel Plot of Effect Size. Once the meta-analyst selects the scatterplot option, a prompt is given to choose the effect-size indicator to be used—Fisher's *Z, r,* or *d.* Next, the name of the predictor to be included is entered, followed by the lowest and highest values in the database for both the

Text continues on page 272.

ADVANCED BASIC META-ANALYSIS DATA FILE IN MEMORY: PPDTEMP

EFFECTS OF PREDICTORS AND MODEL TESTING

EFFECTS OF SAMPLE FOR 17 HYPOTHESIS TESTS
CORRELATION BETWEEN FISHER'S Z AND SAMPLE = −.7972741
CORRELATION BETWEEN R AND SAMPLE = −.8125302
CORRELATION BETWEEN COHEN'S D AND SAMPLE = −.7886403

FORMULA FOR THE BEST FITTING LINE:
FISHER'S Z = .5555048 + (−2.402308E-03) * SAMPLE
R = .5122824 + (−2.113393E-03) * SAMPLE
COHEN'S D = 1.1593 + (−5.130085E-03) * SAMPLE

FOCUSED COMPARISON OF SIGNIFICANCE LEVELS:
Z FOR COMPARISON = 9.343145E-02
ASSOCIATED ONE-TAILED P = .462781
FOCUSED COMPARISON OF EFFECT SIZES:
Z FOR COMPARISON = 3.117001
ASSOCIATED ONE-TAILED P = 9.134625E-04

FIGURE 3 Effects of Predictor, Sample Size, and Model Testing

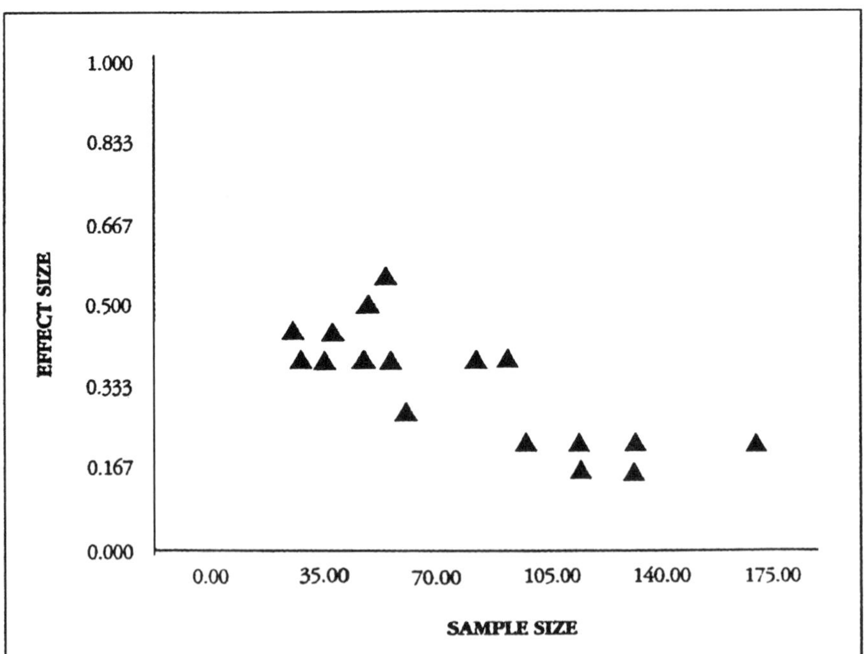

FIGURE 4 Scatterplot of *r* for Effect Size and Sample Size

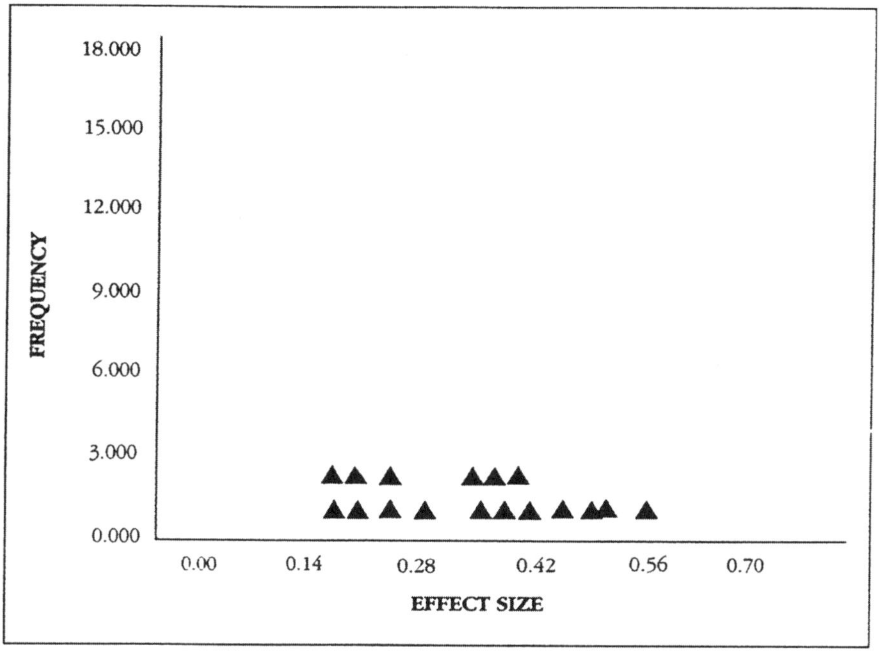

FIGURE 5 Frequency Distribution of *r* for Effect Size of Studies Included in Meta-Analysis

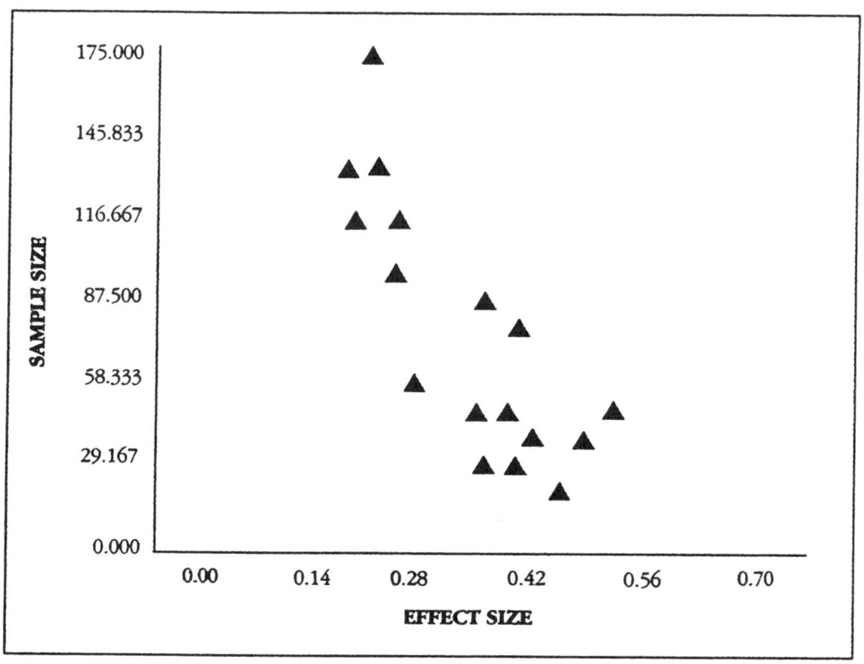

FIGURE 6 Funnel Plot of *r* for Effect Size

effect-size indicator and the predictor. Mullen (1989) warns users that they should not select extremely high- and low-scale values that are well beyond the actual range of values for the effect-size indicator and the predictor. Extreme values will result in the majority of points being placed in a smaller portion of the scatterplot, which will give the appearance of a higher degree of correlation between the predictor and effect size than is accurate. Figure 4 presents the scatterplot of the predictor, sample size, and the effect-size indicator of r for the author's meta-analysis. It illustrates the relationship between the two variables described earlier.

The database system can also generate a frequency distribution for an effect-size indicator as displayed in Figure 5. The meta-analyst is prompted to enter the chosen effect-size indicator and its lowest and highest values.

A third option, Funnel Plot of Effect Size, can be used to determine whether publication bias is distorting the results of the meta-analysis (Light & Pillemer, 1984). In this option, the user chooses an effect-size indicator and then enters the lowest and highest values for that effect size and for the sample size. Ideally, a funnel plot will resemble an inverted funnel. If, for example, a large portion is missing in the lower left quarter of the funnel plot, it can be inferred that hypothesis tests that would obtain small, nonsignificant effects due to small samples have not been included in the meta-analysis. The r index was the effect-size indicator chosen for inclusion in the funnel plot illustrated in Figure 6.

Quantitative research syntheses are gaining in popularity over the traditional narrative as a rigorous method to integrate results from multiple primary studies. It is hoped that meta-analysis will gain increased prominence in nursing research as more nurse investigators become aware of the option of using software systems designed specifically to perform the full complement of meta-analytic calculations.

References

Beck, C. T. (1996). The relationship between postpartum depression and infant temperament: A meta-analysis, *Nursing Research.*

Cohen, J. (1988). *Statistical power analysis for the behavioral sciences.* Hillsdale, NJ: Erlbaum.

Light, R., & Pillemer, D. (1984). *Summing up: The science of reviewing research.* Cambridge, MA: Harvard University Press.

Mullen, B. (1989). *Advanced BASIC Meta-Analysis.* Hillsdale, NJ: Erlbaum.

Mullen, B., & Rosenthal, R. (1985). *BASIC meta-analysis: Procedures and programs.* Hillsdale, NJ: Erlbaum.

Reynolds, N., Timmerman, G., Anderson, J., & Stevenson, J. (1992). Meta-analysis for descriptive research. *Research in Nursing and Health, 15,* 467–475.

Factor Analysis Revisited

Sandra Ferketich ■ **Mary Muller**

Factor analysis is a widely used technique in research. It has proven to be helpful in a variety of situations, such as data reduction and calculation of composite scores. However, in nursing research it is most often used in the examination of instrument validity, which is the focus of this article. Factor analysis is a flexible analytic tool, providing a broad scope of options through the various statistical packaged programs. Unfortunately, many researchers feel overwhelmed by the vast array of options available to them, and without thoroughly understanding the issues they simply choose the program defaults, a statistician's recommendation, or the options appearing most frequently in the research literature. Even more unfortunate is the application of factor analysis to a group of theoretically unrelated variables forcing "them through an arbitrary, meat-grinder computerized approach to finding factors" (Nunnally, 1978, p. 328).

In this article, key decision points, options available for extraction, and rotation of factors and guides to selection of factor analytic options are described. Figure 1 represents a decision tree, illustrating key decision points. Each major decision level is identified. The arrows are guides through the logical decision-making process to assist the researcher in planning a factor analysis.

The initial step in planning a factor analysis, selection of a theoretical model, actually precedes the first choice in the decision tree. This article does not discuss the process of theoretical model selection, but the theoretical model is of major importance to the design of any study. Regardless of the analytic approach chosen for a study, the theoretical model drives the statistical model.

The first decision in this article (Level A) is the choice of psychometric measurement model. This decision concerns the philosophic stance regarding the nature of measurement, in particular, the nature of measurement error. It is difficult to make reasoned choices about factoring methods unless there is some commitment to the role of measurement error in the structure of the instrument. The notion of measurement error is more fundamental than identifying the particular attributes of individual instruments; it concerns the underlying belief in how instruments are able to measure constructs in general. There are basically two models. The first model contends that all measurement error is random and, therefore, all variance is unique to an individual item and not shared with any other item or factor in the instrument. Consistent with other authors, we refer to this as the classic model (Carmines & Zeller, 1979; Nunnally, 1978). The second model recognizes both a random component and a systematic component in measurement error that may reflect common variance attributable to unmeasured or latent factors. This is the neoclassic model. At this point a decision about the nature of measurement error must be made. For most researchers, this decision is made only once. Because the selection of a model is such a fundamental, personal decision—that is neither absolutely right nor absolutely wrong—the reasons for the selection need to be articulated and used to support subsequent decisions in the factoring process. However, some researchers make this decision by default or follow the instructions of a mentor or consultant who has already made the decision.

Choice of the statistical model leads directly to decision Level B. The logical outcome of selection of the classic model is use of principal components analysis. Common factor analysis logically follows from the neoclassic model.

Principal component analysis does not purport to examine the underlying structure of the factors. Rather, consistent with the classic model, it assumes that all error is random and not reflective of an underlying structure. If all error is random and therefore the mean of the error sums is zero, each variable (item) correlates perfectly with itself. Therefore, unity (1.00) is placed on the diagonal of the correlation matrix from which the components are derived. Once the principal components

Sandra Ferketich, PhD, RN, is an associate professor and director, Division of Family and Community Health Nursing, College of Nursing, University of Arizona, Tucson.

Mary Muller, PhD, RN, is an assistant professor, Department of Life Span Process, College of Nursing, Ohio State University, Columbus.

From *Nursing Research,* January/February 1990, 39, *59–62.*

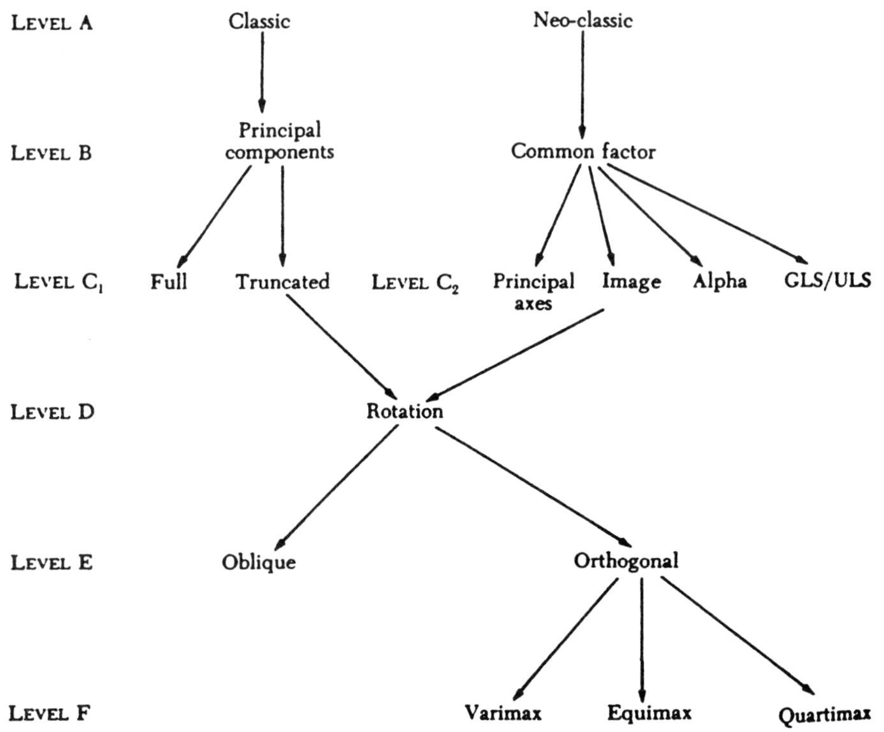

NOTE: GLS = generalized least squares; ULS = unweighted least squares.

FIGURE 1 Factor Analysis Decision Tree

approach has been selected, it is necessary to choose between the two options at decision Level C_1. In a full component model, the number of components are equal to the number of original variables. Each component (variable) is considered a factor. Consequently, the number of components equals the number of items/variables, and also equals the number of factors. Many researchers, however, choose to do a truncated principal components analysis. The smaller components are deleted in an effort to reduce the factor solution to those components contributing most to the explained variance (Gorsuch, 1983). Some researchers mistakenly believe that by deleting the components that contribute the least to the explained variance, they have identified underlying structures that support the components. They may extend the truncated model further and rotate the selected components (usually referred to at this point as factors). As a logical consequence of the error assumptions of principal component analysis, there is no underlying structure to discern and refine through rotation. Therefore, rotation is considered to be inappropriate by some.

The various ways researchers interpret the component solutions reveal that some are cavalier in distinguishing between principal components and common factor analyses. If the distinction is made, it may be murky at best. However, these are indeed two fundamentally different approaches grounded in two fundamentally different psychometric models. The methods do not use the same process to summarize the relationships between variables and do not provide the same information about the data. A principal component is distinguished by the fact that each component is derived from the *real* (measured) data and is not an extension of the underlying structure of unmeasured variables (Harris, 1985; Nunnally, 1978). In contrast, the common factor approaches result in factors that are extensions of the data and represent unmeasured or latent variable(s) discerned from the data.

Common factor analysis organizes the underlying structure of the data recognizing random and systematic measurement error. Therefore, each variable is affected by the independent underlying source (common factor variance), the unique variance of each variable (noncommon factor variance), and distortions caused by random error (Gorsuch, 1983). The systematic portion should reflect a theoretically sound structure. There is, however, a danger that systematic error may reflect the respondents' reaction to stimuli unrelated to factor structure, such as similar wording or items or item position in the instrument.

The choice of common factor approach for factor extraction (Level C_2) is necessary because all variance is not accounted for by each item in this model. Since each variable (item) does not correlate perfectly with itself, unity is not the appropriate estimate for the main diagonal of the correlation matrix. The common factor approaches (principal axes factoring, alpha factoring, etc.) provide different estimates of the variance for each element of the main diagonal. For some approaches, the estimates are the unique variances and for some the common variances.

The most frequently used common factor approach, principal axes factoring, places the squared multiple correlations on the main diagonal. This method has an intuitive appeal in that the squared multiple correlations, representing the correlations among each variable and every other variable in the matrix, seem to best operationalize the theoretical stance that items have a shared common underlying structure. Within prescribed programs (*SPSSX, BMDP*), many statistical computer packages allow the factor analyst to specify other diagonal values. For example, the highest or the lowest correlation of each variable with all others in the matrix may be used. Previous theory and research findings may support the use of specific estimates. The use of the default of the squared multiple correlation is reasonable in the absence of previous definitive findings. In deriving the matrix solution, equations with several unknowns must be solved. However, in the derivation of the matrix solution, the only unknowns in the equation that can vary are the elements of the main diagonal. Therefore, these elements directly determine the eigenvalues. Since many researchers use the Kaiser-Guttman (Guttman, 1954) criteria of an eigenvalue greater than 1 to determine the number of factors to be extracted, the elements of the main diagonal greatly influence the ultimate outcome of the factor solution.

In common factor analytic approaches, once the occupants of the main diagonal have been specified, the computer proceeds to solve for the principal axes in the matrix. The first axis (factor) extracted accounts for the greatest amount of common variance among the variables. This variance is partitioned from the matrix, and the second axis is extracted. Factors will be extracted until the default or preset eigenvalue is reached. The eigenvalue, the sum of the squared correlations of each variable with a factor, identifies the amount of variance explained by that factor. As mentioned above, factors with an eigenvalue of 1 or greater are usually considered nontrivial. The basis for this argument is that the original matrix can be efficiently reproduced by the set of eigenvectors associated with eigenvalues greater than or equal to one. The smallest number of factors is desirable for reasons of parsimony. Guttman (1954) provided three ways to estimate the lower bound for the number of factors needed to reproduce the matrix. These are discussed together for sake of clarity but could be separated for each model. (a) When using principal components where unity is placed on the diagonal, the number of roots extracted with eigenvalues greater than or equal to 1 is the best estimate of the number of factors. (b) On the other hand, when squared multiple correlations are on the main diagonal, the number of nonnegative characteristic roots (zero and all positive numbers) is the lower bound for the number of factors. (c) In practice, however, with sample rather than population models, with squared multiple correlations on the diagonal, using the criteria of greater than or equal to zero may produce an exorbitantly high number of trivial factors. The theoretical and mathematical criteria must then be balanced to solve the dilemma of the number of *real* factors present in the solution. The theoretical considerations should be the driving force behind the interpretation of the numbers.

The second common factor approach available to the researcher is alpha factoring. The focus in most approaches, other than alpha, is the assumption that the universe of items has been identified and therefore no attention need be paid to reliability of the items. Alpha factoring assumes that the items to be factored are only a sample of the universe of items. In addition to extraction of the factors, the solution identifies how well the items represent the universe of items. By definition, the resulting factors are representative of factors assumed to exist in the universe. In practice, the correlation matrix used to obtain the factor solution is generated to maximize the shared portion of the variables in the sample (communalities). The estimate placed on the main diagonal is then a computer-generated mathematical function of the usual correlation matrix, the reliability matrix, and the matrix representing the unique contribution of each item. The outcome of this mathematical function is a matrix corrected for attenuation. For a more thorough discussion of alpha factoring see Kaiser and Caffrey (1965). If further discussion of correcting for attenuation is needed, see

Murdaugh (1981). It seems logical to consider alpha factoring as an extraction approach to be used in the initial stages of instrument development.

Other extraction methods include unweighted least squares (ULS) and generalized least squares (GLS). These approaches use solutions based solely on manipulation of the off-diagonals of the correlation matrix. They differ in much the same way that simultaneous and stepwise multiple regressions differ. In the GLS approach, only one factor is extracted at each step. In ULS there is a simultaneous extraction of the number of factors specified by the analyst. Of course, the analyst must have some notion of the number of factors to be extracted in the ULS approach. For both methods, the criterion used for the matrix solution is the minimization of the residuals between the original correlation matrix and the reproduced matrix. These approaches are particularly appealing because they focus on the minimization of residuals in such a way that the actual values of the main diagonal do not assume such importance in the factor extraction.

Image analysis is based on the attempt to identify the common part of item variance. Multiple regression is used to predict an *image score* for each item from the other items in the matrix. The image scores produce a covariance matrix which is then submitted to a principal components analysis. Regression analysis predicts scores and the consequent matrix directly from the empirical data (Gorsuch, 1983; Nunnally, 1978). This data-driven model, therefore, has the advantages of the principal components approach while recognizing the systematic component of measurement error. Using this method, if the assumptions of the structure of the model are correct, the resulting anti-image covariance matrix will approximate zero. In this way, the analyst has some feedback on the stability of the solution. A major disadvantage, however, is that the method is not consonant with the philosophic notion of the existence of true but unmeasured factors.

The final major decision, at Level D, is determining if the extracted factors are to be rotated. The amount of common variance explained is unchanged; rotation allocates this variance in such a way that the factors are easier to identify and interpret. Thurstone's (1947) ideal simple structure has each item loading on only one factor. All orthogonal rotation methods aim to approach this ideal, but they are rarely successful.

There are two rotation methods, orthogonal and oblique (Level E). Orthogonal rotation is based on the assumption that the factors are uncorrelated, and thus a 90° angle is maintained by the axes in hyperspace that describe the factor's location. Oblique rotations, on the other hand, assume that factors may be correlated with each other and do not require 90° angles between the axes. There are several options for the orthogonal rotations.

The most frequently used orthogonal options are varimax, quartimax, and equimax rotations. Quartimax rotation is used infrequently, however, as it seeks to maximize item loadings on the first factor. The resulting small number of factors are substantively significant, but the loadings for some items may be small.

Varimax rotation is the most frequently used and reported option. It maximizes the sum of the variances of the squared loadings in the factor matrix. This allows for more factors than the quartimax option and tends to clarify the relationship of items to factors by maximizing the loading on one factor and minimizing loadings on all others. The advantage of the varimax is that the extracted factors have a greater number of items that load only on those factors.

The equimax procedure maximizes the variance of the loadings in both the matrix rows (items) and columns (factors). This procedure provides the advantages of the quartimax and varimax options. The disadvantage is that the solutions obtained are not quite as clear as those obtained from either of the other two rotations.

Should the researcher hypothesize the factors as being correlated, an oblique rotation may be chosen at decision Level E. The direct oblimin procedure is the oblique option found in most statistical packages. According to Nunnally (1978, p. 376), "it is intuitively appealing to place factor vectors through dominant clusters of variables, which usually leads to oblique rotations." The resultant solution, however, may be difficult to interpret since the closeness of any two vectors may obscure the distinction between factors.

The factor analyst may choose to implement several options in regard to selection of specific factor solutions. When several rotation procedures are applied to the extracted factors, comparison of the results, particularly from the perspective of the theoretical framework, will result in the strongest final decision. Additionally, "if the simple structure is clear, any of the more popular procedures can be expected to lead to the same interpretations" (Gorsuch, 1983, p. 205). Comparing the results of several rotations and finding strong agreement strengthens the analyst's confidence in the outcome. After all of the decisions have been made and the statistical procedures have been completed, the most difficult task remains: interpretation of the results and planning for a confirmatory analysis. This task is not as amenable to a decision tree and the researcher must fall back on what should have been the original base of the work—the theoretical model. In this way the analyst comes full circle and chooses and interprets results in light of sound theory.

References

Carmines, E. G., & Zeller, R. A. (1979). *Reliability and validity assessment.* Beverly Hills: Sage Publications.

Gorsuch, R. L. (1983). *Factor analysis* (2nd ed.). London: Lawrence Erlbaum Associates.

Guttman, L. (1954). Some necessary conditions for common factor analysis. *Psychometrica, 19*(2), 149–161.

Harris, R. J. (1985). *A primer of multivariate statistics.* Orlando: Academic Press.

Kaiser, H. F., & Caffrey, J. (1965). Alpha factor analysis. *Psychometrica, 30*(1), 1–14.

Murdaugh, C. (1981). Problems in doing nursing research: Measurement error and attenuation. *Western Journal of Nursing Research, 3,* 252–256.

Nunnally, J. C. (1978). *Psychometric theory* (2nd ed.). New York: McGraw-Hill.

Thurstone, L. L. (1947). *Multiple-factor analysis.* Chicago: The University of Chicago Press.

Comparison of Factor Analysis Options Using the Home/Employment Orientation Scale

JoAnne M. Youngblut

Factor analysis is a commonly used technique for evaluating the strength of the relationship of individual items of a scale with the latent concept, assessing content or construct validity of an instrument, determining plausible structures underlying a set of variables, and combining a set of variables into one composite score. In using the technique, the analyst must make decisions about the type of extraction and rotation to request, and about the number of factors to retain. The purposes of this paper are to compare the results obtained with each of the rotation and extraction methods in traditional factor analysis and with LISREL (Joreskog & Sorbom, 1988), and to explore how these results influence the decisions one makes regarding the structure and item composition of a scale.

The decision regarding which type of extraction to use can be based on one's theoretical expectation about the type of error that is present in the scores obtained. The classic model assumes that all error is random where the neoclassic acknowledges both a random and a systematic component (Ferketich & Muller, 1990). Choosing the classic model necessitates principal components (PC) extraction; whereas, principal axes factoring (PAF), image factoring (IF), alpha factoring (AF), generalized least squares (GLS), and unweighted least squares (ULS) are representative of the neoclassic model.

The method of extraction also reflects the analyst's assumptions about the factors obtained (Nunnally, 1978). Principal components extracts "real" factors in the sample, those that are due to optimization of the data at hand. Because these factors are "real" rather than hypothetical, some sources refer to them as components or component factors rather than as factors (Kim & Mueller, 1978; Nunnally, 1978). Maximum likelihood (ML) extracts "real" factors in the population, using the sample correlation matrix to predict the population matrix. In contrast, the PAF, IF, and AF extractions seek to uncover hypothetical factors that are estimated from the observed data but that are not completely defined by those data.

Each of these extraction methods differ mathematically, based on manipulations of the correlation matrix to be analyzed. The PC and PAF methods differ because of the value placed on the diagonal of the correlation matrix. Principal components places a "1" in each of the diagonal spots, whereas PAF places squared multiple correlations on the main diagonal. The IF, AF, GLS, and ULS methods manipulate the off-diagonal elements before extraction. ML adjusts the correlation matrix after each iteration, so that more weight is given to correlations with less unique variance (Kim & Mueller, 1978). In addition, each subsequent factor is tested for significance before extraction (Nunnally, 1978). Thus, nonsignificant factors are not extracted and interpretation is simplified.

The second decision to be made is whether to rotate the extracted factors. Nunnally (1978) recommends that the analyst rotate the factors in order to simplify the interpretation of the factor structure. However, if one chooses PC extraction, rotation may not be theoretically appropriate (Ferketich & Muller, 1990). If rotation is desired, the analyst must decide whether the factors should be orthogonal (uncorrelated) or oblique (correlated).

A third decision in factor analysis is the number of factors to extract. There are many rules of thumb that the analyst may use to guide the decision, or the number of factors may be decided on the basis of the structure that the analyst expects theoretically. Frequently, the number of factors extracted on the first factor analysis is decided either by the analyst theoretically or by the computer empirically. On subsequent factor analyses, the analyst changes the number of factors based either on the values or patterns of the eigenvalues or on the clarity of the factor loadings. For example, if several variables load strongly on two factors, the analyst may decrease or increase the number of factors by one to see if the loadings are cleaner.

Many other technical decisions must be made so that the computer can carry out the procedure. Default set-

JoAnne M. Youngblut, PhD, RN, is an assistant professor, Frances Payne Bolton School of Nursing, Case Western Reserve University, Cleveland, OH.

From *Nursing Research,* March/April 1993, *42,* 122–124.

tings are usually written into the computer program; however, the analyst can override most of them if necessary. For example, in the SPSS FACTOR procedure, the number of iterations, the convergence criterion for extraction and for rotation, and the minimum eigenvalue can be controlled with the /CRITERIA subcommand. In the SAS FACTOR procedure, the subcommands are MAXITER, CONVERGE, and MINEIGEN, respectively.

Despite the many available options and the degree of flexibility, traditional factor analysis does not allow the analyst to specify the exact factor structure of the variables. The analyst may specify only the number of factors to be extracted, not which variables should load on which factors. Looking at the pattern of factor loadings provides an indirect test of the expected model. Unfortunately, problems that affect the interpretation of the factor analysis are often encountered. Variables that are expected to load together, i.e., to represent a particular concept, do not load together. When this happens, the analyst can change the number of factors extracted and hope for the best. Frequently, the analyst runs several factor analyses, manipulating the number of factors extracted and perhaps dropping items that do not load strongly. When several different underlying structures are possible, the analyst is left with the difficult decision of choosing the "best" or "right" solution, often by weighing the positives and the negatives of each.

Confirmatory factor analysis (CFA) with programs such as LISREL (Joreskog & Sorbom, 1988) or EQS (Bentler, 1989) provides the needed control over the analysis in order to directly test the analyst's theoretical expectations about the underlying structure of a scale (Long, 1983). With CFA, the analyst specifies which variables belong to which latent concepts or factors. The program then calculates the parameters based on the hypothesized model and provides measures of fit that help the analyst to see whether the hypothesized model adequately represents the relationships among the variables.

Faced with all the options in traditional factor analysis, Ferketich and Muller (1990) suggest that the analyst try several extractions and rotations. They reason that if the scale holds up under several methods, one can be more confident in the structure of the relationships among the variables. Nunnally (1978) also states that the results obtained with different extraction methods often are remarkably similar.

Instrument

The Home/Employment Orientation (HEO) Scale (Youngblut, Loveland-Cherry & Horan, 1990) was part of a battery of instruments completed by mothers ($N = 110$) in a large, longitudinal study of parents' reactions to the premature birth of an infant. The original scale contained 10 items that mothers rated on an 8-point Likert scale ranging from 1 (strongly agree) to 8 (strongly disagree). Word anchors were not provided for the other six points on the scale. Coefficient alpha for the 10-item scale was .76.

The original scale was designed to measure two related, but distinct, concepts: the mother's orientation toward being employed and her orientation toward staying home with her children. It was expected that these two concepts did not lie on opposite ends of the same continuum, but rather that each was a separate continuum ranging from low to high. Thus, two factors (subscales) with five items each were hypothesized for the 10-item scale.

Analysis Procedures

Each of the extraction methods were used in turn in order to see if the different extraction and rotation methods provided different information about the structure of the scale, the relative strength of the relationship between the items and the underlying concept, and the stability of the items' loadings. Two factors were specified in the procedure since that was the a priori expectation. Varimax rotation was used with all extraction methods. A second PC extraction was done with oblique rotation (oblimin). Since the results obtained with oblique and varimax rotations with PC extraction were identical, other extractions with oblique rotation were not done. Nunnally (1978) suggests that loadings of < .40 are small and warrant caution in interpretation. Thus, items were considered to load strongly on a particular factor if the loading was ≥ .40. Items were considered to load on both factors if the absolute difference between the loadings was less than .20. Items that did not reach the .40 criterion were considered not to load on either factor. Finally, a one-factor solution with PC extraction was requested in order to further assess the strength of each item (Table 1).

Comparison of Methods

Only PC supported the extraction of two component factors. The other six methods supported only one factor. For PC, one item did not load cleanly on one factor and one item did not load strongly on either factor. For AF, two items did not load strongly and one did not load cleanly. For the remaining five methods (PAF, ML, IF, ULS, GLS), there were two items that did not load cleanly and three that did not load strongly. Finding that half of the scale's items did not load strongly and cleanly on a factor suggests that the analyst might consider a one-factor solution.

TABLE 1 Comparison of Factor Loadings

Item	Principal Components	Maximum Likelihood	Principal Axis	Alpha	Image	Unweighted Least Squares	Generalized Least Squares	Principal Components	Principal Components
* Factors	2	2	2	2	2	2	2	2	1
Rotation	Varimax	Varimax	Varimax	Varimax	Varimax	Varimax	Varimax	Oblimin	Varimax
Item 1	F1	F1	F1	F1	F1	F1	F1	F1	F1
Item 2	F1	F1	F1	F1	F1	F1	F1	F1	F1
Item 3	F1	B	B	F1	B	B	B	F1	F1
Item 4	F1	N	N	F1	N	N	N	F1	N
Item 5	F1	F1	F1	F1	F1	F1	F1	F1	F1
Item 6	F2	F2	F2	F2	F1	F2	F2	F2	F1
Item 7	B	F2	F2	B	F2	F2	F2	B	F1
Item 8	N	N	N	N	N	N	N	N	N
Item 9	F1	B	B	F1	B	B	B	F1	F1
Item 10	F2	N	N	N	N	N	N	F2	N

NOTE: F1 = Factor #1; F2 = Factor #2; B = Both Factors; N = Neither Factor.

Factor analysis can be used to identify psychometrically weak items, i.e., those that do not load strongly in a one-factor solution. Items 4, 8, and 10 did not perform well on many of the extractions. These same three items did not load strongly in the one-factor solution.

LISREL VII (Joreskog & Sorbom, 1988) was used to test the proposed theoretical structure of the HEO. Results of the LISREL test are presented in Figure 1. Although the chi-square is significant, the goodness-of-fit index of .89 is very close to the recommended .90 criterion for good fit of the model to the data (Boyd, Frey & Aaronson, 1988). However, inspection of the parameters raises some questions about the adequacy of the theoretical model. First, the residuals for five indicators are high (> .60) and all are significant ($p < .01$). Thus, the factor to which the indicator is tied does not account for a major part of the variance in these indicators. Second, three of the indicators are not tied strongly to the theorized factor. Since the parameters on the arrows between the factor and the indicator are analogous to factor loadings, criteria established to evaluate strength of a loading in factor analysis can be used to evaluate the tie

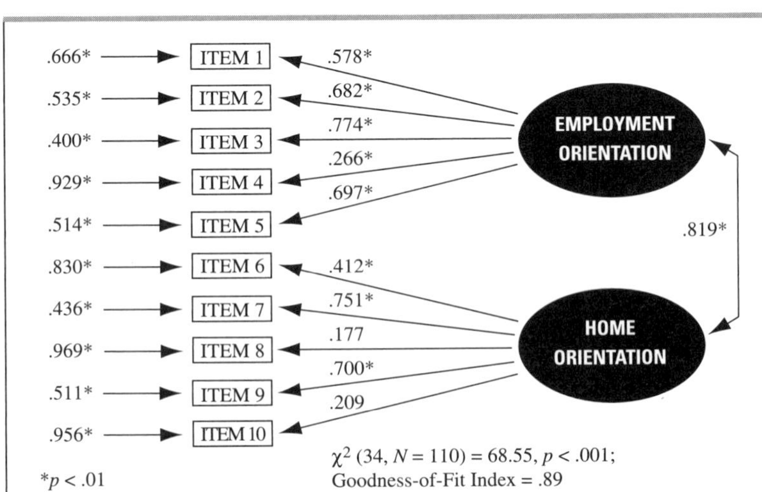

FIGURE 1 Testing Factor Structure with LISREL

between the factor and the indicator (Long, 1983). Thus, items 4, 8, and 10 do not load strongly. Finally, the strength of the correlation ($r = .82$) between the two latent factors indicates that the two concepts are redundant. Perhaps a one-factor solution would be more suitable in this case.

Conclusions

The patterns of loadings were remarkably similar across the different types of extractions and rotations available in traditional factor analysis. Items that were strong with one extraction tended to be strong across methods. The same was true for weaker items. In addition, confirmatory factor analysis supported the results of the traditional factor analysis. While this may be unique to the scale used, it is likely that these similarities indicate that the HEO scale has a strong factor structure (Nunnally, 1978).

Factor analysis often is used to provide information about the composition of a scale. In order to decide which items to keep and which items to drop from a particular scale, the researcher generally combines the information obtained from a factor analysis and a reliability analysis. This study indicates that the researcher's decision may be facilitated by comparing an item's performance on several factor analyses with different extractions. In addition, CFA with programs such as LISREL or EQS can further substantiate the researcher's ideas about scale composition and factor structure.

References

Bentler, P. M. (1989). *EQS Structural Equations Program Manual.* Los Angeles: BMDP Statistical Software.

Boyd, C. J., Frey, M. A., & Aaronson, L. S. (1988). Structural equation models and nursing research: Part I. *Nursing Research, 37,* 249–252.

Ferketich, S., & Muller, M. (1990). Factor analysis revisited. *Nursing Research, 39,* 59–61.

Joreskog, K. G., & Sorbom, D. (1988). *LISREL VII.* Mooresville, IN: Scientific Software.

Kim, J. O., & Mueller,.C. W. (1978). *Factor analysis: Statistical methods and practical issues.* Beverly Hills: Sage.

Long, J. S. (1983). *Confirmatory factor analysis.* Beverly Hills: Sage.

Nunnally, J. C. (1978). *Psychometric theory.* New York: McGraw-Hill.

Youngblut, J. M., Loveland-Cherry, C. J., & Horan, M. (1990). Factors related to maternal employment status following the premature birth of an infant. *Nursing Research, 39,* 237–240.

Canonical Analysis in Nursing Research

Richard L. Wikoff ■ **Patricia Miller**

Canonical analysis was derived more than 55 years ago (Hotelling, 1935, 1936), but because of its complexity, it has not been used much until recently. With the development of sophisticated computer program packages, the original work of Hotelling has been extended and many proofs of the technique have been offered.

The purpose of this article is to present the canonical model and discuss its use and interpretation. This will be done using data collected for an article previously published in *Nursing Research* (Miller, Wikoff, McMahon, Garrett & Ringel, 1988). The mathematical bases of canonical analysis will not be presented. Such information may be found in several textbooks, including Anderson (1958), Cooley and Lohnes (1971), Morrison (1976), and Tatsuoka (1971).

Canonical analysis is appropriate when one is interested in the relationship between two sets of continuously measured variables. Since canonical analysis is based on the general linear model, it requires the same assumptions as multiple correlation, regression analysis, and factor analysis. This includes linearity of variables, homoscedasticity, and at least interval data if the notion of variance is to have any meaning. If inferences are to be made from the results then the assumption of multivariate normality must be met. For further discussion of these assumptions, see Pedhazur (1982) and Stevens (1986). Variables should be measured reliably and the range of scores not restricted, as either of these will attenuate the results.

Miller et al. (1988) reported the results of a longitudinal study of patients who had suffered a myocardial infarction (MI). They were evaluated in the hospital and again at 30 days, 60 days, 1 year, and 2 years following the MI. At each time period, each patient was given a battery of tests, including the Health Behavior Scale (HBS), a 5-point Likert type scale designed to measure patient adherence to the medical regimen. "If I am at home I will follow my diet" is an example of the type of item. The scale has five subscales, one for each of five regimen prescriptions (diet, smoking, activities, medicine, and modification of stress response). Each subscale has four items: one for each of four situations (home, work, sports, or social). The subscales (20 points possible) were used to measure medical regimen adherence (MRAS) for each prescription. In order to assess the validity of the subjects' responses, the subject's spouse or significant other was asked to complete a modified version of the HBS. For example, the item above was reworded, "If my spouse is at home, he/she follows the prescribed diet." This scale will be referred to as the Medical Regimen Adherence-Significant Other (MRAO). In the discussion that follows, the MRAO scales are the predictors and the MRAS scales the criteria. Data from the two-year follow-up are used to illustrate canonical correlation. Because there were so few smokers, the smoking subscales were not included.

The most important question in this illustration, since we are interested in the validity of the patients' responses, is, "Is there a significant overlap between the patient and significant other responses, or are they significantly different?" However, we might ask several other questions. For example, How strong is the relationship between patient and significant other responses? How many canonical functions are necessary to account for the shared variance between these two sets of responses? What are the relative weights of the different subscales in this relationship? How much variance in each set can be accounted for by virtue of the correlation with the other set? How much of the variance of the patients' responses is predictable from the spouses' responses?

Canonical analysis rests on an analysis of a correlation matrix containing the intercorrelations of two sets of variables. The two sets of variables may be labeled X (predictors) and Y (criteria). Each set consists of two or more variables. There are p variables in X and q variables in Y. Each subject is measured on each of the $(p + q)$ variables. Next, all possible intercorrelations are deter-

Richard L. Wikoff, PhD, is professor, Department of Psychology, University of Nebraska at Omaha, Omaha, NE.

Patricia Miller, PhD, RN, is a professor at Briarcliff College, College of Nursing, Sioux City, IA.

From *Nursing Research,* November/December 1991, *40,* 367–370.

TABLE 1 Intercorrelation Matrix

	MRAS				MRAO			
	1	2	3	4	1	2	3	4
MRAS 1	–	.59	.45	–.04	.54	.30	.42	.09
MRAS 2	.59	–	.72	.34	.22	.38	.43	.41
MRAS 3	.45	.72	–	.44	.04	.11	.30	.48
MRAS 4	–.04	.34	.44	–	–.04	–.06	–.02	.82
MRAO 1	.54	.22	.04	–.04	–	.68	.46	.08
MRAO 2	.30	.38	.11	–.06	.68	–	.56	.08
MRAO 3	.42	.43	.30	–.02	.46	.56	–	.08
MRAO 4	.09	.41	.48	.82	.08	.08	.08	–

NOTE: $r \geq .14$, $p < .05$; $r \geq .18$, $p < .01$; 1 = Diet, 2 = Activity, 3 = Stress, 4 = Meds

mined to form a $(p + q)$ by $(p + q)$ matrix (**R**). This matrix (**R**) can be partitioned into four submatrices. $\mathbf{R}_{xx}$ contains the correlations among the X variables, $\mathbf{R}_{yy}$ the intercorrelations in the Y set, and $\mathbf{R}_{xy}$ and $\mathbf{R}_{yx}$ the intercorrelations of the X and Y variables. This provides two kinds of information, the pattern of interdependence within each of the sets and the pattern of correlations between the two sets. The problem is to determine the pattern of these between-sets correlations. The intercorrelation matrix for the regimen-adherence data is presented in Table 1.

The analysis is accomplished by determining pairs of linear combinations of the original variables called canonical variates such that in each pair the resultant linear combination of the X variables is maximally correlated with the linear combination of the Y variables. Each variate extracts the maximum amount of variance possible and each succeeding variate is orthogonal to the preceding one. The procedure is similar to principal components analysis except for the restriction that the sets of weighted variables be maximally correlated for each variate pair. The weights applied to the linear combinations may be determined in a form to be applied to raw scores (similar to b coefficients in regression analysis) or in standardized form to be applied to z scores (similar to the β weights of regression analysis). The raw and standardized canonical coefficients are presented in Table 2 for the predictor variables and in Table 3 for the criterion variables.

If the coefficients are multiplied times the scores for the corresponding variables and summed, the result is a canonical score. For example, to get the canonical score

TABLE 2 Raw and Standardized Canonical Coefficients for the MRAO Variables of the MI Data

	RAW CANONICAL COEFFICIENTS FOR MRAO VARIABLES			
	Function			
Variable	1	2	3	4
Diet	.01608	.28531	.17023	.04866
Activity	.02306	–.13333	–.21408	.22736
Stress	–.02609	.08751	–.15098	–.27451
Medication	–.55862	–.01726	.02773	.05797
	STANDARDIZED COEFFICIENTS FOR MRAO VARIABLES			
Diet	.06418	1.13896	.67957	.19427
Activity	.09748	–.56364	–.90497	.96114
Stress	–.09683	.32479	–.56038	–1.01889
Medication	–.99768	–.03082	.04952	.10353

TABLE 3 **Raw and Standardized Canonical Coefficients for the MRAS Variables of the MI Data**

	RAW CANONICAL COEFFICIENTS FOR MRAS VARIABLES			
	Function			
Variable	*1*	*2*	*3*	*4*
Diet	.00791	.29511	.09904	.01395
Activity	.01051	−.05753	−.27123	−.19152
Stress	.03830	−.05062	−.00200	.34020
Medication	.30804	.05472	.19560	−.15468
	STANDARDIZED COEFFICIENTS FOR MRAS VARIABLES			
Diet	.03131	1.16773	.39190	.05522
Activity	.04774	−.26125	−1.23170	−.86973
Stress	.16005	−.21157	−.00837	1.42188
Medication	.89602	.15917	.56895	−.44992

for subject *i* on the predictors for Function 1, multiply as follows:

$z_{xi} = .06418DO + .09748AO - .09683SO - .99768MO$

The formula for the criteria is:

$z_{yi} = .03131DS + .04774AS + .16005SS + .89602MS$

The correlation between z_y and z_x is the canonical correlation (R_c). It is a product moment correlation and indicates the degree of correlation between the weighted MRAO variables and the weighted MRAS variables. The square of the canonical correlation (R_c^2) is the eigenvalue and gives the percent of variance in the weighted MRAS set accounted for by the weighted MRAO set.

Successive canonical variables are determined as long as the relationships are significant or until the number of variates equals the number of variables in the smaller set, since at that time 100% of the variance of that set will have been extracted (Stewart & Love, 1968). The variates are similar to the components of principal components analysis. Table 4 shows the canonical correlations, eigenvalues, lambdas, and probability levels for the MI data.

TABLE 4 **Eigenvalues, Canonical Correlations, and Tests of Significance for the MI Data**

Root No.	R_c	R_c^2	Lambda	F	p
1	.840	.705	.098	8.722	<.001
2	.695	.483	.333	6.334	<.001
3	.547	.299	.645	5.156	<.001
4	.284	.081	.919	3.769	.059

Lambda is a multivariate test of significance. It is an inverse measure of the proportion of variance accounted for by the variates. A lambda of 1.00 means that there is no discriminating information in the variate. Because its distribution is so complicated, it is usually transformed either to chi square or *F*.

The canonical functions are tested for significance using a series of hierarchical tests. The first *F* test indicates whether any of the canonical functions reported are significant (1 to 4). If *F* is significant, then at least the first function and its corresponding R_c are significant. After the first function has been removed, a test is made of the remaining functions (2 to 4). If this *F* is significant, then at least the next function is significant. Testing continues in this stepwise manner until all of the functions have been removed. In the MI data, the first three functions were significant beyond the .001 level, and the probability level of the fourth was .059.

The correlations between the original variables and the variates can be calculated and the resulting matrix is known as a structure matrix. This matrix is shown in Table 5.

The variates represent derived variables similar to the components of principal component analysis, and the correlations are similar to loadings. The squares of the loadings are coefficients of determination. They indicate the proportion of variance in each of the original variables accounted for by each of the canonical variables. For example, the correlation between MRAS-Activity and canonical Function 1 was .475. This value squared is .226. Thus, 22.6% of the variance in this subtest is

TABLE 5 Correlations Between Original Variables and the Canonical Variables

Variable	CANONICAL VARIABLE 1	2	3	4
	MRAO VARIABLES			
Diet	.003	.911	.163	.380
Activity	.006	.364	.763	.535
Stress	−.094	.521	.752	−.393
Medications	−.992	.044	.012	.115
Sum L^2	.993	1.236	1.174	.598
Var. Ext	.2482	.3090	.2935	.1495
	MRAS VARIABLES			
Diet	.081	.945	.289	.130
Activity	.475	.269	.838	−.018
Stress	.598	.107	.458	.649
Medications	.981	−.066	−.137	−.120
ΣL^2	1.552	.981	1.014	.453
Var. Ext.	.3880	.2453	.2535	.1132

accounted for by Function 1. The column sum of the squared loadings of variables (ΣL^2) within a set for each variate gives the variance extracted from the set by the variate. When this is divided by the number of variables in the set, the resulting value is the proportion of the variance of the set extracted by the canonical variate. For example, for Function 1, the total variance extracted from the MRAS variables was 1.552. This value divided by 4 (the number of variables) is .3880. Thus 38.8% of the variance of the MRAS variables was accounted for by Function 1.

The square of the canonical correlation for a variate (R_c^2) is the proportion of variance in one of the weighted variable sets predictable from the other weighted variable set. However, each variate accounts for only a part of the variance of the set of original variables. The total proportion accounted for by all the variates will be less than 100% of the variance in the larger set, and less than 100% for the smaller set unless the number of significant variates equals the number of variables in the smaller set. If the proportion of variance in the criterion variables extracted by a variate is multiplied times R_c^2 for the variate, the result is the proportion of variance in the criterion variables explained by the predictor variables in variate *i*. Similarly, the variance in the predictors, which is accounted for by the criterion variables, can be calculated for each of the variates. These values are referred to as the redundancies (Stewart & Love, 1968). The variances accounted for and the redundancies are shown in Table 6.

The R_c^2 for Variate 1 was .705. The proportion of variance accounted for in the MRAS variables by Variate 1 was .3880. Multiply .705 times .3880 and the result is .2735. Thus, a little over 27% of the variance of the MRAS variables is accounted for by the MRAO variables. The proportion of variance in the MRAS variables accounted for by Variate 2 was .2453. The R_c^2 for Variate 2 was .483. The redundancy equals .483 times .2453 = .1185. The redundancy for all four variates given the MRAO variables was .4770. Given the MRAS variables, 42.41% of the variance in the MRAO variables is redundant. Note that the redundancy is asymmetrical.

The canonical variables are similar to components in principal component analysis. Because of the restriction that the correlation between the two sets of weighted variables be maximized, these dimensions are not always interpretable. It would be possible to rotate them to a meaningful solution. However, to do so would reduce the canonical correlations, thus defeating the purpose of canonical analysis.

The results of the canonical analysis indicate significant agreement between the patients' and spouses' responses. Approximately half of the variance of the patients' responses (47.70) was explained by the responses of the spouses. Four canonical variables are necessary to

TABLE 6 **Components of Redundancy Measure**

Canon Funct.	R_c	R_c^2	Var. Ext.	Cum. Var.	Red.	Prop of Total Red.
			MRAO SET			
1	.840	.705	.2482	.2482	.1750	.1750
2	.695	.483	.3090	.5572	.1492	.3242
3	.547	.299	.2935	.8507	.0878	.4120
4	.284	.081	.1495	1.0002*	.0121	.4241
			MRAS SET			
1	.840	.705	.3880	.3880	.2735	.2735
2	.695	.483	.2453	.6333	.1185	.3920
3	.547	.299	.2535	.8868	.0758	.4678
4	.284	.081	.1132	1.0000	.0092	.4770

* Due to rounding errors

account for the relationship between the two sets. This makes sense as the four scales measure different concepts.

It is often necessary to use data reported by the patient when examining many of the factors of interest to nurses, such as those that affect compliance behaviors for cardiovascular disease patients. But, if the question raised has to do with whether patients are truthfully reporting their behavior, the use of canonical correlation as illustrated in this study provides independent affirmation of patient compliance. Canonical analysis has applications in many fields. The technique is not limited to any one discipline. When one is interested in the relationship between two sets of continuously measured variables, canonical analysis is the procedure to use.

References

Anderson, T. W. (1958). *An introduction to multivariate statistical analysis.* New York: Wiley.

Cooley, W. W., & Lohnes, P. R. (1971). *Multivariate data analysis.* New York: Wiley.

Hotelling, H. (1935). The most predictable criterion. *Journal of Educational Psychology, 26,* 139–142.

Hotelling, H. (1936). Relations between two sets of variables, *Biometrika, 28,* 321–377.

Miller, P., Wikoff, R., McMahon, R., Garrett, M., & Ringel, K. (1988). Influence of a nursing intervention on regimen adherence and societal adjustments postmyocardial infarction. *Nursing Research,* 37, 297–302.

Morrison, D. F. (1976). *Multivariate statistical methods* (2nd ed.). New York: McGraw-Hill.

Pedhazur, E. J. (1982). *Multiple regression in behavioral research* (2nd ed.). New York: Holt, Rinehart & Winston.

Stevens, J. (1986). *Applied multivariate statistics for the social sciences.* Hillsdale, NJ: Lawrence Erlbaum Associates.

Stewart, D., & Love, W. (1968). A general canonical correlation index. *Psychological Bulletin,* 70, 160–163.

Tatsuoka, M. M. (1971). *Multivariate analysis.* New York: Wiley.

Discriminant Analysis

Geraldine E. Edens

As nursing research increases in complexity, nurse researchers often find univariate statistical techniques inadequate. As Goodwin (1984) discussed, there are distinct advantages in choosing a single multivariate statistical technique to test a research hypothesis, such as controlling alpha or the probability of committing a Type I error, increasing power, and increasing efficiency in analysis and interpretation. One multivariate statistical technique, discriminant analysis, provides a means for establishing significant group differences, explaining those differences, and classifying future individuals believed to belong to one of the groups represented (Tatsuoka, 1971).

When the dependent or criterion variable is dichotomous in nature (i.e., defined by membership in a particular group), and the research question is concerned with identifying the characteristics associated with group membership, discriminant analysis is the appropriate statistical technique to use. Once characteristics of group membership are known, discriminant analysis can also be used to classify future cases into the identified groups.

Like regression analysis, discriminant analysis allows the researcher to identify what independent or predictor variables (also referred to as discriminating variables) are related to the criterion variable and, in addition, predict values on the criterion variable when given values on the independent or predictor variables. The major difference in discriminant analysis is that the researcher predicts group membership instead of a continuously scaled score that may assume a wide range of values. Groups are identified by the researcher and discriminating variables are chosen that measure characteristics on which the groups are expected to differ.

Several published nursing studies have used discriminant analysis as a primary or a secondary form of data analysis. For example, Trainor (1982) sought to identify characteristics that differentiated two groups of individuals enrolled in a self-help group for ostomates, those who visited other ostomates and those who did not. The discriminating variables age, type of ostomy, and length of time since the first ostomy surgery were included in the analysis. Smith and Shamansky (1983) randomly sampled 239 households to determine potential users of family nurse practitioner (FNP) services. The sample was divided into two groups, potential users and nonusers. Discriminant variables were then chosen to differentiate characteristics associated with the two groups. From the analysis the researchers obtained a profile of potential users of FNP services as an aid in the development of marketing strategies. Greenleaf (1983) used discriminant analysis to identify characteristics associated with women who participated in the labor force in nursing and other comparable professions. The dependent variable was made up of two mutually exclusive groups, in the labor force and out of the labor force. The discriminant variables were age, family income, educational preparation, children in the household, and general happiness.

Underlying Assumptions and Mathematical Formulations

For results of discriminant analysis to reflect reality, several underlying assumptions should be satisfied. First, the research problem must define at least two cases per group. Tatsuoka (1970), however, recommended that the total sample size be *at least* two or (preferably) three times the number of discriminating variables used. Thus, if five variables are used in the analysis, a sample size of 10 to 15 is required. Second, the number of discriminating variables to be included in the analysis cannot exceed the total number of cases minus two ($n - 2$), nor should they be fewer than the number of groups being compared. These variables must be measured at the interval level. Third, no discriminating variable can be a linear combination of other discriminating variables. Fourth, the covariance matrices for the groups must be equal. Finally, each group must be drawn from a population with a multivariate normal distribution on the discriminating variables. Not all aspects of discriminant analysis require that all these assumptions be met. Violations,

Geraldine E. Edens, PhD, RN, is an assistant professor in the School of Nursing, University of Miami, Coral Gables, FL.

From *Nursing Research,* July/August 1987, *36,* 257–261.

however, result in reduced efficiency and accuracy (Klecka, 1980).

Discriminant analysis attempts mathematically to weight and linearly combine the discriminating variables in such a way that maximal group differences are obtained. This is done through the formation of one or more linear discriminant functions (LDFs). Symbolically an LDF, for a composite of measures of p discriminating variables, for individuals in K criterion groups, can be expressed as $Y = v_1 X_1 + v_2 X_2 + \ldots + v_p X_p$ where Y is an individual's score on the first discriminant function, the vs are the weighted coefficients, and the Xs are the standardized values of the p discriminating variables used in the analysis. Mathematically, this linear combination of discriminating variables maximizes the ratio of the sum of squares and cross-product matrix among groups (H) and the sum of squares and cross-product matrix within groups (E). The discriminant coefficients (v) are derived by computing the largest characteristic root or eigenvalue (λ) of E^{-1} H and then solving a set of p equations to find the associated eigenvectors (Huberty, 1975). The result produces a number of uncorrelated and hierarchically ordered discriminant variates that maximize between group differences. The number of possible LDFs is equal to p (the number of discriminating variables) or $K - 1$ (the number of groups minus 1), whichever is smallest.

Describing Group Differences

Discriminant analysis is a versatile analytical strategy. It can be used to interpret multiresponse data in descriptive research studies. If significant group differences exist, discriminant analysis enables the researcher to gain a full understanding of the data set by answering the following questions: (a) How many dimensions are represented by the multivariate differences between groups? (b) How can these underlying dimensions be interpreted? (c) How can the groups be spatially represented? (d) What are the individual contributions of the original variables to the underlying dimensions? (Borgen & Seling, 1978).

Establishing Significant Group Differences

The first step in discriminant analysis is to determine if the discriminating variables are able to differentiate among the groups. Unless the researcher is assured group differences exist, it is meaningless to seek a linear composite of the discriminant variables for further analysis. Establishing separation is equivalent to significance testing using one-way multivariate analysis of variance (MANOVA). The omnibus null hypothesis is tested, using a multivariate test of significance (e.g., Wilk's lambda, Hotelling's T^2, Bartlett's V), to determine whether the group centroids or the imaginary points, which multidimensionally represent the groups' means on each of the discriminating variables, are equal to one another. If Wilk's lambda is used, for example, the value obtained is transformable to an F value for deciding whether to reject the null hypothesis. For a comprehensive discussion of MANOVA the reader is referred to Tatsuoka (1971).

Explaining Significant Group Differences

When significant group differences exist, a follow-up technique can be performed that enables the researcher to examine the number of dimensions on which the groups differ and to determine which discriminating variables contribute to the separation. Linear discriminant functions are derived using the best set of discriminating variables that define group membership. This is determined by controlling the order in which the discriminating variables enter the LDFs.

As in multiple regression, this is accomplished by employing stepup, stepdown, or stepwise procedures. If the order of entry can be determined a priori, a stepup or stepdown procedure is recommended, because the discrimination obtained at each step can be examined. When the order of entry is not specified a priori, a stepwise procedure should be used to look at all possible combinations of the variables. Criteria for inclusion and removal must be specified so that maximal group separation is obtained, such as minimizing Wilk's lambda. This procedure may be costly and time-consuming when the number of variables is large, because it tests all possible variable combinations. Variables may be eliminated and stepwise procedures repeated until the best subset of discriminating variables is obtained.

Once the LDFs are formed, the next step is to decide how many LDFs to retain for analysis. In the two-group case this is not an issue, as only one LDF is derived. In the multigroup case, however, there may be as many LDFs as there are discriminating variables or as many LDFs as the number of groups minus one, whichever is smaller. If the derived LDFs are viewed as axes in geometric space on which individual scores can be plotted, the higher the spatial dimension, the more difficult the interpretation of those scores becomes. Thus, the researcher should eliminate any LDFs that are judged not to contribute to group separation.

Elimination can be done several ways. Klecka (1975) suggested examining the eigenvalue and the canonical correlation associated with each LDF. The eigenvalue is a measure computed in the process of deriving the LDFs. The sum of the eigenvalues represents the total variance of the discriminating variables. Expressing each eigenvalue as a percentage of this sum yields the relative contribution of each LDF to the total variance and, thus, can be a basis for judging its overall worth. The canonical correlation provides a measure of the strength of association between each LDF and the criterion group variable. Squaring the canonical correlation coefficient can be interpreted as the proportion of variance in the LDF explained by the groups. Thus, the lower the canonical correlation, the lower the overall ability of the LDF to discriminate among the groups.

Another means of judging the value of a LDF is through tests of significance. Although Huberty (1975) noted the literature on these procedures lacks clarity, the computation of Wilk's lambda is provided in several computer packages and thus warrants explanation. Wilk's lambda tests the statistical significance of the variance *un*accounted for by the independent variables that are included in the LDF. It is computed as each function is derived, beginning with zero functions, and can be transformed into a chi-square statistic to obtain significance levels. The larger the Wilk's lambda, the less the unexplained variance. Therefore, when Wilk's lambda is no longer significant, the information contained on remaining functions is of little importance to the analysis.

For example, a researcher investigated whether students who chose one of four specialty areas for practice after graduation from a baccalaureate school of nursing could be differentiated from one another on the basis of age, grade point average (GPA), assertiveness, ego development, and critical thinking ability. A random sample of 80 graduating seniors were divided into four groups based on their choice for nursing practice after graduation: Group 1, medical-surgical; Group 2, maternal-child; Group 3, mental health; and Group 4, critical care. A four-group discriminant analysis was performed using five discriminating variables.

Using Wilk's lambda as a test of significance, separation was found to exist among the groups. A value of .1023 was obtained that, when transformed to an F statistic, $F = 17.042$, was significant at the .01 level. Three LDFs were then derived from the data and yielded values as shown in Table 1. In this example, Function 1 explained the greatest proportion of variance (eigenvalue = 4.33) of the discriminating variables. Both Functions 1 and 2 were strongly associated with the groups (canonical correlations = .901 and .631, respectively). Function 3 accounted for a small percentage of the variance and was not strongly associated with the groups. The Wilk's lambda of .909, obtained after Function 2 was derived, was not significant, indicating little need for additional functions. Thus, Functions 1 and 2 should be retained for further analysis and Function 3 should be eliminated.

Graphic Representation of Linear Discriminant Functions

Once useless LDFs have been eliminated, the next step is interpretation. Graphic representation of the LDFs is often helpful. Figure 1 plots the four criterion groups on the two LDFs that were retained. Each LDF represents a separate dimension on which individual discriminant scores can be plotted. For comparative purposes, group centroids on each of the discriminant functions are computed and plotted. In this example the first LDF separated Groups 1, 2, and 4 from Group 3 and the second LDF separated Groups 1, 2, and 3 from Group 4. Thus, the analysis suggests to this point that students choosing to practice in medical-surgical, maternal-child, and critical care areas differed from students choosing to practice in mental health, and students choosing to practice in medical-surgical, maternal-child, and mental health areas differed from students choosing critical care.

Determining Variable Contribution to the Linear Discriminant Function

Given this information, the next task is to interpret on which discriminating characteristics the groups differ. By examining coefficients associated with each LDF, a determination of what the LDFs mean, in terms of the original variables, can be made. Functions are often named on the basis of this interpretation. Two types of coefficients

TABLE 1 Values of Linear Discriminant Functions, Using Wilk's Lambda

Linear Discriminant Function	Eigen-value	Percentage of Variance	Canonical Correlation	After Function	Wilk's Lambda	Chi Square	Sign
				0	.102	169.8	.00
1	4.33	85.03	.901	1	.546	45.0	.00
2	.66	13.03	.631	2	.909	7.0	.15
3	.09	1.95	.300				

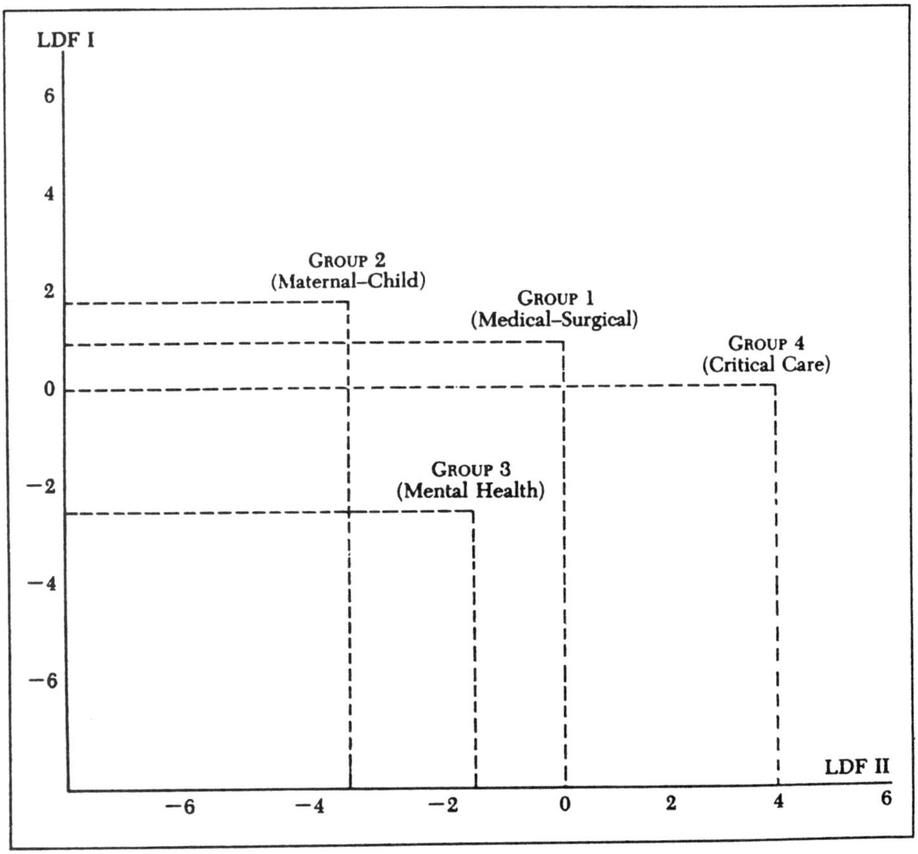

FIGURE 1 Graphic Representation of Two Linear Discriminant Functions (LDFs) with Four Group Centroids Plotted

should be examined in relation to each LDF, standardized discriminant function coefficients and structured coefficients.

Like beta weights in regression analysis, standardized coefficients represent the *relative* contribution each variable makes to an LDF and thus to calculating individual discriminant scores. Interpretation, however, can become a difficult task, especially when the variables correlate highly with one another. To minimize this problem, discriminating variables should be selected carefully, preferably on some theoretical basis. Researchers should not include a large number of variables simply because they are available and then attempt to derive meaning based on the results.

When collinearity does exist, examination of the structured coefficients assists with interpretation. These coefficients are simply product moment correlations between each variable and each LDF. Thus, they indicate individual variable strength without the confounding effects of the other variables.

Extending the research example illustrated in Figure 1, Table 2 presents the standardized discriminant function coefficients and structure coefficients obtained for each of the five variables included in the analysis. On Function 1, ego development has the largest standardized coefficient (.761) of all the variables; on Function 2, critical thinking (.893). The other variables have relatively small coefficients in comparison on both functions. Because standardized coefficients indicate the *relative* contribution of an individual variable to an LDF, ego development and critical thinking are the variables that contribute most to Functions 1 and 2, respectively. Both ego development and assertiveness, however, have high structure coefficients on Function 1, indicating they are both strongly related to the function. This should alert the researcher to examine the correlation matrix to

TABLE 2 Standardized and Structured Coefficients of the Discriminating Variables

	Standardized Coefficients		Structured Coefficients	
Variables	*Function 1*	*Function 2*	*Function 1*	*Function 2*
Age	.251	.343	.071	.315
Grade point average	–.202	–.351	–.021	–.215
Assertiveness	–.321	–.227	.744	–.301
Ego development	.761	.019	.758	.010
Critical thinking	.102	.893	.113	.835

determine if collinearity exists, which, in this example, it does. Ego development makes a large positive contribution to Function 1, but assertiveness makes a small negative one. The net effect represents the true effect on each discriminant score (Klecka, 1980).

In this example it can be concluded that the first and largest discriminant function separates Groups 1, 2, and 4 from Group 3 on ego development and assertiveness or that students choosing to practice in mental health areas scored higher on these attributes than the other groups. The second function separates Groups 1, 2, and 3 from Group 4 on critical thinking ability, indicating students who chose to practice in critical care scored higher on this attribute than the other groups. Age and GPA were not strong discriminating variables and could be eliminated from further analysis.

To this point discriminant analysis has been discussed as a technique for interpreting group membership. There are times, however, when the researcher will want to classify cases for the purpose of either predicting group membership or validating the discriminating power of the LDF(s).

Predicting Group Membership

The original purpose for discriminant function analysis, proposed by Fisher (1936), was to provide a means for classifying individuals or objects into two or more defined groups. Given measures on p-identified discriminating variables, membership in K mutually exclusive groups is predictable. Prior to deriving any classification functions, however, it is important that the assumption of equal covariance matrices be met. This can be tested using Box's (1953) M statistic, which is available on several computer packages.

If LDF analysis is to be used for prediction purposes, some estimate of its power to do so is essential. When significant group separation is found, an estimate of intergroup distances can be obtained through a pairwise comparison of groups using Mahalanobis' (1936) distance statistic or D^2. D^2 can be converted to an F statistic to determine statistical significance and thus provide a clearer picture of where separation is occurring. The strength of the relationship between the discriminating variables and group membership also provides an index of discriminating power. Huberty (1975) discussed several statistics that can be used for this purpose, including an extension of Hays' (1973) omega squared. These indexes are analogous to the eta statistic used in analysis of variance.

Another index of discrimination can be obtained by classifying the cases used to derive the LDFs. By constructing a *confusion matrix*, predicted group membership can be compared to actual group membership, yielding the proportion of correct classifications along the principal diagonal. When compared to expected percentages based on random assignment, the LDFs' discriminating ability can be estimated. These percentages, however, tend to overestimate discriminating power because they are based on the same data used to derive the functions. An alternative is to use a cross-validation method. When sample size is large enough, the sample can be randomly divided in half and one subset used to derive the functions and the other subset used to test the classifications.

Classification Functions

Several mathematical procedures may be used to determine classifications. They all, however, involve defining the distance between an individual case and each group centroid. Classification may be based on the discriminating variables themselves or on the derived LDFs.

Using the discriminating variable directly, a linear classification function is calculated for *each* group that maximizes group differences while minimizing variation within the groups. For each case, classification scores are derived and the case is classified in the group yielding the highest value. Another classification method is to use

Mahalanobis' (1936) D^2 to determine the closest distance between an individual case and group centroid. The smaller the D^2, the closer the individual to that group centroid.

Both of these methods of classification can be converted to probabilities of group membership, denoted as Pr(X/G), where the probability that an actual member of group K is as far from the group centroid as observation X is. Using these probabilities, decisions can be made as to the group in which each case should be classified. There are times, however, when classification is not possible, such as when discrimination is low and the groups overlap considerably or when a case is so far from all group centroids that classification is meaningless. These probabilities are simply distance estimates from the data point to the group centroid and will not sum to 1.0 for any given case. If, however, it is assumed that every case must belong to one of the groups, the probability of group membership for each group can be calculated. Denoted as Pr(G/X), these *posterior probabilities* will sum to 1.0 over all groups.

For example, assume that the researcher wanted to use the discriminating variables, ego development, assertiveness, and critical thinking ability, to predict students' preference for nursing practice. Distance probabilities and posterior probabilities were derived from the data set (Table 3) for three individual cases. The posterior probabilities for Cases 1 and 2 are high for Group 1 (medical-surgical) and Group 3 (mental health), respectively. The distance probabilities for these cases, however, are relatively small, indicating that although they are closest to the groups indicated, they might not belong to the population from which the original groups were drawn (Klecka, 1975). In this situation the decision as to which group, if any, the cases should be assigned must be weighed carefully. Case 3 has high probabilities in both areas, and can be safely classified into Group 2 (maternal-child).

These probabilities are based on the assumption that each group has an equal chance of having a case classified, given the discriminating characteristics. There are times, however, when parameters of the population are known that would influence group classification. For example, if in a given population 25% of individuals are depressed and 75% are not, then based on discriminating characteristics alone a researcher would not want to take an equal chance (50–50) of classifying an individual as depressed or nondepressed. In this event, *prior probabilities* can be incorporated into the analysis. Prior probabilities can also be used when the *costs* of misclassification are known. For example, it may be three times as costly (in terms of harm to the individual being classified) to falsely label a depressed individual as nondepressed as it is to label a nondepressed individual as depressed (Afifi & Clark, 1984).

Guidelines for Use

Considerations for using discriminant analysis should be based on the specific purposes of the research and whether the assumptions can be satisfied.

Description

To describe and explain group differences:

1. Determine if the groups are separated from one another using a multivariate test of significance.

2. If separation exists, derive the linear discriminant functions. Use a stepping procedure to determine the best combination of variables, unless the hypothesis being tested specifies specific variable combinations.

3. Determine which LDFs are the best discriminators and eliminate those that are not.

4. Examine the standardized and structure coefficients to determine *meaning* of the LDFs. Weak variables should be eliminated and stepping procedures repeated until the best subset of discriminating variables is found.

TABLE 3 Distance and Posterior Probabilities of Group Membership

	Distance Probabilities Pr (X/G)				Posterior Probabilities Pr (G/X)			
Cases	*Group* 1	*Group* 2	*Group* 3	*Group* 4	*Group* 1	*Group* 2	*Group* 3	*Group* 4
1	.168	.102	.009	.142	.655	.000	.000	.344
2	.063	.004	.260	.029	.386	.001	.587	.024
3	.122	.894	.007	.002	.001	.997	.006	.000

Classification

To predict group membership:

1. Test for the equality of the covariance matrices, using Box's (1953) *M* statistic; violation of this assumption will distort group membership probabilities.

2. Estimate the discriminating power of the LDFs by using (a) Mahalanobis' (1936) statistic, (b) some measure of association, (c) the percentage of correct classifications (confusion matrix), and/or (d) a cross-validation methodology.

3. Determine whether prior probabilities should be incorporated into the classification functions based on known parameters of the population and/or the costs of misclassification.

4. Classify cases into the groups after carefully examining all probabilities of group membership.

References

Afifi, A. A., & Clark, V. (1984). *Computer-aided multivariate analysis.* Belmont, CA: Wadsworth Publishing Co.

Borgen, F. H., & Seling, M. F. (1978). Uses of discriminant analysis following MANOVA: Multivariate statistics for multivariate purposes. *Journal of Applied Psychology, 63,* 689–697.

Box, G. E. P. (1953). Non-normality and tests on variances. *Biometrika, 40,* 318–335.

Fisher, R. A. (1936). The use of multiple measurements in taxonomic problems. *Annuals of Eugenics, 7,* 179–188.

Goodwin, L. D. (1984). Increasing efficiency and precision of data analysis: Multivariate vs. univariate statistical techniques. *Nursing Research, 33,* 247–249.

Greenleaf, N. P. (1983). Labor force participation among registered nurses and women in comparable professions. *Nursing Research, 32,* 306–311.

Hays, W. L. (1973). *Statistics for the social sciences* (2nd ed.). New York: Holt, Rinehart and Winston.

Huberty, C. J. (1975). Discriminant analysis. *Review of Education Research, 45,* 543–598.

Klecka, W. R. (1975). Discriminant analysis. In N. Nie and others, *SPSS: Statistical Package for the Social Sciences* (pp 434–467). New York: McGraw–Hill Book Co.

Klecka, W. R. (1980). *Discriminant analysis*. Beverly Hills, CA: Sage Publications, Inc.

Mahalanobis, P. C. (1936). On the generalized distance in statistics. *Proceedings of the National Institute of Sciences of India, 12,* 49–55.

Smith, D. W., & Shamansky, S. L. (1983). Determining the market for family nurse practitioner services: The Seattle experience. *Nursing Research, 32,* 301–305.

Tatsuoka, M. M. (1970). Discriminant analysis: The study of group differences. *Selected Topics in Advanced Statistics,* No. 6. Champaign, Il: Institute for Personality and Ability Testing.

Tatsuoka, M. M. (1971). *Multivariate analysis: Techniques for educational and psychological research.* New York: John Wiley & Sons.

Trainor, M. A. (1982). Acceptance of ostomy and the visitor role in a self-help group for ostomy patients. *Nursing Research, 31,* 102–106.